T0291787

THE DIGESTIVE TRACT

THE DIGESTIVE TRACT

A Radiological Study
of its Anatomy, Physiology,
and Pathology

By

ALFRED E. BARCLAY

O.B.E., M.A., M.D. (Cantab.), D.M.R. & E. (Camb.), M.R.C.P., F.A.C.R.

Honorary Radiologist to the Nuffield Institute for Medical Research, Oxford

Formerly Lecturer in Medical Radiology, University of Cambridge, Hon. Medical Officer in charge of the X-Ray Department, Manchester Royal Infirmary, and Lecturer in Clinical Radiology, University of Manchester. Sometime President, British Institute of Radiology; Electro-Therapeutic Section, Royal Society of Medicine; Roentgen Society; and Electro-Therapeutic Section, British Medical Association

SECOND EDITION

CAMBRIDGE
AT THE UNIVERSITY PRESS
1936

CAMBRIDGE
UNIVERSITY PRESS

University Printing House, Cambridge CB2 8BS, United Kingdom

Cambridge University Press is part of the University of Cambridge.

It furthers the University's mission by disseminating knowledge in the pursuit of education, learning and research at the highest international levels of excellence.

www.cambridge.org
Information on this title: www.cambridge.org/9781107494909

© Cambridge University Press 1936

First edition 1933
Second edition, revised 1936
First paperback edition 2015

A catalogue record for this publication is available from the British Library

ISBN 978-1-107-49490-9 Paperback

To
MY WIFE

NATURE

Her one unswerving purpose is the fulfilment of her needs: in many different ways she attains her ends.

We watch the unwearying and persistent resource with which, setting precedent at naught, she strives to maintain effective service.

She disdains the formulae and standards of mass production, providing instead a kaleidoscopic panorama of balanced form and function.

She obeys the inexorable laws of science, yet is unfettered by their compelling force. She enslaves such science as we know.

Life, that unfathomable mystery that can make the dead bones of science live, life is her servant.

Of the mystery of life we know nothing, and, in all humility, we seek to learn the secrets.

A. E. B.

PREFACE TO THE SECOND EDITION

This new edition embodies a number of changes, especially in the addition and rearrangement of matter to keep abreast of the latest research. Some new work on the quantities of radiations to which the radiologist is exposed in diagnostic procedures has been added and, in the chapter on radiological risks, measurements in international r units have been substituted for those which were originally given in fractions of the Unit Skin Dose, the only method available at the time of the investigations. The figures approximate very closely to those of Zuppinger, which are given for comparison. Both sets of figures are reassuring and indicate that the operator and staff run very little risk in a well ordered and equipped department.

Cinematographic X-ray records have now become possible and a few observations based on this method of investigation have been included. Gastric peristalsis and the way in which the pylorus acts are reviewed in detail and the latest researches on the subject are summarised. When writing the first edition I still held that, although the majority of long stomachs were normal, yet I was willing to accept that there was such a condition as gastroptosis. Since then I have become convinced that there is no such thing as gastroptosis in the generally accepted sense, and give the reasons for this opinion.

The section on pathology has been extended and certain conditions which have recently received considerable attention are now included or extended, particularly hypertrophic stenosis of the pylorus and duodenitis.

Two new appendices have been added, the one on the photographic measurement of small intensities of radiations such as those to which the radiologist is exposed in the course of his work and another on the legal ownership of films.

A considerable number of new illustrations have been added and some old ones have been replaced.

There is a background for every serious endeavour. In this case it is a questioning of the authority of tradition. Many of the accepted fundamentals of student days have been found fallacious in practice. This note has unconsciously found its way into these pages and has called forth an answering chord not only in the letters of private correspondents but also in the reviews, which have been so generous. These include such phrases as: "the old clinical teachings", "the old anatomical 'facts'", "the sometimes preposterous physiological explanations", "stimulus to further lines of research". To accept the authority of tradition is a most comfortable way of passing through life, but it is not the way of progress. Radiology has made it possible to study the inner workings of living mechanisms, and we are no longer entirely dependent on pure hypotheses and deductions from experimental methods that may, or perhaps must, be subject to grave fallacies.

I maintain that the set descriptive type of anatomy and physiology is often merely a dangerous half-truth. Nature has no set forms, no fixed methods and no set formulae; she has many alternative ways of attaining the same results and these she balances according to her needs. One mechanism at a time may perhaps be described in set terms, but we must realise that, given any slight difficulty or alteration in conditions, she is capable of producing the same result in other ways that are still within what she regards as normal limits. We are far from finality in our knowledge of very large sections of both the anatomy and the physiology of the alimentary tract. This is particularly so as regards the fundamentals which are still unquestioningly accepted in spite of the introduction of new methods of investigation. Research workers have used these newer methods for turning over the virgin soil of relative details, rather than directing their endeavours to the less congenial task of questioning fundamentals that are strongly entrenched in tradition.

We are forced to recognise that Nature will not conform to cut and dried descriptions. We describe one form or one function as the normal, and Nature alters that form or that function on the most trivial of pretexts—a door bangs and the tone of the stomach alters and changes its shape; a fragment lodges in the vallecula, or there is a slight sore throat, and perhaps the whole complex mechanism of swallowing is altered. For every function in the digestive tract there are a number of mechanical and chemical forces available; each is a variable and Nature can balance these variables one against the other to produce the same result. The resource of Nature in order to overcome difficulty and perform function seems at times to be almost inexhaustible, and who shall say when the bounds of normality pass to the sphere of pathology? The borderland is indeed wide.

I wish to urge that we cannot stereotype a description of any mechanism as Nature's normal method; there is an average mechanism that is usually employed, but it may vary not only in each individual but also with the slightest alteration in conditions. To one the prospect of a race or of an interview brings an acceleration of intestinal movement and even diarrhœa, while in the majority it induces a loss of visceral tone that results in a sinking sensation and marked diminution of intestinal activity. In yet others no disturbance is noted.

Many anatomical and physiological conceptions, even the most plausible, may be open to question. Take, for instance, the evidence of tissue culture. If a small nest of undifferentiated cells representing that part of a chicken embryo which should develop into the femur is allowed to grow in suitable media, a perfectly-formed miniature bone is produced. This artificially-nurtured bone shows those prominences, curves, and internal architecture that have been regarded as the results of imparted strains and stresses. Yet this little bone has never experienced any of these stresses. We have perhaps too readily accepted the apparently obvious explanations that have been put forward—it is easier to accept than to disprove such things.

The subject is of far more than academic interest, for in my view it has led to some of the most disastrous chapters in the chequered history of medicine. We may smile at the indiscriminate blood-letting of our grandfathers, but that phase was relatively harmless compared with the much more recent operative procedures that were undertaken on the assumption that the descriptive teaching of anatomy and physiology represented the truth, the whole truth and nothing but the truth.

Up to the time of Lister the accepted anatomy was that of the dead body, and it was assumed that when the abdomen was opened the viscera would be exposed according to the text-book pictures. The pre-Listerian surface markings are still current in most text-books and in some of the schools of anatomy. Yet what do we see in the operating theatre? An incision is made, the bleeding is stopped, the peritoneum is opened. Then with calculated thoroughness the experienced surgeon examines the presenting viscera. Not till he has identified these does he think of proceeding with his operation. He knows that he can take nothing for granted. The last thing he is justified in accepting is that he will find the viscera arranged according to the surface markings. The living anatomy that he exposes is as foreign to the descriptive anatomy of the dissecting-room as is the flexibility of the Chinese ideography to the set rectitude of the Roman alphabet. On the other hand, the inexperienced operator has not this knowledge and has to learn in the school of experience. Much of what he has seen in the dead subject in the dissecting-room is useless and very definitely misguiding. Many mistakes have been made by inexperienced surgeons who had not yet realised the facts, and some of the cases of the war period bore painful testimony to this.

Some thirty or forty years ago there was a school of thought, voiced by Glénard and many others, which attributed symptoms to looseness and displacements of viscera. Visceroptosis had become a fashionable complaint, gastroptosis was a very definite condition, and later on loose kidneys and the mobile proximal colon came into the limelight as sources of symptoms. The teaching of the physicians, based on their recollections of the anatomy of the dead subject, was definite. They palpated and percussed out the air that happened to be in the stomach and, naturally, had no idea of the fallacies on which they were relying.

They were dogmatic, for nobody could gainsay them—the patient had certain symptoms and these were due to ptosis. Then it became possible to open the abdomen with relative safety. The only anatomy that the surgeon knew was that of the dead subject, for he had no experience of what was and what was not normal in the living abdomen, and he looked to see whether the viscera occupied the positions described in the text-books. If the patient had symptoms that seemed to originate from some organ and he found it mobile, that organ ought to be fixed. He tried all sorts of devices to fix the viscera into a pattern such as he had been taught to consider the one and only normal. He found a long stomach: that must be gastroptosis, and he hitched it up or even excised a portion. This phase did not last long, because the results were so disastrous. Then symptoms were attributed to the kidneys that were loose, the proximal colon that was mobile, and the caecum that was sloppy. One remembers the various ligatures that were tried—silk, silkworm gut, catgut, kangaroo tendon, metal wire—but none of them was effective. Eventually it was realised that fixation resulted only when sufficient local damage was done to produce adhesions.

But the results! What a tale of tragedy it all was—surgeons persistently attempting year after year to make the viscera conform to the pattern of the dead and not realising that what they were attempting was diametrically opposed to the conditions that Nature insistently demands: absolute freedom of movement and an entire absence of fixed points. It was a long time before it was realised that in these operations the one thing to be feared was the production of adhesions, fixed points. It was not till the experience had been bought, at the price of human suffering, that it was realised it was not only futile but wrong practice to make the living anatomy conform to the dead pattern. The clinical result was only too often a failure, the last state being infinitely worse than the first.

This type of operation has not even yet completely died out, and from time to time one comes across the tragic results of this sad conception in surgery. The procedures adopted were perfectly logical but the foundations of the anatomy on which they were based were those of the dead and not of the living.

Physiology was to blame for another equally tragic and almost as widespread, but shorter-lived, phase of surgery: the colectomy and short-circuiting operations. The text-books suggested that the caecum and colon were merely cesspools, relics of antiquity, for "the absorption is practically complete by the time that the food has arrived at the lower end of the ileum". If these organs were of this type, surely toxic absorption must occur, and, naturally, a search was made for possible effects. Some radiologists took a very leading part in this phase of medicine and there are many descriptions of stasis in various parts and of the "kinks" said to be responsible for it. Looking back, one sees a substratum of truth and an overwhelming superstructure of hypothesis erected on it. One remembers particularly the cases of ileal stasis and the symptoms attributed to it. Yet the chief exponents of these theories admitted that the radiological appearance of ileal stasis disappeared if the patient took a purgative. He could only show ileal stasis radiologically if he withheld purgatives! Almost any condition might be due to stasis: amongst other supposed effects of this hypothetical toxic absorption, many will remember trying to detect the "precancerous" breast condition that was described. The argument was carried to extremes, logical but misguided extremes, and the colon was short-circuited, or, with extraordinary technical skill, removed.

The story of this phase of surgery with its appalling mortality and the wreckage of so many of those who survived, is still fresh in the memory. It does not concern the present argument except in that it emphasises the lesson that it would have been better not to teach anything of the physiology of the colon, to admit ignorance in fact, rather than to mislead those who were responsible for its clinical application. We still know very little about the physiology of the colon. There is nothing so dangerous in medicine as a half-truth that is capable of neither proof nor disproof. It was on physiological half-truths that the fixation and colectomy operations were designed.

In other spheres, as in that of the abdominal surface markings, accepted teaching is now obviously contrary to facts, and we are asked, "But if this teaching is not correct, what is the explanation? What must I teach?" It is better to teach nothing at all, or even to acknowledge complete ignorance, rather than propagate that which is unproven or even definitely wrong. Yet if the teacher takes this line, examiners may not share these views and will blame him for the apparent ignorance of the candidates. That this is so is shown by the fact that the old abdominal surface markings have survived a quarter of a century of known fallacy. To accept them is the line of least resistance, for it is easy to teach the descriptive anatomy of the dead abdomen but extraordinarily difficult to give students an adequate idea of the fluid anatomy of the living subject. And how can an examiner find out whether a student knows his subject when almost any answer may be correct? To take an extreme instance: a perfectly normal, healthy medical student happens to have a long stomach that extends to the level of the symphysis pubis, and that student, on being questioned, answers quite correctly that his own stomach is perfectly normal (just as his long nose is perfectly normal), and that in the standing position it is in relationship with the caecum, bladder, and perhaps the sigmoid!

It cannot be overemphasised that Nature has no set forms and no standardised functions. She has at command a variety of forms that merge one into the other and, in function, the bewildering way in which she is able to balance up the many factors she uses, even in a simple act, makes standardised descriptions merely half-truths. The more we see of Nature's ways the more misleading and dangerous are these half-truths.

But, clearly, students must be taught something, for they must have pegs on which to hang their knowledge. How are they to be given an understanding of the fluid character of the anatomy and physiology of the living subject? The only solution, a makeshift, is to increase X-ray demonstrations and X-ray cinematograph lectures so that the students can endow the pictures they see in the text-books and in the dissecting-room with the attributes of life, as is being attempted in some schools. Incidentally, those who demonstrate in the X-ray room must be as familiar with the radiographic appearances as they are with the shrivelled, toneless caricatures of the living which they demonstrate in the dissecting-room. For obvious reasons it is a great mistake to send an untrained demonstrator of anatomy into the X-ray department and expect him to demonstrate the living subject, for (a) he is ignorant of the risks of X-ray work and how they can be avoided; (b) he will not be familiar with either the methods or technique; (c) he will be inexperienced in the wide variations that are compatible with normality.

The lot of an examiner dealing with these problems is indeed hard, for he cannot look for the cut-and-dried answers to questions that have been current through the centuries. How is he to determine the standard of knowledge a student has attained if almost any answer to a question on the form, position, and relationships of the viscera may be correct? Nevertheless, it is more important that the student should realise the truth than that the ways of the teacher and examiner should be smooth.

OXFORD
1936

ACKNOWLEDGMENTS

My debt to fellow-workers is immeasurable, for, apart from direct contributions and quotations from their writings, one constantly absorbs ideas, and frequently the source of the inspiration is forgotten. It is with the intention of acknowledging this in some small measure that I have invited some of my friends to allow me to reproduce illustrations of phases of the work with which their names are associated. Naturally this is a very incomplete and unsatisfactory way of acknowledging my debt; it is nothing more than a gesture. Moreover, some—notably Russell D. Carman, Preston M. Hickey, Martin Haudek, Guido Holzknecht and Albers Schönberg—have passed away from us. I must, however, especially acknowledge the inspiration of such men as my friends A. F. Hurst, W. C. Alvarez, Gösta Forssell, Hans Berg, A. W. George, L. G. Cole, F. Haenisch and F. M. Groedel.

I owe much to the encouragement I have always received from my surgical and medical colleagues in Manchester, particularly A. H. Burgess and George Murray, and especially to those closely associated with me in the radiological department: J. M. Woodburn Morison, R. S. Paterson, E. W. Twining, E. D. Gray, J. F. Bromley, J. B. Higgins; and also to H. M. Meyrick-Jones, who has worked with me in Cambridge. They have helped me in many ways, but especially with the illustrations.

I very gratefully acknowledge the invaluable assistance of Sir Humphry D. Rolleston, who has read through the MS and proofs and clarified many ambiguous points, making suggestions both for omission and inclusion.

For much of the material in the chapter on the gall-bladder I am indebted to L. A. Rowden. Professor Lovatt Evans has looked through such physiology as is involved in this section. The physics in Chapter I has been discussed with G. Stead, who has kindly written a brief appendix on secondary radiations. I am indebted to Miss D. E. Shillington Scales for secretarial assistance, and to H. P. Hudson of the Department of Pathology for collaboration in the photographic technique of Plate I.

My thanks are due to the editors of *The Quarterly Journal of Medicine* and the Oxford University Press for the use of most of the illustrations in Chapters VI, VII and VIII; to the editor of *Acta Radiologica* for figures illustrating the mechanism of swallowing; to Messrs Sherratt and Hughes for supplying blocks which were used in my early book *The Alimentary Tract*; to Oxford Medical Publications for supplying the two colour plates from Hurst and Stewart, and to *The Lancet* for illustrations which have appeared in that journal.

Much of the material incorporated in this volume has been published in journals, particularly in *The British Journal of Radiology* and its predecessor, *The Archives of the Roentgen Ray*; *The British Medical Journal*; *The Lancet*; *The Quarterly Journal of Medicine*; *The British Journal of Surgery*; *Acta Radiologica*; *The American Journal of Roentgenology*; *Radiology*; and elsewhere.

All except a very small number of radiographs are untouched. The few that have been reinforced are from blocks that have been used in journals in which art paper was not available and in which this procedure was necessary to show the details. Some of the radiographs are very old; many are pre-war and are not up to modern standards of technique, but they are retained because they illustrate my meaning. The line drawings are mostly direct tracings from actual radiographs.

Mr D. H. Kitchin and Dr Kathleen Kitchin have acted as editors and have been very largely responsible for bringing scattered material into ordered form. They have also verified the references and compiled the index. It gives me much pleasure to record my appreciation of their services. The support of the Syndics of the University Press, and the painstaking co-operation of the staff of the University Printer, have made the labour of producing the book a pleasure.

Finally, the volume is dedicated to my wife in acknowledgment of her unfailing helpfulness and co-operation in my work, particularly in the laborious task of proof-reading.

In the preparation of this second edition I have received assistance from many colleagues, particularly E. W. Twining, whose work on hypertrophic stenosis of the pylorus is included, and S. C. Shanks, who has allowed me to publish his findings in 150 consecutive cases of gastro-enterostomy. The appendix on the photographic measurement of small intensities of radiations is from the work of G. E. Bell of the National Physical Laboratory and that on the legal ownership of films has been contributed by D. H. Kitchin, a member of the bar who has made a special study of the law relating to medical practice.

Finally I must acknowledge and thank those who have reviewed the first edition for the way in which they received it. Their commendations have been an inspiration to further endeavour, as have been the many letters I have had from friends all over the world.

TABLE OF CONTENTS

Part II. THE RADIOGRAPHIC EXAMINATION OF THE "NORMAL" GASTRO-INTESTINAL TRACT

SECTION I: ANATOMY

THE ANATOMY OF THE "NORMAL" STOMACH AND THE INHERENT MOBILITY AND ADAPTABILITY OF THE ABDOMINAL VISCERA

CHAPTER XVIII

THE SMALL AND LARGE INTESTINE

LIST OF ILLUSTRATIONS

INTRODUCTION

This work has grown out of an M.D. thesis published in 1912 and elaborated and brought out in book form in 1915 under the title of *The Alimentary Tract*; much of that book is incorporated, but in the main the present work is the substance of lectures delivered to students preparing for the Cambridge Diploma in Medical Radiology and Electrology.

Hidden away in journals, often in articles long since forgotten, are many observations which have accumulated in the course of time and become merged in what is now common knowledge. These tags of memory, many of them subconscious, often make the diagnosis of the experienced clinician much more valuable than the logical conclusions of one less experienced. Readers of these pages will find in them all that I can pass on as the result of many years of groping, often by tracks that have now become well-worn highways with milestones, sign-posts and danger-signals erected one by one by the pioneers as they passed forward. There is little encouragement to short cuts but instead, I hope, the means, the technique and the experience with which to interpret what is seen.

Some of the views expressed may not be in accordance with accepted tradition. I can only say that they are founded on personal experience, backed by knowledge of the similar experience of other radiological workers.

What is Radio-diagnosis?

Radio-diagnosis is not a new branch of medicine but a new outlook on medical problems. It is a clinical method, and the essential pre-requisite of the radiologist is a sound knowledge of anatomy and clinical medicine. Without these, no elaboration of radiographic technique, no shining splendour of apparatus and perfection of X-ray pictures, can make his opinion more valuable than that of the technician. His special training, knowledge and experience in interpreting the meaning of shadow pictures in terms of clinical medicine alone justify the medical man in following the specialised calling of radiology. Essentially, the radiologist must be a clinician, and the wider his knowledge and experience of clinical medicine, the greater will be his advantage as a radiologist. He is a specialist in the application of a particular method of investigation, a method which opens up certain fields that are entirely closed to other clinical methods.

When X rays were first applied to medicine, they were regarded as a new application of photography, and it was not realised that the interpretation of the shadow pictures required any special skill or experience. Hence X-ray departments were housed in basements and put in the charge at first of porters or nurses, later of medical men who had often had no special training. Even now we suffer from the handicap that this early lack of foresight imposed on those who became specialists in the use of this new method and who expanded its application. By sheer weight of clinical worth and progress they brought radiology out of the basement and into the position of a department which is now a keystone to efficient medical and surgical service; so much so that when the radiological service in a hospital is poor, the medical and surgical efficiency of that hospital is usually of the same calibre.

Occasionally medical men still display an outlook on radiology so narrow that they think each member of a hospital staff might do his own X-ray work. A cottage hospital installs a portable X-ray outfit. The general practitioners who staff the hospital suggest that each of them should radiograph and examine his own cases—and why not? All the details of exposure, etc., are set out on the card of instructions, and any yokel can turn on a switch. Therefore, why not? Simply because the application of X rays and the interpretation of X-ray pictures require special knowledge and experience. Anyone, by following instructions, can produce a radiograph, but the ability to do this does not make a radiologist, nor is this the service which makes radiology valuable.

This volume is a summary of the personal and acquired experience of a quarter of a century of fluoroscopic and radiographic examination of the alimentary tract. That is a long time, and the novice may therefore expect to find in these pages a dogmatic "Yes" or "No". Dogmatism in diagnosis is a cloak that every novice (including the author) unwittingly assumes as soon as he has become familiar with the shadow of the opaque food in the stomach. Later he finds his mistakes and, as his experience matures, he becomes, far more often than he cares to admit, unable to give a definite answer no matter how he gathers the remnants of his cloak around him to keep out the chill knowledge that he has not always been right in his deductions. Radiology is all a matter of deduction. There is one and only one safe guide, one key to radiological inter-pretation—knowledge of the normal.

This book is mainly concerned with the study of the normal. The physio-logical rather than the pathological is stressed, for it is always far more difficult to recognise and make a diagnosis of the normal than of the definitely patho-logical. For both the novice and the experienced, the most difficult diagnosis is: "No pathological condition present". The normal has so many possible variations and mutations that an attempt to catalogue them, to picture them in an atlas, would be futile. The only road to follow is the main road in which the student learns the why and the wherefore, the physiology of the normal, so far as it is known; and when he has learnt this he will have less difficulty in recognising what is and what is not a pathological condition. It should then be a very short journey to arrive at a correct diagnosis—provided that he has the essential basic knowledge of morbid anatomy.

Radiological Anatomy and Physiology

Radiology has been so successful in the diagnosis of pathological conditions that there is a tendency to overlook its applications to physiology and to anatomy. The early workers were faced with the fact that the orthodox anatomy and physiology of the alimentary tract were hopelessly at variance with what they saw. By degrees they worked out the normal as far as they could, and to-day the radiologist turns to radiological works and not to the text-books of physiology or anatomy for help in interpretation. He sees the living anatomy and living physiology, which have not yet found their way into the text-books. It is a fact that a text-book of physiology published in 1929 quotes Beaumont and his experiments on Alexis St Martin (1833) as the last word on the form and function of the stomach, and speaks of it as a bilocular organ consisting of an upper part, a hopper, and a lower part, a mill. There is no reference to the pioneer work of the radiologists. Doubtless this book is an extreme example, but it is written for students of medicine. Moreover, the author attempts to give the student a grasp of human physiology in the simple terms of chemistry and physics. I believe this plan is ill-advised. As Alvarez says, "The most paralysing thing in scientific work is a facile explanation which puts a stop to curiosity without really advancing our knowledge of the subject".

To keep pace with the increase of knowledge, universities have naturally had to divide and sub-divide the various branches of study included in the training of the medical student. Artificial bounds have arisen, and in the schools anatomy represents form, physiology has charge of function, and pathology deals with disease. But in life these three melt imperceptibly into one another and, to the radiologist who studies living conditions, there is no artificial dividing line. His is a living picture in which there are no sharp divisions, no walled-off departments, for he sees anatomy, physiology and pathology as one whole. The form, the shape of the stomach is anatomy, yet a slight deficiency of tonic action—a physiological change—may alter the picture completely, while the presence of a contraction may be pathological or merely a physiological response to some stimulus.

The domain of the radiologist is the study of the living, functioning human being. It is for him to take the bare facts of descriptive anatomy and clothe them with the attributes of life; to take the observations of the physiologist and show whether the deductions from the laboratory and animal experiments are applicable to the living subject; and to interpret the changes in the normal shadows that are the result of disease. The waywardness of Nature, the entire absence of standards both in form and functions, make it impossible for medicine ever to be an exact science. What a dull business it would become if it could be reduced to formulae! For many of us it would cease to have any attraction. The incalculability of the human element, the balancing of a hundred bits of insufficient, and perhaps contrary, evidence call up in us that indefinable instinct that goes by the name of clinical sense. It is this that makes medicine such a fascinating study, one in which the greatest masters are ever students, learning by experience to their last days. The radiologist must study medicine and its auxiliary branches from his own angle, and the wider his clinical knowledge, the more valuable will be his opinion. But above all things, and particularly in gastro-intestinal work, he should try to cultivate clinical sense—that indefinable but invaluable asset closely allied to common sense.

Many attempts have been made to schedule medical diagnosis, to tabulate signs and symptoms, and numerous atlases of radiographic appearances have been published, but all such attempts at short cuts to knowledge must fail, for the diagnosis of disease and its significance is and always must be an art. The faculty, the intuitive gift, of knowing whether a patient is or is not really ill is often the essential factor in deciding whether some unusual appearance indicates an anatomical peculiarity, a physiological anomaly, or a pathological manifestation.

The question whether radiology is a specialist subject or merely a technique is frequently raised. My views on the matter are very definite. It is and must be a specialist subject for many years to come, both by reason of the technique involved and the wide divergence in outlook that is not readily grasped by those who have not extensive experience in the methods involved. The parallel between surgery and radiology is a close one, and is a very strong argument for developing radiology as a specialist subject. Could surgery have developed as it has done if it had not become a separate department of medicine? Yet surgery is as much a technique as is radiology. If radiology is subservient to other departments, it may, in some instances, develop satisfactorily so far as one or two departments are concerned, but in others it will be neglected and fall into disrepute, mainly from the lack of a competent radiologist. It seems to me that the greatest value for all branches of medicine and of the sciences is that the radiological service should be centralised and serve all branches. When any of these finds that it needs, and can maintain, a separate radiological installation (including a radiologist) of its own, then and not till then should there be decentralisation.

There is comparatively little in the whole range of clinical medicine that does not come into the radiologist's purview, and the ideal radiologist would have an all-round knowledge so vast that no single brain could compass it. Most of us have to be content with gathering together as many as we can of the fragments of knowledge which appear to be of primary significance. Hence this volume is necessarily a collection of those points which the writer believes to be of importance in the radiological study of the alimentary tract.

PART I

TECHNIQUE

CHAPTER I

ROUTINE AND TECHNIQUE

THE IMPORTANCE OF ROUTINE

A great deal could be profitably written on the pitfalls into which the radiologist may be led in the performance of his duties. Only by following a well-tested routine can he avoid the snares that are set for him, not only by Nature —who has not labelled each disease with a series of signs and symptoms that would make it unmistakable—but also by the clinician who, for one reason or another and with the very best of intentions, restricts the exercise of a routine which, unfettered, will almost automatically give the answer to the problems that are sent to the radiologist. Everyone knows that the case which goes wrong is the special case, the important patient who expects peculiar consideration, and this is nearly always because routine is disturbed. The radiologist reports a normal stomach and misses a malignant growth of the small intestine because the patient cannot wait for routine observations. He misses obvious gall-stones because the general practitioner is with the patient and thinks it is a case of duodenal ulcer and wishes for a report before he takes the patient home.

Routine may cause apparent delay but, unless there is some urgent reason to the contrary, the radiologist is well advised to insist that his routine shall take its course. He will thus inevitably avoid many mistakes that come of haste and lack of thoroughness.

Routine is the essence of successful work. This, however, does not imply that there is one and only one routine, or that the routine that I myself use and recommend is the best. "There are nine and sixty ways of constructing tribal lays, and every single one of them is right." The point is that, subject to the general principle that the examination should show the whole tract as far as possible, every worker must develop his own routine to suit the requirements of his own conditions of work. He may spend his whole time at the hospital or in his private practice, or divide his time between the two. If his whole time is available in one place, he may develop a technique by which he follows one meal all the way through. This may seem the obvious course, but in practice I have found that it does not usually work out satisfactorily. There are three reasons for this: first, the times of the various necessary observations may be inconvenient; secondly, for the examination of the stomach the ordinary opaque meal—which is not a food but only a suspension of opaque salt—is unsatisfactory, as it cannot be relied upon for information about the rate of emptying; and thirdly, this method does not give adequate opportunities for confirmation of observations; the possible variations within the normal are so wide that this is a very great disadvantage. Some form of "double feeding" is, in fact, almost universal, and this routine certainly lessens the chance of missing an abnormality. Even at the present time, as in the early days, some observers give an opaque meal five hours before the X-ray examination begins, in order to determine the question of delay in emptying. Haudek of Vienna was the originator of this method. We gave it an extended trial, but abandoned it because we so frequently found difficulty in interpreting the tangled shadows in the intestine and elsewhere; in fact, it was often necessary to re-examine from the beginning, after this first meal had been cleared out.

Whatever routine is adopted, I consider it essential that X-ray observations should be made while the first mouthfuls of opaque "food" are canalising the stomach, before there are any other shadows in the abdomen to complicate the picture, and that the examination should be continued from time to time as necessary until the observer is satisfied concerning the stomach, duodenum and small intestine. Further, to obtain information as to the rate of emptying, a second meal, consisting of a *real* food mixed with opaque salt, is given five hours before the patient is seen on the second day.

It does not greatly matter what routine is followed provided the observer knows it so intimately that he practises it almost automatically. He must learn to observe accurately, and to record his observations before passing on to the next stage; otherwise he will have to ask the patient to return so that he can confirm observations of which he is not quite certain, or observe essential points that he has missed. He should never depart from his routine, no matter how tempting it may be to jump to conclusions and focus his attention on some particular part, even if this is suggested by the clinical data.

Obviously there are occasions on which the routine must be varied because something unusual is noted that requires special investigation. The routine must be automatic and yet so elastic that it allows for digressions as necessary. The radiologist should work so automatically within this routine that his mind is free to observe, to investigate, to follow like a sleuth-hound any slight variation from the normal that he may detect. Mind and body, eyes and fingers must all be at his disposal to take advantage instantly of every slight indication, for it is often on quite trivial observations that the ultimate diagnosis rests. For instance, a small fleck of opaque food may be noticed in one spot high up on the stomach wall as the first mouthful enters; the observer seizes upon it and attempts to palpate it out. Perhaps, by getting his fingers high up under the costal margin, he may detect a tender spot related to the now suspected point, although the on-coming opaque food has obliterated it. He has, however, noted its appearance and he turns and twists the patient, re-feeds him, examines him standing, lying, tilted, or in any other position until he has convinced himself that his observation is or is not confirmed. He should have things so arranged that he can at any time and without delay expose a film to record what he sees. His radiographic technique should be so standardised that failure is practically impossible, for he may never have the opportunity of recording the appearance again. When the observation is made and, if necessary, recorded he must return to his routine. These side excursions must never become side tracks, and the routine must be picked up again exactly where it was left.

Prejudgment

One of the chief values of a conscientious routine is that it guards the observer from bias and prejudgment, very grave dangers to accurate diagnosis. If the radiologist knows the clinical diagnosis, his observation will necessarily be biased. Yet he should know everything vital in the case history, in order that his examination may be made on right lines. In chest cases particularly the danger of prejudgment is so great that the benefit to the patient if the clinician does his own radiology is doubtful. In this branch the only satisfactory procedure is for the radiologist and the clinician to examine independently and to come to conclusions by consultation. It is from the correlation of the two methods, each worked out independently, that the most satisfactory conclusions will be evolved. The same principle applies to gastro-intestinal examinations, but the bias produced in the radiologist's mind by the necessary information which the clinician gives him can be largely counterbalanced by the routine examination, which ensures attention to every part of the alimentary tract, however much the symptoms may have stressed one particular region.

The Importance of Complete Examinations

When asked to examine and report on a patient who presents clinical indications of a lesion in some part of the alimentary tract, it is more than probable that the radiologist will be requested to confine his examination to this part on one of the following grounds: (1) that in the circumstances it is unnecessary to do a complete examination because the clinical indications are so localised; (2) that by curtailing the usual routine the patient's pocket will be saved; and (3) that time presses and the surgeon cannot wait. The most reasonable arguments will be adduced to deflect the radiologist from the strict path of a routine which experience teaches him is essential. For instance, if the observer does not examine the chest as a routine procedure, he will inevitably miss a certain number of cases of phthisis in which the symptoms are so predominantly gastric that the chest is entirely unsuspected. This I have seen on a number of occasions. Moreover, in a certain number of cases gastric symptoms are due to cardiac lesions; hence it is always advisable to observe the heart for any signs of gross disorder of rhythm or enlargement. Once in the very early days I had just completed an oesophageal examination, with a negative result, when a visitor came to see me. For his benefit the patient consented to swallow some more opaque food, again with negative result but with the perfect demonstration of an hourglass stomach due to an unsuspected ulcer.

The number of cases in which gastric, duodenal, gall-bladder and appendicular lesions have been clinically interchangeable and misleading are so numerous in the experience of every worker that no comment is needed in stressing the rule that a complete investigation is essential if we are to avoid missing things. The way in which small intestine and even colonic, to say nothing of hepatic and pancreatic, lesions refer their disturbances to some other part, particularly to the stomach, is now well recognised. One can hardly believe that a carcinoma of the rectum could refer its main symptoms to the stomach, yet I have seen such a case, and at the operation within an hour or so, dictated solely by the radiological finding, an extensive rectal carcinoma and a length of black and almost gangrenous gut were found.

Hospital Routine

The large number of cases that have to be examined in a hospital X-ray department is one of its very serious difficulties, and something has to be done to bring it within practicable limits. It is only human for the clinician, who is similarly over-burdened, to refer as many cases as he can to other departments in the hope that they may point out a short cut to the diagnosis.

In the early days in my department we had to press clinicians to send cases for examination, but before long we had more than could be managed, for the department was small and the staff limited. We soon found that the least satisfactory cases from every point of view were the gastro-intestinal outpatients. We therefore restricted the opaque meal service to in-patients, and insisted that any patient to be examined should be admitted to the wards. There was much grumbling from some of our colleagues, but they acquiesced, and we have never ceased to be thankful, especially when we hear of the wholesale unsatisfactory work that is imposed on some radiologists by those in charge of out-patients who refer any and every case "for opaque meal". There are many radiologists still struggling to give a good gastro-intestinal service but finding it impossible to do so owing to the indiscriminate way in which cases are referred to them. In Manchester, the question of the examination of outpatients has been before the medical board on several occasions within recent years, owing to the size of the waiting list and the complaint that so many of the beds are occupied by patients undergoing opaque meal examinations. The arguments used in favour of extending the service to out-patients are:

(1) That it relieves the pressure on beds.

(2) That it is not necessary for patients to be in hospital for this purpose.

(3) That, if necessary, the radiologist staff should be increased and the department extended.

The arguments against are:

(1) That to increase the work by including out-patients would inevitably diminish the efficiency of the service to in-patients, for no radiologist can do more than a limited number of cases.

(2) There is not an unlimited supply of men who are competent to do this work, for they must be highly trained and experienced if their reports are to be of any value.

(3) The examination of out-patients is, *per se*, unsatisfactory, because

(*a*) they will not strictly observe the necessary preparation;

(*b*) they frequently fail to attend for continued observations, or appear on any other day that suits them better, the opaque food having meanwhile passed on;

(*c*) they are invariably, and rightly, sent for another examination when they are taken into the wards, probably some months later, for medical or surgical treatment.

On these arguments the medical board agreed that it was inadvisable to accept patients for opaque meal examination direct from the out-patient departments and that all such cases should be admitted to the wards.

THE OPAQUE MIXTURES

The Food used for the First Meal

The bulk of the first opaque meal is in liquid form, and may consist of any one of the numerous satisfactory preparations on the market; the two main requirements are that it shall be palatable and that the opaque salt shall not settle rapidly. For those, however, who wish to make their own opaque food, the following recipe is recommended:

Three to six ounces of barium sulphate are mixed with a salt-spoonful of tragacanth; a small quantity of boiling water is poured on to the mixture, which is worked into a smooth paste. The tragacanth must not touch cold water or it will form gummy lumps. A flavouring agent, generally raspberry syrup or cocoa, is mixed in. Up to about half a pint of milk is added and the whole is thoroughly stirred, preferably by a mechanical mixer. The mixture remains in suspension for about one hour and is not unpalatable, a point of considerable importance, since foods which are disagreeable to the patient are apt to produce a greater or lesser degree of atony.

The mixture should be made first thing in the morning so that the opaque salt has time to settle in the glass. The thick sediment at the bottom, composed almost entirely of the opaque salt, is just what is wanted for the preliminary examination of the mucosa (p. 23); the patient is given a spoonful from the bottom of the glass. When the observer has obtained all possible information from manipulating this in the stomach, the mixture in the glass is stirred up and the patient, under the instruction of the observer, drinks as much as may be necessary. I seldom find that more than a third of a pint is wanted.

Barium sulphate has superseded the various bismuth salts because of its relatively low cost, but larger quantities, roughly 50 per cent. more by weight, are required to obtain an equal density of shadow.* A thorium dioxide preparation called umbrathor, which gives a perfect colloidal suspension, shows up the gastric mucosa very well; 20–30 c.c. is sufficient.

In Brisbane Dr B. W. L. Clarke showed me particularly beautiful mucous membrane patterns. The routine food he has selected, after many experiments, consists of 3 or 4 oz. of barium sulphate mixed with two or three tablespoonfuls of gelatinous marmalade. Boiling water is poured on this; it is allowed to stand for a few minutes, and is then put through a strainer. For enema work the same proportions are used. The mixture is cheap, palatable, does not settle out and evidently adheres most satisfactorily to the mucous membrane, better in fact than most of the proprietary and expensive preparations that are on the market.

The Food used for the Second Meal

This is a more natural meal than the first, and in private practice it is made up at home by the patient and taken nineteen hours after the first meal, i.e. five hours before the second-day examination. The basis of it is a real food and may be either bread and milk or porridge, into which 2 oz. of bismuth carbonate is mixed. In private practice the patient purchases the salt himself. I continue to prescribe bismuth carbonate for this purpose because pure barium sulphate is not always stocked by the chemist to whom the prescription is taken, and also because the bismuth salt gives a rather smoother mixture. Moreover, cases are recorded in which the deadly and soluble barium sulphite was dispensed instead of the sulphate, with fatal results. The psychological effect of spending, say, 3s. or 5s. on the opaque salt and preparing this meal is to make the patient less critical of the radiologist's mixture and more respectful of the opaque food that costs so much! For those who dislike bread and milk or porridge, the bismuth can be mixed into a corn-flour blancmange just before it sets, and this, according

* The atomic weights and densities of the various substances used in X-ray work are as follows, and it is on the atomic weight and the density that the opacity of the shadow depends:

	Atomic weight	Density		Atomic weight	Density
Aluminium	27	2·7	Tungsten	184	18·8
Chlorine	35	3·23	Platinum	195	21·5
Copper	64	8·93	Gold	197	19·32
Zinc	65	7·1	Lead	207	11·37
Bromine	80	3·1	Bismuth	208	9·80
Silver	108	10·5	Radium	226	?
Iodine	127	4·95	Thorium	232	11·3
Barium	137	3·75			

to some patients, is the least unpalatable way of taking it. There is no reason why the patient should not have other food with the opaque meal, but he should not take any subsequent meal before he comes for examination.

The Opaque Enema Mixture

An opaque enema is made up of 8 or 10 oz. of barium sulphate with a teaspoonful of powdered tragacanth well mixed in. About half a pint of boiling water is poured on and the mixture is stirred to a smooth paste. To this is added warm water up to a quart. A comfortable temperature is 90° F. This quantity, if the patient is postured, should be enough to fill the colon and caecum in almost any circumstances, apart from idiopathic dilatation.

For the technique of a double contrast enema (the injection of air after an opaque enema) the ordinary opaque enema mixture is not very satisfactory as it does not adhere to the mucous membrane. Umbrathor sticks to the mucosa and outlines it well so that, combined with the inflation of air, it gives good results, especially for Fischer's technique for the inflation of the colon.

X-RAY CINEMATOGRAPHY

Ever since X rays were invented various workers have tried to capture X-ray appearances in a series of exposures in order to reproduce movement, but it has only recently been possible to take pictures in rapid enough succession to make a true moving picture. The direct method is to expose a succession of films of comparatively large size in place of the ordinary radiographic film; this requires an expensive and cumbersome apparatus, because it is technically very difficult to stop and start a large band of film between eight and sixteen times a second, the minimum rate required. The indirect method is to use an ordinary motion picture camera and photograph the image on the fluorescent screen. Until recently this has been impossible because the screen would not give enough light to make a sufficient impression on the film. Now, however, manufacturers have succeeded in making brilliant screens, fast lenses and highly sensitive emulsion, so that it is possible to illuminate the screen sufficiently brightly without using a current so heavy that it will burn out the tube and harm the patient. Ingenious methods of cutting off the current when the camera shutter is closed have also economised energy.

The outstanding exponents of the direct method are perhaps Jarre(184) and his colleagues in America. For their studies of the urinary tract they only require exposures of about four a second, but their Cinex camera can work considerably faster. I(52) have devised an apparatus which works quite well at about the same rate for studying the movements of the colon. Van der Maele (317a) in Belgium also claims to have overcome the mechanical problems of the direct method. The best results by the indirect method have been obtained in this country by Russell Reynolds(280a) and in Germany by Janker(183a). Jarre has summarised the history of the subject, beginning with McIntyre(227), who in 1897 forecast the possibility of cinematographing the screen image.

CHAPTER II

TECHNIQUE OF SCREENING, PALPATION
AND REPORTING

Historical

The opaque meal method of examination began to come into use about 1905, and about this time also the dangers of X rays were definitely appreciated, even by the dabblers. In the early days a large proportion of the X-ray work was done by entirely unskilled persons, for of course there was no training available and workers felt their way as best they could, more often than not with the sketchiest knowledge of the fundamentals of electricity and physics. In most of the big hospitals there were X-ray installations, and these were usually under the control of medical men who might or might not have some special knowledge and interest. The X-ray department had no standing, and when the medical officer in charge raised his voice about the dangers of X rays, there was more than a tendency to take no notice. In fact, it was not until the calamities of the War and the prominence of all X-ray work in that period that the dangers were appreciated by the medical profession and the responsible authorities. Hence, in the early days, many workers had become thoroughly afraid of the agency with which they worked, and when the opaque meal method of examination was mooted, the obvious advantages of watching the fluorescent screen over examining the photographic record of one particular phase were discounted.

Of course the controversy was not as simple as this. The apparatus was feeble, X-ray tubes most fickle, and a satisfactory screen examination such as we know it to-day was the dream of the seer. A glimpse one had perhaps, and then the dark—a tube showing the blue cathode stream that indicated overheating! Then we changed to the reserve "cranky tube" and hoped for luck, but never to the pet tube that on no account would we allow to be used for screening. Screening was certain to wreck any and every tube in the department and leave the radiologist at his wit's end to know how he was to produce any sort of a radiograph, even of a simple bone case. The X-ray department was not popular, for it was terribly expensive and the demand for new X-ray tubes was met with the reply: "What has happened to the new tube for which we paid five pounds six months ago?" Do the managers of those days ever think of the struggles of the early workers who tried, and succeeded, in "delivering the goods" of a new and wonderfully efficient method of diagnosis, on an expenditure that would to-day be sanctioned out of petty cash? Little did we, newcomers to the ranks of radiology, realise how in time all that which we achieved so precariously would become standardised and as simple as A B C! We were concerned first, last and all the time with our apparatus, and we were very lucky if we could get sufficiently detached from it to make observations on what we occasionally saw. Those were the days of adventure and discovery. Every time we saw the shadow it was an adventure, and everything we saw was a discovery. We took untold risks both knowingly and unknowingly. Upright screening stands had hardly been thought of; each one manufactured was to the design of this or that worker, and probably never repeated. For some years I had no upright screening stand: the patient held the screen! Eventually one was made to my design by the hospital carpenter.

Such was the atmosphere of "screening", and very often one had to give up and acknowledge failure. Moreover, when we did make a diagnosis—hour-glass stomach or carcinoma—we often had no radiograph to show, and, naturally, the surgeon wanted to see a picture. Anyway, we had to try to obtain pictures as well as giving our report of the screen examination, and we succeeded reasonably well. But we maintained that the fluorescent screen examination was the one essential technique for making the diagnosis. By degrees, conditions of screening became easier, but there was always a school of radiologists who held that the radiograph was the thing. This was particularly so in the United States of America, where the pendulum had swung from utter foolhardiness in screening to an excess of precaution. They bent all their energies to perfecting a method that would give them as many radiographs as were necessary to obtain a series of pictures of all phases of the gastric cycle—serial radiography. As this radiographic school developed their technique, they expended perhaps eighty $10'' \times 8''$ pictures on glass plates in the examination of each case! The elaboration of apparatus to produce these results, to say nothing of the cost, made the adoption of this technique quite impracticable. Moreover, those of us who practised the screen method gradually discovered that we were possessed of an exceedingly powerful ally if we employed palpation while we did our screen observations. This was so obvious that we quickly gave up all ambition to pursue the costly radiographic method, which could not give us any of the information as to fixation and many other things that were only obtainable by the combination of sight and manipulation. At first it was merely manipulation of the shadowed organs, but later the sense of touch was added and it became a three-fold process of sight, manipulation of shadows, and touch. We therefore maintained that the screen method was the method of choice, while the advocates of the radiographic method were just as insistent that their procedure was the more effective. Time has shown that, up to a point, both views were right, and the most effective routine is an intensive screen examination combined with the taking of as many films as may be necessary, to record those things which have been noted on the screen and to clear up any points that have not been quite satisfactorily observed.

The observer who does not make full use of the screen misses much, both in the examination of the chest and of the gastro-intestinal tract. In the former he misses the available information as to the movements of the diaphragm, the air entry, etc., while in the gastro-intestinal tract he misses that intimacy of contact with the shadows on the screen that gives not only information but confidence. In recent years, however, serial radiography has become much more efficient. The serial pictures are now not only positioned by screen observation but the degree and direction of pressure can be regulated and the time lag before a film is exposed is now reduced to a matter of a second or so. In fact, serial radiographic methods have invaded the field that was formerly held exclusively by those who practised palpation.

Some of those who use the serial radiographic methods most effectively realise its limitations, but their followers are apt to use this technique exclusively and to neglect screening with detailed palpation. The film records should be supplementary and not an alternative to palpation. There is little doubt that some have neglected to cultivate skill in screen examinations, particularly in palpation, from lack of knowledge of the risks involved and of the means by which palpation can be safely employed (see pp. 18 and 38).

ROUTINE FOR EXAMINATION

The following scheme is suggested as a guide; I believe that it gives a more satisfactory result than following through with a single meal, and it has the great advantage that every observation can be confirmed if necessary.

[An appointment is made for 2 p.m. on Monday.]

Saturday night	Purgative.
Sunday	Enema if necessary; normal food.
Monday	Light breakfast; no food after 11 o'clock.
2 p.m.	History taken. Examination with *first opaque meal*. Patient carries on normal life and takes no purgatives.
Tuesday, 9 a.m.	*Second opaque meal* of ordinary food. No further food until—
2 p.m.	Examination. If examination complete, purgative: if incomplete—
Wednesday	Further examination, without further preparation or opaque food. A purgative or enema must follow.

Preparation of the Patient

If sufficient notice is given, all metallic drugs should be discontinued for a week. It may take a long time for the intestine to rid itself of opaque salt; I have seen the appendix still filled with barium more than three weeks after the patient had been examined.

The usual practice, to which I still adhere, is to give a purgative thirty-six or forty-eight hours before the examination. The type of purgative is immaterial, provided that it does not upset the patient. If he is of constipated habit an enema is also recommended twenty-four hours before the examination. The patient pursues his normal life, except that he takes no food or drink for at least three hours before the examination, to make sure that the stomach is empty. It is essential to examine the alimentary tract under conditions as nearly normal as possible; therefore, the effect of purgation should have passed off before the examination begins. If the purge is still acting when the patient is seen, there may be increased activity of peristalsis, increased rate of emptying and apparent irritability. Castor oil has a peculiar constipating after-effect, reducing gastro-intestinal activity. Purgatives upset many patients and cause abnormal phenomena such as nausea, and many workers have abandoned the use of purgatives as a routine thirty-six hours before the examination and advise giving two drachms of magnesium sulphate about an hour before the last meal on the night before the examination. This salt has no action on the stomach, and the lower bowel and appendix should be cleared by nine o'clock next morning. Some workers maintain that the appendix is visible in a greater percentage of cases with this routine. Others give magnesium sulphate *after* the barium food, but this is only advisable if the object of the examination is to visualise the appendix (see pp. 96 and 169).

The History

The examination should always begin with an inquiry into the history. By taking the clinical history the radiologist attains three main objects:

(*a*) He can obtain personal knowledge of the illness; frequently his experience indicates leading questions which bring out suggestive data, entailing variations in routine without which the diagnosis might be missed. As a simple example, a note that only certain types of food produce a sensation of oesophageal obstruction at once suggests that the type of opaque food employed should correspond as nearly as possible to that which causes the trouble.

(*b*) He has the opportunity of getting to know something of the patient's mentality.

(*c*) An opaque meal cannot but be an ordeal to some patients, and a chat beforehand provides an opportunity for allaying quite natural nervousness. It is important to remember that the patient is often alarmed, sometimes literally "scared stiff", and a little reassurance and an explanation of the procedure will secure the necessary relaxation.

The main points in the history are:

The duration of the symptoms;

The periodicity of attacks;

Pain: its character, time, relation to food, duration, and what measures relieve it;

The vomit: its character, frequency and time of onset;

Haematemesis;

Appetite;

Loss of weight;

Bowel action;

Jaundice;

The condition of the teeth—a radiographic examination of the teeth is very often indicated as part of the routine examination.

History of abdominal and gynaecological operations.

Intensity of Radiation for Screen Examinations

The radiologist must constantly think of the danger to which he is exposed, and the question that the novice always raises is how much current (milliamperage) he should use in a screen examination. The answer cannot be given in definite figures, because it will vary not only with the size of the patient and the thickness of the parts under examination, but also with the individual apparatus. The right quantity to use is the *minimum* that will give satisfactory illumination, and this can only be found by experience. To gain that experience, the observer must be certain that his eyes are in the most sensitive condition to appreciate the screen image.

For ordinary purposes, he will find that 2 or 3 ma. gives fairly satisfactory illumination with thin subjects, but that he will have to use up to perhaps 5 ma. or even 7 ma. for stout people. For chest work 60 K.V. will probably be sufficient. For abdominal work under ordinary conditions 80 K.V. (approximately 5 in. spark-gap) is needed to give satisfactory illumination, but for very stout subjects 90 K.V. may be necessary, and even so the radiation coming through is so diffused by scattering that the image is extremely blurred. It is in these conditions that the Potter-Bucky grid or the Schonander screen are of value.

In abdominal work 90 K.V. with 50 ma. usually gives a satisfactory exposure for films in about a quarter to half a second. There is no appreciable movement during so brief a period. If a Potter-Bucky diaphragm is used the exposures will be about three times as long. With the use of a finer focus tube, possibly of the rotating anode type, great improvement in detail can be obtained. The milliamperage can be much increased while the voltage can be correspondingly reduced, thus giving not only finer detail and greater contrast in the film but also shortening the exposure.

Preparation of the Observer's Eyes

It is essential not to start screening until the eyes are properly prepared. The time taken in accommodating varies with the brightness of the day and with the health of the observer. The radiologist can save a great deal of time if he wears red goggles while he interviews his patients and writes his notes, especially if the light is fairly strong. The best shade of red approximates to crimson lake. It need not be too dark to see reasonably well; with the goggles that I employ I can read or write, provided the light is good. Goggles may be replaced by a simple and effective eyeshade (Fig. 1) cut out of coloured celluloid. It is fastened with paper clips to an elastic band to go round the head. If coloured celluloid is not available, an ordinary X-ray film will serve. It is cleared in hypo and then stained with carbol fuchsin or similar stain. For comfort, the upper edge of the celluloid can be bound with adhesive plaster.

A very simple instrument for testing the eyes is the retinometer designed by Dr A. Howard Pirie (Fig. 2); it consists of three little radium studs (a half-inch triangle, an eighth-inch spot and a point of about a sixteenth of an inch) behind a shutter that is opened by a string of a certain length. At first the radiologist will not be able to see even the large triangle, but as accommodation improves he can see the middle stud and is able to start observing; but his eyes are not in the best condition until he can see the smallest stud at a distance of about a yard. The luminous dial of a wrist-watch can also be used for this purpose, but is not a standard measure.

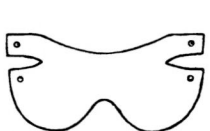

Fig. 1. Pattern for eyeshade cut out of red celluloid (7½ in. width).

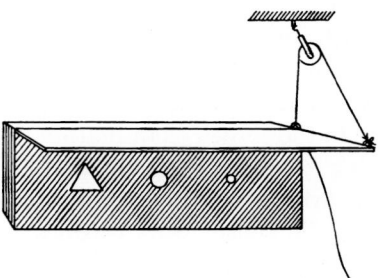

Fig. 2. Howard Pirie's retinometer.

"*Visual Anaesthesia*"

A fact of great importance and a real danger in screening is that the observer can very easily sit in front of the screen watching the image without observing; particularly when he is getting tired he is apt to go on staring at the screen while thinking of something entirely different; he may not even be conscious of the screen image. All radiologists have probably been guilty of this form of carelessness. Immediately the observer finds that he is not observing rapidly and accurately, or not observing at all, he should switch off. On these occasions he should follow his train of thought to its conclusion and then return to the screen examination, for he can then make his observations rapidly and accurately without being distracted by a half-completed line of subconscious thought in an entirely different direction. The observer who allows his mind to wander while the tube is running exposes both his patient and himself to unjustifiable risks.

RADIOLOGICAL PALPATION

Gloves

For many years, in order to protect the hands, I used gloves with the ends of the fingers cut out. The protective material was only in the back of the glove! There is, however, a psychological factor at work when gloves of any kind are used. The observer sees the shadow of the glove on the screen and it gives him an illusion of security, although he knows quite well that the protection is only partial and is practically negligible on the exposed palmar surface. Personally, I feel far safer without gloves, for I am fully aware of danger if my fingers get into the beam of the rays even for a moment; hence I am constantly on guard.

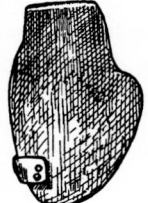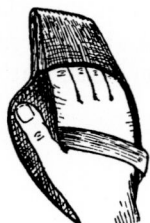

There is absolutely no reason why the fingers should ever get into the direct beam, for the thickness of the abdominal wall is always between them and the organ they are palpating. To push and prod the organs with a wooden spoon, or to manipulate them with the hand sheathed in a thick glove (Fig. 3), certainly helps in the screen examination, but anything coming between the skin and the palpating hand, even a silk nightdress, interferes with the tactile sense.

Fig. 3. Glove for manipulation. This is made out of X-ray-proof rubber of ½ to 1 mm. lead equivalent.

Soft washleather gloves have been used extensively (Cilly, Leddy and Kirklin (97)), as they were supposed to diminish the risks, but they are useless for this purpose (p. 34).

The Technique of Palpation

In palpation one does not press straight in, but obliquely from below upwards, and the fingers may be an inch or more below the horizontal level of the part they are palpating (see Fig. 7, a–d). It is therefore possible so to manipulate the diaphragm that the fingers are always just below the illuminated area and are never exposed. The technique requires considerable practice and patience, but is essential if the greatest possible amount of information is to be gained without taking undue risks. Palpation, even of the appendix, is not necessarily in the direct line of the rays, for the observer can palpate just as well obliquely, using the interposed thickness of the abdominal wall as the margin of the illuminated field. Moreover, not only has he the diaphragm for protection but he can "hide" behind the opaque food, as, for instance, when he palpates the duodenum, and particularly when he wishes to push food through the pylorus.

A thorough examination involves far more than the mere taking of a few films and watching the shadow of the opaque food as it passes on its way, for this could be done as effectively by a technician, using serial radiography. A screen examination is essentially the personal work of an experienced medical man. It is not just a less costly substitute for an expensive serial film or cinematographic method. It is the method of choice, and we use it because of the unique assistance in diagnosis given by manipulation and palpation.

It is doubtful if the value of this intricate procedure is even yet appreciated by the majority of workers, although Carman and his successor Kirklin, Gilbert Scott and some of the Continental writers—notably Berg—have laid considerable stress on it. Radioscopic palpation involves far more than mere manipulation. It is a complex art, and one that is not acquired without much patient practice. It is so trying that only a limited number of cases can be thoroughly investigated in a given time. Berg even maintains that six cases a day is the limit for one observer if the work is done conscientiously and thoroughly.

Radioscopic palpation is not the same thing as the clinical art, a delicate sense of touch learnt at the bedside, but something much more intricate, depending on a co-ordination of the two senses of touch and sight. J. E. Adams (2) has said: "If an abdominal surgeon is really a physician who can work with his hands there is no doubt that constant practice will almost endow him with eyes at the tips of his fingers." The radiologist who is palpating under fluorescent screen control must have these finger-tip eyes. His right hand must have nothing else to do but to rest or to press on the abdomen as necessary; his brain must be focused on the co-ordination of his vision with his tactile sense, and his left hand must take its part automatically and as far as possible unconsciously, raising and lowering the tube, opening and closing the diaphragm, protecting his right hand from danger by keeping the beam of rays off it, and coming to its assistance at need. At times both hands are necessary to exert pressure in two places at once when, for instance, the observer tries to block the descending loop of the duodenum with the left hand while pushing food out of the stomach with the right (Fig. 7d), or for separating out superimposed coils of intestine. In fact, both hands are needed in so many cases that it would be an advantage to set the left hand entirely free by instituting foot control for the tube and diaphragm movements. Hence the simpler the apparatus employed the better, provided that it is efficient. The apparatus that is an assembly of clever and complicated devices is the last one to choose for this type of work, for the radiologist must manipulate both the patient and the controls himself. Only by so doing can he co-ordinate the illuminated field with the area that he is investigating by his palpation.

It is quite hard work to feel and manipulate the opaque food in a stomach that is separated from the observer's fingers by a strong abdominal wall with its 2 in. or 3 in. of resistant muscle and fat. In fact, palpation is often quite a violent form of exercise both for the operator and for the patient, especially if the latter does not relax efficiently. The fingers and wrist quickly tire. Powerful wrist muscles are certainly an advantage, but much can be done to strengthen the palpating finger by using the middle finger only and reinforcing it by overlapping the index and ring fingers behind it (Fig. 4). This is a particularly useful method for pressure on deep-seated spots in order to determine accurately the point where the pain originates. In the upright position, employed so largely in radiographic examinations, palpation and manipulation are much more difficult and awkward than with the patient lying on a couch, but they yield far more information, for the factor of gravity comes to the observer's aid by drawing the

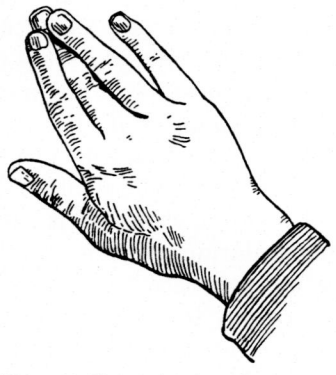

Fig. 4. The palpating finger supported for determining the exact point of origin of pain on deep pressure.

viscera downwards against his manipulation as he presses them upwards.

Radioscopic palpation is, in my opinion, the greatest ally we have in detecting the finer pathological changes in the stomach and other organs. It is, of course, essential for revealing the contour of the furrows of the mucous membrane in which the smaller pathological lesions may be tucked away. Obviously it is exceedingly dangerous in the hands of those who do not understand the art, for even in expert hands it necessarily entails comparatively prolonged examinations involving exposure of both patient and observer. Nevertheless, for those who study the method and realise the danger to themselves of ignorance and carelessness there is, I believe, no risk whatever, and the increased accuracy of diagnosis is so great that no conscientious radiologist can afford to neglect the art. The only radiations to which the hand need ever be exposed are those which are scattered in the patient. The hand must never be in the path of the direct rays, i.e. in the illuminated area. Measurements of the intensities involved confirm these views and will be found on p. 44.

Pressure Sense in Palpation

Considerable stress must be laid on the importance of the tactile sense, though it is difficult to express it in words. Constantly an opinion is given quite as much on what is felt as on what is seen. The relation of the movement to the degree of pressure exerted is brought to the senses by the touch in a way that gives meaning to the underlying condition. A relatively large aperture is used to study the general effect of pressure, but for detailed study a smaller area is illuminated.

The observer estimates the force needed to displace the shadows and at the same time he is *feeling*, sensing resistance not only by touch but by the way in which shadows move both relatively to the pressure and also in relation to each other. He estimates the finer details, particularly in the study of the mucous membrane pattern, not so much by what he actually feels as by gauging, by sense of touch and the visible effect on the shadows, the exact amount of pressure and how to apply it in order to produce a certain result. It is a question of craftsmanship. It is not the strength of the pressure but the quality and method of application. As Berg says, there are among riders those with rough and those with light hands. The skilful horseman guides his mount with a velvet touch and never hurts his horse's mouth; so also the skilled radiologist guides and controls his manipulation so that there shall be no pain, unless there is an actual tender spot for which he is testing. It is from the alternate compression and release that he obtains his results, utilising at the same time the patient's respiratory movements. He employs every movement and combination of movements that he can think of: direct pressure, gliding pressure, retaining and relaxing pressure as the patient breathes, jabbing in suddenly, smoothing or ironing out shadows that are too heavy, separating details with finger-tip pressure, turning the patient this way and that, using the vertical and horizontal positions, or any other device that his ingenuity suggests to unravel the detail that without this technique is merely a confused jumble of superimposed opacities.

THE TECHNIQUE OF THE FIRST EXAMINATION

After a preliminary survey of the chest and mediastinum—which must be a part of the routine of every gastro-intestinal in-vestigation—the patient is rotated slightly with the right shoulder forward. The optimum angle for this right oblique position is that in which the posterior mediastinum is best seen between the shadows of the heart and the vertebrae. In this position the whole length of the oesophagus is under observa-tion, and the first opaque food swallowed should always be watched as it passes down to the stomach, even in cases where there is no clinical suggestion of trouble in this region.

For satisfactory palpation and manipulation of the stomach it is essential to make observations with the minimum amount of opaque food, for it is almost impossible to obtain any detail of the gastric mucosa when more than a small quantity has

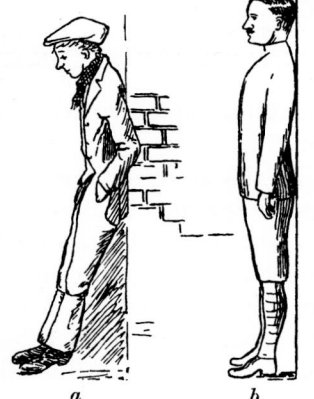

a   *b*

Fig. 5. The right (*a*) and wrong (*b*) postures for palpation in the upright position.

entered the stomach. The patient is therefore given a very thick emulsion, practically pure opaque salt, for the first mouthful. He stands in the upright screening stand on a platform about a foot high, leaning back with his feet well in front and his chin dropped, so that the abdominal muscles are relaxed as far as possible (Fig. 5). The operator sits on a stool at such a height that the patient's stomach is just above his eye level, for in this position he can use most easily and to the best advantage whatever degree of force may be necessary.

If the observer is not entirely satisfied that he has obtained all possible detail in the upright position, the patient is transferred to the couch. In the recumbent position details can often be brought out more easily than in the upright posture, but the observer loses the co-operation of the action of gravity on the opaque food, which he can balance against the pressure he exerts on the abdomen. All observers tend to use one posture more than the other, but the

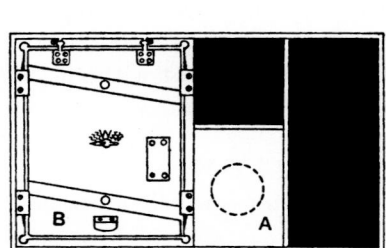
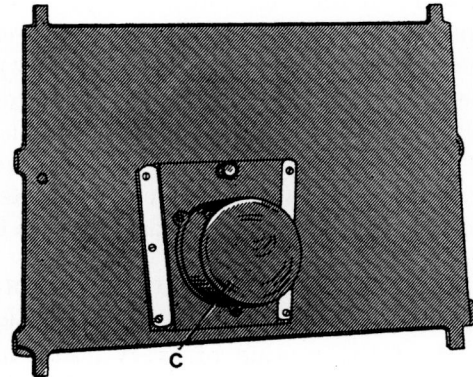

Fig. 6. Diagram of Berg's compressor screen for pressure manipulation and radiography of a viscus. *A*, Fluorescent screen. *B*, Cassette. *C*, Tubular compressor.

maximum of information is obtained by the worker who, as a routine, employs both.

In the study of the mucous membrane, the duodenal cap and all the finer details revealed by fluoroscopy, it is often difficult to obtain film records of what is seen, for, in placing the film in position, time is lost or the pressure is altered and the film picture fails to show the appearance noticed. Several workers, notably Åkerlund and Berg, have designed apparatus to overcome this difficulty. It consists of a small tubular diaphragm fitted with a pad at one end and a fluorescent screen at the other, with a device for exposing serial films as necessary (Fig. 6). It is by the use of such apparatus that these two workers have been so successful in the study of the duodenal cap and mucous membrane respectively. Chaoul employs a band diaphragm for the field under observation. Several pieces of apparatus for this purpose are now fitted with film-changing devices. It is essential that the exposure be made under direct screen control. I myself have not used this apparatus, but can quite appreciate that it is likely to give much more uniformly satisfactory results. Åkerlund (6) says: "A series of X-ray films exposed under such conditions yields more information than the most thorough fluoroscopy; the detailed checking of the film by screening is a necessary condition in obtaining such a series."

The Study of Mucosa

The most important and instructive palpation of the stomach is that which is done while the first mouthful of very thick opaque food passes down. As it enters, the observer presses on the stomach and holds the food up for a moment, gradually allowing the hand to move down so that the shadow follows slowly, outlining the rugae (Fig. 7 a–d). He can push the food up and down between

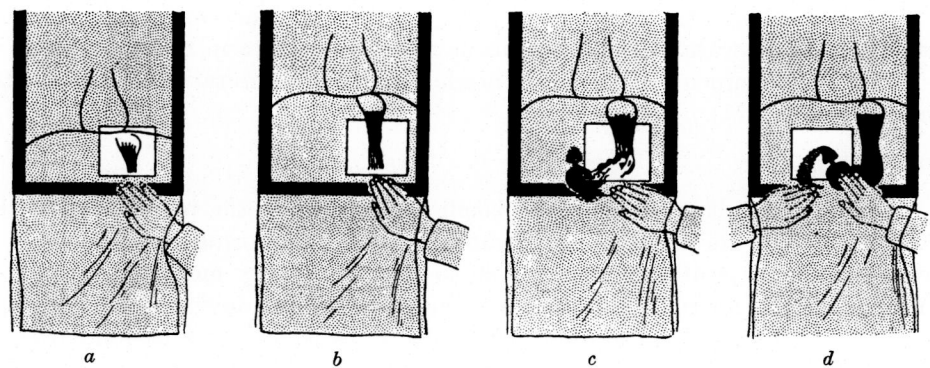

Fig. 7. a. The first mouthful of opaque food held up. The palpating hand is not in the direct beam of X rays. Note the rubber apron hanging from the screen. b. The hand sliding down just below the illuminated area and allowing the opaque food to canalise the empty stomach, outlining the rugae of the mucous membrane. c. Palpation with the stomach half filled, the contents being divided by the pressure. d. Using both hands, the right pushing food through the pylorus and shielded behind the food in the stomach, the left holding back the food in the second part of the duodenum.

the rugae quite easily in thin subjects, and even with a powerful abdominal wall this "combing out" is usually possible if the abdomen is thoroughly relaxed and the left hand is used to reinforce the right. In this manner he can detect the craters of small ulcers on the anterior and posterior walls that cannot be found by any other means, for such ulcers may not show any "niche" on the outline and frequently give no incisura with the fluid meal.

Posturing of the patient, by laying him on the couch, raising him up, and turning him on one or other side, is of great value in association with palpation, and every means should be adopted to make a thin layer of the emulsion flow between the rugae of the whole of the stomach so that the observer obtains a clear idea of their formation.

The demonstration of the patterns of the mucous membrane is tedious and painstaking work. It reveals conditions which might not even be guessed at by any other method. It is of very great practical importance and may in time be the means of accurately diagnosing abnormal conditions of the mucosa. Much has been done by Forssell, who initiated this work, and by Baastrup, Chaoul, Berg, Albrecht, Åkerlund and others, and I hope that these investigations will be continued, but that observers will refrain from laying down hard and fast lines of diagnosis until a very solid foundation of observations of the normal has been laid. We should hesitate long and be very sure of our ground before we stress variations in the mucous membrane pattern, lest they prove as misleading and as obstructive to future progress as the legacy which radiologists have received from the descriptive anatomist. The variations of the mucous membrane pattern may be like those of gross anatomy: endless and indefinable.

The new intragastric photography may be of assistance in interpreting the radiographic appearances of the mucous membrane pattern, but the technique is difficult and much experience is needed in the interpretation of the photographs (see p. 271).

Pylorus

In many cases it is not easy to visualise the rugae in the pyloric end of the stomach. They are usually best demonstrated by posturing the patient in a semi-recumbent position on the couch, so that the heavy mouthful gravitates into the pyloric antrum, and then making him lie right down, thus letting the bulk of the opaque food gradually slide back, assisted by palpation, towards the cardia, leaving a film between the rugae and outlining them. If the pylorus is rather to the right of the middle line, it may be necessary to rotate the patient to the left side.

Duodenal Cap

After the gastric mucous membrane has been explored as far as possible, more food is given, say a cupful, and observation is concentrated on the pylorus and the duodenum. In the first instance this is done on the upright screening stand. If the food will not go through the pylorus, an attempt should be made to push it through by pressure from the right hand, which is held "hidden" behind the opaque food in the stomach. This method usually fills the duodenal cap quite satisfactorily (Fig. 7 d). If, in spite of persistent manipulation, the food will not leave the stomach, the observer should wait with his hand on the abdomen until a wave of peristalsis comes along and should press suddenly as it approaches the pylorus. In some cases, however, the duodenal cap fills more readily in the recumbent position, especially if the patient is kept on the right side for a few moments. When the duodenum is irritable and the food races through without filling the duodenal cap satisfactorily, it is generally possible to block the second part of the duodenum by pressure with the left hand while urging the food through the pylorus with the right. It is important, however, not to be over-persistent with palpation, as the patient may feel bruised and will then resist.

A point in the technique that is often overlooked is that one view of the duodenum is not sufficient. The duodenal cap may appear regularly and perfectly formed in one plane, but persistently deformed in another at right angles. The patient should be examined not only in the postero-anterior plane but also in the lateral, and not only in the standing but also in the recumbent position. I prefer to have him lying on his back, as this makes palpation and manipulation easy, but I think that the duodenum fills more readily if he lies on his face. Some observers develop a technique for taking serial views of the duodenum under visual control in this position and, in fact, I did so myself for a time, but gradually abandoned it because it did not fit into my routine and absorbed more time than could be spared. There is, however, a great deal to be said in favour of this position, provided that serial films can be exposed under visual control. A mirror system is often employed for the purpose. I used to employ a simple lead-covered tunnel, with a gap of 6 in. × 5 in. through which the duodenum was screened from below and four exposures made on a 12 in. × 10 in. film with the tube above, the change-over being effected in a few seconds and a series of exposures completed in less than half a minute.

After the first food has passed the duodenum, the patient is kept under intermittent observation for about an hour until the observer has satisfied himself that there are no accumulations which might indicate obstruction in any intestinal coil.

When this examination is completed, the patient resumes his normal life and is told not to take any aperients.

The technique of the second examination

The second examination is usually timed for twenty-four hours after the first and the patient is given instructions to take the second meal five hours before he presents himself. Usually this should all have passed out of the stomach and should be in the terminal coils of the ileum, the caecum and proximal colon, while the rest of the colon is outlined by the meal given on the previous day. More often than not, however, the bowels have been moved, and the colon is only outlined as far as the splenic flexure. The presence of residual opaque food in the stomach calls for comment. In practice, if the stomach is empty, it is usual to give another mouthful or two in order to confirm what has been seen on the previous day and to make sure that no suggestion of any pathological condition has been overlooked. The examination of the caecum, appendix and colon is best carried out on the couch, as manipulation is so much easier. If the appendix is seen and palpated, the examination is now complete, unless the radiologist desires to make further observations on the large intestine. If the appendix is not seen, or if the shadows in the pelvis cannot be disentangled, the patient should come again on the following day without preparation and without having taken a purgative. A larger proportion of appendices are found filled on the third than on the second day. If the appendix is satisfactorily visualised, it is usually only of clinical interest from the point of view of adhesions, as its X-ray appearance seldom gives information about pathology. The indirect evidence of appendicular pathology is far more important than the visualisation of this wayward relic of antiquity. The technique for the visualisation of the appendix by means of magnesium sulphate is referred to on p. 169.

When the examination is finished, a purgative or enema must be ordered. Barium which stays in the intestine for a few days settles into a consistency not unlike plaster of Paris, and the patient will be very uncomfortable if it is not cleared out as soon as possible. I have been told of cases of actual obstruction, and I have personal knowledge of a number of instances in which the rectum has had to be relieved by a Volkmann spoon.

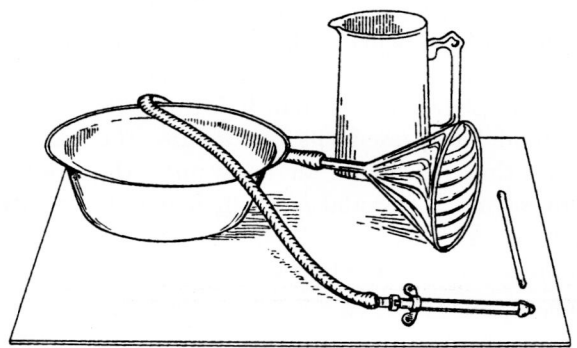

Fig. 8. Apparatus for opaque enema: basin, two-pint jug, glass funnel, rubber tube and enema nozzle.

THE TECHNIQUE OF THE OPAQUE ENEMA

For convenience and safety in palpation, the patient's left side should always be next to the observer. It is of the first importance to have a good view and be able to palpate effectively the upper sigmoid and descending colon as the enema passes up. In order to bring the caecum out of the pelvis—a manœuvre on which he places considerable stress—Courtney Gage instructs the patient to come for examination with the bladder as full as possible. It is of course essential to have the bowel thoroughly cleaned before the opaque enema is given. I prefer a wash-out to castor-oil. The only disadvantage is that it is apt to leave the bowel wet, which may interfere with the demonstration of detail as the opaque enema flows. Those who use the double contrast method prefer castor-oil. The patient should lie on his back with the pelvis tilted if possible. A mechanically-tilting couch is a great help to satisfactory work, but in its absence the pelvis can be raised on cushions; and, if the enema does not flow easily, a strenuous but satisfactory procedure is for the observer to join one hand with his assistant's under the patient's buttocks and raise them as necessary, while employing the other hand for manipulation and palpation. In view of the definite risks from scattered radiations, the observer should always wear a protective apron or take other measures to protect himself (see pp. 38 and 45).

For the actual injection an ordinary glass funnel with a rubber tube half an inch in diameter is satisfactory. This is connected to a specially designed metal cannula, half an inch wide and six inches long, fitted with a round-nosed trocar that is removed after insertion and before the rubber tube is attached (Fig. 8). I have recently designed a new type of trocar and cannula, which eliminates the disadvantages of the existing type (Fig. 9). It consists of two tubes, one sliding in the other; the inner tube bears a round nose with a flange against which the outer tube engages when at its full distance of travel inwards. The inner tube is pierced just below the nose with a series of slots for the fluid to pass through. The outer tube has at its further end a rounded conical collar to assist in its introduction

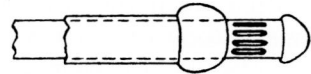

Fig. 9. Diagram of enema nozzle with sliding outer sheath.

and retention, and its rear end is fitted with a wing-nut to make it easier to hold. The inner tube is attached to a rubber feedpipe. For insertion the outer tube is pushed forward until it engages with the nose of the inner tube, the nose of the inner and the collar of the outer together forming a truncated cone to facilitate entry. When it is properly inserted, the outer tube is pulled back, exposing the slots; the fluid can then be introduced. The whole apparatus can be taken to pieces for cleaning purposes. It obviates the difficulty of attaching the tube to the cannula after this has been inserted, the slots do not tend to get blocked by folds of mucous membrane, and the rubber tube is not likely to come away from the cannula, even when it perishes.

If the barium does not flow, there is either an air-lock in the tube, or—with the old type of tube—the nozzle is pressing up against a fold of mucous membrane. To release the air-lock, the tube is nipped by the fingers below the funnel and squeezed with the other hand a few times. If this procedure does not renew the flow, the cannula, which may be held in position by the patient, should be drawn back an inch or so to make sure that it is not blocked by a fold of mucous membrane. Care must be taken that it does not slip out—the results are disastrous! The control should be in the hands of the observer and not left to an assistant, for it is helpful to him to be conscious of the degree of pressure that he is employing, particularly when there are obstructions in the rectum and sigmoid. For this purpose the funnel and rubber tube are admirably suited.

A call to stool is especially apt to occur if the pressure is increased unduly in order to promote the flow; it is at once relieved by lowering the funnel and allowing some of the injection to flow back into a basin. Some workers still use a Higginson's syringe but, apart from the difficulties of keeping it clear, only an experienced observer has any idea how much pressure he is exerting. Moreover, when the patient is disturbed by a call to stool, he cannot be relieved by simply drawing off as much as is necessary to reduce the tension.

The pressure at which the enema is given can be regulated by raising and lowering the funnel. It must always be given slowly and the patient should hardly feel it. If it enters too rapidly, irregularities in the wall may be missed. A certain degree of control of the flow can be exercised by posturing the patient. At the start the couch should be tilted foot-downwards and the patient rotated a little on to his right side, so that the enema always tends to run uphill. This prevents it from filling the whole sigmoid and passing into the descending colon before the observer has had a chance of making observations.

Often when the shadow reaches the brim of the true pelvis it halts and appears to be obstructed. If dropping the head end of the couch is not successful in helping the enema over the bony prominence, posturing may be needed, perhaps to the extent of rolling the patient almost on to his face. Again, when the head of the enema reaches the splenic flexure it may be arrested, and rolling the patient on to his right side may help its progress and, incidentally, give the observer a better view of the splenic loop.

Palpation is of course of great assistance, and full use should be made of it as soon as the shadow reaches a point at which it can be employed, i.e. at the upper limit of the sigmoid. The tortuous disposition of the sigmoid renders it very difficult, if not impossible, to visualise the whole course, even by rotating the patient; for this reason abnormalities are very frequently missed. The same difficulty applies at the splenic flexure, but this loop can always be visualised satisfactorily by rotating the patient to the right.

In the examination of the colon, palpation is chiefly of the manipulative type and the tactile sense can only be employed where the gut can be rolled under the fingers with the resistance of the ilium behind it; here thickenings are detected with comparative ease and certainty.

When the examination of the left side is completed, the patient should be turned round on the couch so that the right side is next the observer, who can thus manipulate the caecum. Palpation of the far side of the abdomen is very unsatisfactory and also tends to unnecessary exposure of the hands. A further observation after the patient has been to stool is a necessary part of the routine and particularly useful in cases of diverticulitis.

THE RADIOLOGIST'S REPORT

The radiologist's study of X-ray technique, his radiographic results and his special knowledge of interpretation are all a means to an end—namely, *the diagnosis*. His opinion on a case is often so important that both radiologists and clinicians now speak of the "X-ray" or "radiological" diagnosis. It is, however, only in part an "X-ray diagnosis". Radiology can show but one side of the picture—that which deals with gross outline and density. The radiologist relies on his clinical knowledge for the interpretation of the shadows he sees. To take an extreme instance: the X-ray diagnosis of "coin in the oesophagus" is made, not because of any positive evidence that the shadow is that of a coin, but because of the history and the radiologist's experience that such shadows are almost invariably due to swallowed coins. Or, to take a finer point, his only justification for suggesting that mottling seen in a chest is due to tuberculous disease is his clinical experience.

The report should be on definite lines. Starting with the salient features of fluoroscopic observations and with references to the points shown in the radiographs, it should end with the conclusions that are reached and the points in differential diagnosis. The writing of a positive report on a definite pathological condition is easy, but a negative report, especially when unusual conditions are present which may or may not be related to the symptoms, is exceedingly difficult, and particularly so if we do not know the clinician for whom the report is written. To some surgeons we do not mention anything of which we do not know the interpretation lest they should insist on an opinion for guidance in which we are not justified; while to others we know that we can express our doubts and fears freely, in the knowledge that they know our work and will not lay more stress on the points raised than is justified by the clinical picture.

There is always a very strong tendency to throw unsought and unjustifiable responsibility for the diagnosis upon the radiologist. The implication that in a difficult case he is regarded as a final court of appeal must never draw him into guessing beyond the limits of what he has seen. He must base his report absolutely and entirely on what he sees, and not on what he imagines he ought to have seen. He should make up his mind definitely as to what he has seen. It is only in the interpretation of what he has observed that the clinical side of the picture should in any way influence his judgment. In fact, he should write his report *before* looking at the clinical diagnosis. In many departments the radiologist first reads the clinical report and then turns to his pictures to see how far he can make his X-ray report harmonise with the clinical. This is an entirely wrong attitude. His mind is prejudiced and his report is biased. On the other hand, no matter how confident he may be in what he has seen and his interpretation of it, he must remember that the X-ray evidence is but one piece of a jigsaw puzzle, which must fit, even if this means re-arrangement. I recall two extreme examples. In one, a radiologist made the startling diagnosis of a laryngeal displacement that was incompatible with life, and yet the patient was sitting in comfort in the waiting-room! In the other, because the patient could eat ordinary food, his physician would not accept the radiologist's diagnosis of a typical chronic gastric ulcer. In the first instance the radiologist had no clinical sense, and in the second the clinician was so obsessed with the time-honoured conception of the clinical picture of a gastric ulcer that he could not accept radiological evidence that was absolutely definite. To make the picture complete, the clinical and the radiological evidence must be set in order side by side.

A vital part of the routine is ample time for examining films carefully on a good viewing box; to examine them casually in a dark room or against a cloudy sky is to court disaster. Until he has studied his film records carefully and compared them with his notes, the radiologist should never express an opinion either to doctor or patient. In practice it is often very difficult to refrain, for both patient and doctor are apt to worry him into expressing opinions before he is ready.

The radiologist often comes across abnormal conditions that have no relation to the symptoms, and may have to exercise self-restraint to avoid calling attention to something that would be better overlooked. He can, unintentionally, be just too clever, for the patient is not in a position to appreciate that the human body can show many harmless deviations from what is called the normal. The radiologist's first purpose is to help to cure the patient, and the mental impression he conveys is of the greatest importance. To hedge, even slightly, over some anomaly that is of scientific interest but of no clinical importance may have a disastrous mental effect on the patient in whose outlook the radiologist's opinion may be the deciding factor. I remember cases in which, finding some interesting condition such as a displaced stomach, a duodenal pouch or a transposition of viscera, I have allowed the patient to see my interest—sometimes by calling in my partner—with the result that, in spite of my assurances, the patient was convinced that I was hiding something from him. In this way I may have done incalculable harm.

The diagnosis of gastro-intestinal conditions, particularly of the stomach and duodenum, should be made primarily on the fluorescent screen, the films being merely records of what has been observed. In most departments, and also in private practice, it is still customary to send out a number of films or prints with the report. The question of the ownership of these films is dealt with in Appendix VI (p. 387).

PRECEPTS FOR EXAMINATIONS

"DON'T"

Don't undertake the examination at all unless you can do it properly and in the way which you think will give a reliable result.

Don't start your examination with the intention of finding something pathological.

Don't focus your attention on the lesion which you think ought to be present; follow your routine, and if it is there you will come to it in due course.

Don't be "jockeyed" out of your routine—including the preparation—by anybody, particularly by surgeons who are in a hurry to clear the beds. Short cuts over strange country are often the longest way—they are dangerous and likely to lead you astray.

Don't try to make a diagnosis until you have completed the whole examination and can sit down at leisure to go through your clinical and radioscopic notes with the films you have taken.

Don't try to demonstrate to anyone until you have already made your examination and know what you are going to show; you need all your faculties for observation.

Don't puzzle about what you see; just record the fact and wait till you have made all your observations before you worry about the interpretation.

Don't be afraid of saying that you do not know the interpretation of what you see.

Don't jump to conclusions and don't guess.

Don't expose yourself or the patient unnecessarily.

"DO"

Adhere rigidly to your routine, both in technique and in the sequence of observations.

Make certain of each observation, note it and pass on rapidly to the next point.

Make notes of what you see as you go along, whether you understand it or not.

Make your report out in ordered sequence of your observations, followed by your deductions.

Make certain that your deductions are reasonable in comparison with the clinical picture.

Repeat any observation of which you are not certain. Even if you are certain, it is advisable to confirm.

Remember that the majority of cases, particularly those in private practice, are normal, or not grossly pathological, and come for examination because of the fear of cancer.

Remember that disordered physiology may give rise to symptoms identical with those of pathological lesions.

CHAPTER III

RADIOLOGICAL RISKS AND THEIR AVOIDANCE

A. *RISKS OF THE RADIOLOGIST AND HIS STAFF*

Radiology is not a profession for the careless or ignorant worker. The protection of the operator and his staff from the dangers to which they are exposed is of paramount importance and the welfare of those who work in X-ray departments is the responsibility of the radiologist in charge. He can call to his assistance the expert advice of the electrician on electrical risks, and that of the physicist on the protective value against radiations of the materials used, both in the structure of the building and in the apparatus itself, but he cannot throw his responsibility on to their shoulders. It is his duty to see that working conditions are such that neither he nor any of his assistants is exposed to any unnecessary risk or unduly exposed to any necessary one.

In the very early days the worker was entirely unprotected; the X-ray tubes, held in wooden clips, were bare and, in order to test the quality of the rays emitted, the radiologist often used the shadow of his own hand on the fluorescent screen! During the war the problem of the protection of the worker became a very pressing one. It was accentuated by the fact that a large proportion of those who did this work in the Army were quite inexperienced and had no knowledge either of the dangers or of how to avoid them. Also, the protection on the apparatus supplied was, for the most part, hopelessly inefficient. The results were sometimes disastrous, and a number of workers suffered from more or less acute burns. A much-needed alarm was sounded. The X-ray and Radium Protection Committee was formed* and drew up the first schedule of recommendations in 1921.

No one can doubt the dangers of radiations, and the Committee took up the attitude that, since they did not know how much can be tolerated by the human body without ill effect, it was their duty to devise a condition of absolute protection: not one ray, whether direct or scattered, was to be allowed to reach the worker if it could possibly be avoided, no matter what the cost to diagnostic efficiency. Measurements of intensities suggest, however, that the massive and unwieldy apparatus which was evolved in response to these early recommendations erred on the side of timidity. The problem is not now so important, as the modern tube is self-protected. There is, however, no need to provide

* On the initiative of Dr Stanley Melville, with the co-operation of Dr Robert Knox, Dr G. W. C. Kaye and Prof. S. Russ, under the chairmanship of Sir Humphry Rolleston. The latest schedule of Recommendations is printed in Appendix V, p. 383.

protective material on the walls of radiographic and radioscopic rooms to shield passers-by, and only a very small lead equivalent is necessary even on the adjacent dark-room walls to protect photographic material. (These remarks do not, of course, apply to treatment installations.)

The real danger lies in the cumulative effects of many small "accidental" doses of direct radiation. Very many of the early workers, especially those who tested their tubes with their hands, suffered from chronic dermatitis of the backs of the hands or other exposed parts, though even the slight protection afforded by the clothes saved the arms. Many of the men damaged in this way have died, warts developing in the scar tissues and eventually becoming malignant. An actual X-ray burn is not necessary to produce this chronic dermatitis; in fact, it has been seen slowly developing for years after all exposure had ceased.

Conditions that have been tolerated

X-ray departments are improving so rapidly that soon there will be none of the old bad conditions left under which workers suffered loss of health and life. It is, therefore, well that present-day workers should realise the quantities of radiation to which their predecessors were exposed. Without such knowledge the demand for protection may be carried to such an extreme that future workers may think themselves in danger from an intensity of radiations that has proved harmless in practice. The efficiency of the work must not be impaired by unnecessarily clumsy apparatus. I do not for one moment wish to minimise the danger inherent in X rays. Without incessant watchful care, efficient diagnostic screen examination cannot be made safe, but there is inevitably a residue of radiation from which the observer can only be completely protected by precautions that would make observation prolonged and tedious and diminish diagnostic efficiency. I have always maintained that the radiologist's first object must be to make an efficient examination, and that in order to attain it he must, if necessary, take some risk. The question is where to strike a balance between the two factors of efficiency and risk.

In order to obtain biological material for this purpose, Miss S. F. Cox and I tried to measure the quantity of radiations to which workers were exposed under the old conditions.* This work was done before the introduction of the international r unit and the measurements were assessed according to the practice then in routine use. The r unit values have now been added; they vary with the kilovoltage, and for the purposes of this book the value of 450 r per U.S.D. has been taken, this being the value between 80 and 100 K.V. We measured and estimated the average daily dose received by two workers. The first was a woman who supervised X-ray therapy in a small basement room where three Coolidge tubes were in constant use, worked at 7 in. spark-gap and held in open-

* This paper is republished in Appendix II, p. 363.

topped glass bowls. When exposed in the place occupied by this operator, a radiographic plate darkened in a few minutes, yet she had been there many hours a day for some years, apparently without suffering any ill effects. Her blood count was normal. Every day she received about $\frac{1}{140}$ or 0·007 of a unit skin dose. This represents about 3·15 r units. Though this is a very small quantity, in seven years she must have received a total of 17 or 18 unit skin doses (10,200–10,800 r units). In the second case we could only compute a part of the exposure, but in the aggregate it had been considerably larger than that of the first case.

Since the first worker showed no ill effects, we held ourselves justified in assuming that the amount of radiation she had received daily for seven years could not be much, if at all, beyond the safety limit. Nevertheless, in order to be unquestionably on the safe side, we decided to fix as our general safety limit an intensity of $\frac{1}{25}$ of this dose, i.e. 0·00028 of a unit skin dose (0·126 r units) per day. This dose does not affect a Sabouraud pastille or any of the ordinary instruments for computing dosage, but causes considerable darkening of an X-ray film.*

The Safety Limit

As the result of further experience and the observation of working conditions in many centres where no ill effects have occurred I am now convinced that we were over-cautious in taking such a high figure as $\frac{1}{25}$. I now maintain that $\frac{1}{5}$ of the known tolerated dose is more reasonable, i.e. 0·63 r (0·0014 U.S.D.).

For the last seven years at the Mayo Clinic palpation in the direct beam has been the rule, and the workers must have sustained a dosage that was very far beyond the standard now laid down (0·63 r). True, they wore washleather gloves, but Cilly, Leddy and Kirklin[97] have proved conclusively that these have no protective value. That these workers, who palpate every case and do a most unusual amount of screen work, should have escaped injury, is no argument that others less skilled should take risks. It does, however, strongly confirm my contention that a daily safety limit of 0·63 r leaves an adequate margin of safety.

There is no sense in unnecessarily taking even the semblance of a risk when dealing with such an insidious source of danger as that involved in exposure to X rays, and I fully realise that I am taking a great responsibility in urging that the accepted daily tolerance dose is unnecessarily high. I feel, however, that safety lies in knowledge of the facts and that no useful purpose is served by maintaining a standard which is constantly disregarded. No standards or

---

* In the first edition a figure was included indicating the blackening of X-ray film with intensities of radiations of the order of the daily safety limit. This figure is now omitted; X-ray film is not necessarily standard and the figure might well be misleading.

recommendations will protect the foolhardy and ignorant worker. Safety lies in knowledge, not in respectful fear of the unknown.

It is therefore suggested that the worker should prepare his own scale, using standard photographic materials, on the basis of the following figures kindly prepared for me by Miss Cox*:

Find the time required for the U.S.D. under the average conditions of radiography and screening, but using only so much current as the tube will stand, e.g. 90 K.V., 2 ma., 1 mm.Al. Suppose that this gives the U.S.D. in five minutes at 9 in. The effect of the distance factor will be to reduce 1 U.S.D. to 0·0014 U.S.D. (0·63 r units) at a distance of 20·1 ft. This of course would be an inconvenient way of making the scale, and the same effect can be produced at a shorter distance by reducing the exposure. If the film is exposed for twenty seconds at 5 ft. (i.e. 1/15th of the time required for U.S.D. at 9 in.), it will represent the photographic effect of 0·0014 U.S.D. As the efficiency of apparatus varies, the figure of five minutes is not likely to be correct for other outfits working on the same factors, so that each worker must determine this basic figure for himself. He can then divide this time by 15, and this will be the correct exposure to give 0·0014 U.S.D. (0·63 r units) at 5 ft.

The dangers in an X-ray department fall under three heads: those arising from (1) the X rays, (2) electrical shocks and (3) the conditions of work.

(1) DANGERS FROM EXPOSURE TO X RAYS

Inspection of Equipment

A systematic inspection of accommodation, apparatus and working conditions by an experienced radiologist or a specially trained physicist is highly advisable, particularly when the department is new. In addition, the radiologist should test periodically by means of a fluorescent screen every place where he and his staff work. For this purpose the room must be perfectly darkened and the eyes of the observer suitably prepared. He should also make periodic tests by placing X-ray films in the positions usually occupied by workers, who should themselves carry dental films in a pocket-book or elsewhere for a few days. I wish to emphasise the value of this very simple test, which is not only useful and reliable, but is sometimes also a guide to the way in which an assistant carries out his work. Carelessness tells its tale. These films should show only a faint trace of exposure after some days, even when carried by those who do fluoroscopy, if they work conscientiously and carefully.

Even though the apparatus has been tested by a physicist, the radiologist should always be on the look-out for dangers. Recently I found that a piece of protective material had become detached inside a tube box, allowing a stream of rays to pass out in a very dangerous manner. I have seen a number of X-ray burns on the legs produced by leaks in under-couch tube boxes; in one instance the protective material had come away from the box and in others, under war conditions, ordinary glass instead of lead glass had been used.

* The value of the photographic method of measurement of small intensities of X rays is dealt with in Appendix II, p. 363.

Working Precautions

Four essential points must be remembered in considering protection from X-ray dangers.

(*a*) The direct radiation, i.e. the primary beam arising from the focal spot on the target of the tube, is extremely dangerous. On no pretext whatever should the radiologist allow any part of his person to be exposed to it. Such exposure is entirely unnecessary and unjustified. Nothing will save from accident those who allow the primary beam to pass over the edge of the fluorescent screen and then get into it. To safeguard such workers is impossible, and to attempt to do so not only makes apparatus unnecessarily clumsy and expensive, but hampers the intelligent worker in the service of the patient.

(*b*) The intensity of the rays varies inversely with the square of the distance. (Photographic tests, which were confirmed by a special iontoquantimeter, suggested that this law did not apply to the secondary radiations that are given off from the primary beam. The apparent discrepancy is due to the fact that they do not arise from a point, but are complicated by back-scattering from walls and other surfaces. The blackening of a photographic film may therefore be much greater than it should be according to the inverse-square law.)

(*c*) The quantity of the rays received by a worker varies directly with the duration of his exposure.

(*d*) The protective value of any material is the same whether it is close up to the anti-cathode or at a distance.

No protective devices will save the man who wantonly exposes himself—perhaps on the score of absorption in his observations. The risks to the observer are naturally greatest in screening, for he must be close to, if not actually in the direct line of the rays for some minutes, and the intensity of radiation employed in screen examination is very considerable. In a large department, where a great deal of gastro-intestinal work is done, the radiations measured at 9 in. from the anti-cathode amounted to an average of 17·6 unit skin doses (7920 r units) a day, a figure that is now probably nearly doubled because of the increase in the volume of work. In order to keep a check on the exposure of the assistants during their screen examinations, we had a recording clock that registered only when the tube was in operation. We found that each gastro-intestinal examination took an average of four minutes' screening. Inexperienced workers will, however, take more time, and far more than they realise.

It is inevitable that the observer should be exposed to some extent in the screen examinations which are essential in thoracic and abdominal diagnosis. The first concern of the radiologist must be the patient. If he is going to place his personal safety in the forefront and is not ready to take such very slight risks as are unavoidable, he had better look out for some other field for his activities. This, however, is not to suggest that he should take no precautions at all. On the contrary, he should take every precaution that is compatible with efficient service for the patient.

SECONDARY RADIATIONS*

The observer must realise that X rays are comparable to light rays, and that as soon as any opening is made in the X-ray-proof box, the rays will escape and scatter just like rays of light coming from an incandescent bulb placed in the same position as the X-ray tube. There is the direct beam that comes through the diaphragm and is, or should be, completely stopped by the patient's body and by the lead glass of the fluorescent screen, and there are the secondary radiations shooting out from the primary beam in all directions. The intensity of this type of radiation diminishes proportionately with the smallness of the diaphragm opening; therefore the minimum opening should always be used. Incidentally, this has also the advantage of giving sharper detail in the screen picture.

When an X ray is stopped, it breaks up, generating new rays. Some of these are of the same penetrating power as the original beam, but a large proportion are much softer and appear to have very little penetrating power. The problem of protection from secondary radiations is an exceedingly vexed one. Some people regard these rays as extremely dangerous but, in my opinion, if ordinary working precautions are observed, they need not cause anxiety. At the same time it is desirable that the radiologist should realise the existence and intensity of the secondary rays to which he is exposed. Personal experiment is the method by which he will best understand the problems.

He will probably have had a guarantee that all his apparatus is of a certain degree of protective value. Having tested out roughly with a screen† to see if this guarantee is correct and that there are no leaks when the tube box is entirely closed, he should then open the diaphragm, and he will find that the larger the opening the greater will be the illumination of his fluorescent screen at any point in the room. Holding the screen in various positions, he will discover that this secondary radiation is coming not only from the direction of the tube box but also from the ceiling and floor. A convincing demonstration is, with the tube below the couch, to hold the screen upside down above the head: it is illuminated by rays that are obviously reflected from the ceiling. With the diaphragm wide open and passing the current he uses for radiography, he can see not only the illumination of the screen, but even the bones of his hand held behind it, almost

---

* See Appendix III, p. 379.

† A ladder of increasing thicknesses of $\frac{1}{8}$ mm. of lead foil is easily made for the purpose. If such foil is not available, the backing of a dental film may be used. This has a thickness of approximately 0·2 mm.; it is not pure lead and approximates sufficiently to $\frac{1}{8}$ mm. of lead for a rough test.

anywhere in the room. The more penetrating the quality of the rays and the larger the diaphragm opening, the brighter becomes the screen illumination. As he closes the diaphragm, the lighting of the screen diminishes. The intensity of this radiation is by no means negligible. Under the conditions of barium enema work the observer may be exposed to an intensity of radiation equal to 3 per cent. of the primary beam and having a similar penetrating power. The brightness of the image when making an exposure with, say, 50 ma. at 80–90 k.v. is enough to frighten anyone into taking precautions (see Figs. 10 and 11).

Another interesting and enlightening experiment is to get an assistant to move across the direct beam of radiations while the observer stands at one side holding the screen. Immediately the assistant's body begins to pass across the beam, the screen illumination brightens markedly; it fades as the whole beam passes through his body (the secondary rays being absorbed), increases again as he passes across the edge of the beam, and diminishes when the rays are no longer scattered by his body. The experiment shows that the operator is particularly exposed to this type of ray when standing beside the screening stand or couch, notably in barium enema work.

Precautions against Dangers arising from Secondary Radiations

It is the primary beam of rays which must be guarded against with constant vigilance; these secondary rays are as the spray compared with the waterfall. If the whole waterfall is enclosed in a tube, there will be no spray, but the amount increases proportionately with the quantity that is allowed to tumble down the rock face. So also, when the primary beam is enclosed inside the ray-proof tube box, there is no secondary radiation. The amount that escapes into the room depends entirely upon the quantity of the primary radiation that is allowed to pass out of the tube box. Therefore the radiologist should always use a completely enclosed type of tube box or a self-protected tube (metalix type) for all screen work, and should persistently and conscientiously keep the diaphragm opening down to the smallest aperture that he can work with.

Even so, a certain amount of "spray" must inevitably escape, but it is very doubtful whether this is sufficiently intense under ordinary working conditions to produce any ill effects. My hands must have been bathed in this type of radiation year after year, yet I have no indication that they have suffered. It is doubtful if any worker has suffered from secondary radiation alone. I believe that palpation with the bare hands is perfectly safe for any man who recognises the risk of letting them get into the direct beam and who has never suffered from X-ray dermatitis. For those who have so suffered, no form of glove or other device can make even occasional palpation a safe proceeding, and they should leave the method entirely alone.

It was my practice for many years to sit within 4 or 5 ft. of a Coolidge tube when it was in use for treatment on a 7 in. spark-gap. I was only protected from the direct radiations by a very inadequate half-open type of tube box and was literally bathed in secondary radiations, a dental film in my pocket being completely blackened in an hour. Yet neither skin, hair, nor sweat glands showed any changes. This fact affords no proof whatever that these rays are not a definite danger, but it proves that quite a large quantity can be tolerated for a prolonged period without ill effect—at any rate on the skin.

There are, however, two positions of real danger from this type of radiation. The first is that of any person standing beside the couch, as a glance at a fluorescent screen held beside the patient will show (Figs. 10 and 12). The second position of danger is that of the assistant standing beside the observer at the upright screening stand (Figs. 14 and 15). The amount of this type of radiation that reaches the observer is almost negligible, for he is protected not only by the patient but by the lead glass of the screen, but the assistant who operates the switchboard (which is usually mounted on a trolley) often stands just beside the observer, exposing himself to the full force of these secondary rays (Fig. 14).

The radiologist will have to tolerate a certain amount of this X-ray "spray" all his life and there is no sense in taking unnecessary risks. Although elaborate precautions are unnecessary it is worth while for both observer and assistant to wear X-ray-proof aprons. In the screening room of a department where no effort is made to cope with the problem of secondary radiations, dental films showed only a trace of blackening when worn under a lead rubber smock equivalent to $\frac{1}{4}$ mm. of lead, even by the man who did all the screen examinations.

That some have been fortunate does not justify others in taking risks. Personally I attribute my freedom from trouble rather to good luck than to good management, for good fortune dictated the saving factors: *speed* in observation was the only way to get through the day's work; the sharpness of the shadows was increased by using a *small diaphragm*; the tubes would not stand up to prolonged work and had to be conserved, so that the *minimum of current* was always used.

Can Fluoroscopy be reasonably safe?

I have no hesitation whatever in answering in the affirmative. I can speak from an experience of many years' almost continuous screen work, during many of which protection was almost negligible. One well-known radiologist who has screened every case that he has seen since 1898 is absolutely free from any indication of ill effect, and has become the father of a large family. Up to 1918 he wore neither apron nor gloves of protective material, yet his hands have escaped completely, probably owing to his early appreciation of the value of a small diaphragm opening in giving detail in the screen picture. Consequently

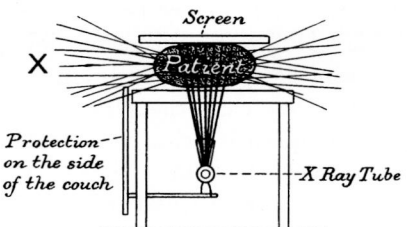

Fig. 10. Diagram to illustrate the danger to the observer in screening at the couch, particularly in barium enema work.

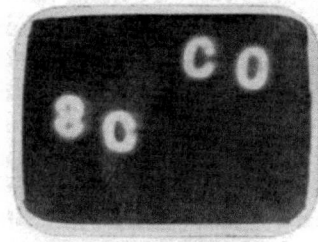

Fig. 11. A dental film exposed at X in Fig. 10, i.e. in the position of the abdomen of an observer during an opaque enema examination with 90 K.V., 4 ma. for five minutes, with an aperture wide enough to cover a 12×15 film.

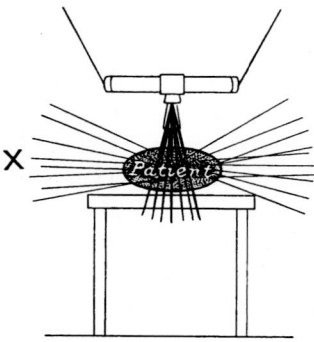

Fig. 12. Diagram to illustrate the danger to an assistant standing beside the couch during radiography.

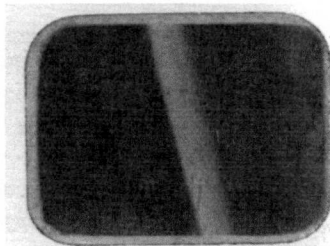

Fig. 13. A dental film worn by an assistant (X in Fig. 12) during a morning's work.

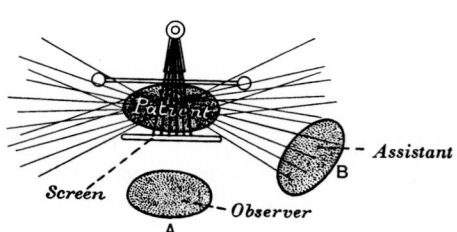

Fig. 14. Diagram to illustrate the safety of the observer, A, and the danger of his assistant, B, during observations in the upright screening stand.

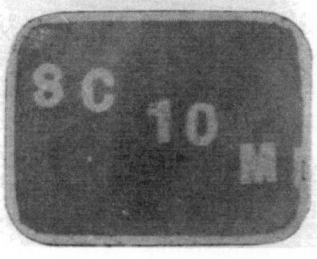

Fig. 15. Dental film exposed in the position occupied by assistant (B in Fig. 14) during two opaque meal examinations. The film worn by the observer at A was so little affected that the lead letters placed on it did not show.

he probably never exposed himself to direct radiation. His only protection since 1918 has been a light rubber coat.

The Upright Screening Stand

The fluorescent screen *must* be of adequate size, it *must* be covered with good X-ray-proof glass, and it *must* have an X-ray-proof apron hanging from it. The size of the screen must be not less than 12 in. × 15 in. and should preferably be 14 in. × 17 in., so that the observer can, if necessary, see in his field the whole width of the abdomen or chest, and particularly the whole width of the patient's diaphragm.

The question of X-ray-proof glass is difficult and one for compromise. Glass of the protective value of 1·5 mm. of lead was recommended by the Protection Committee, but is heavy and expensive. The protective value of the glass that I had in use for many years was only about $\frac{1}{2}$ mm. of lead, and this was approximately the maximum obtainable up to about 1920. I never heard of any observer sustaining any damage to his face when using this value of lead glass. I am absolutely confident that glass of 1 mm. lead equivalent is fully adequate, but even this thickness makes the fluorescent screens very heavy. This weight is unimportant in the upright screening stand, where it is counterbalanced, but is a grave disadvantage in the screen that is used in conjunction with the couch and which, for the sake of convenience, habitually rests upon the patient's abdomen. Moreover, such a heavy screen tends to hamper observation and is far more liable to accident. In many modern couches, however, it is supported on a carrying arm, and some workers suspend the screen above the couch.

Side wings, to limit the scattering, have been recommended for upright screening stands, but they can only partially fulfil this object. Moreover, they make the apparatus clumsy and increase the cost quite disproportionately. I do not think they are at all necessary.

Although the observer conducting fluoroscopic examinations with the upright screening stand is in the direct line of a beam of enormous destructive power, he will be perfectly safe if his ordinary position is at least 4 ft. from the anti-cathode and he is protected by lead glass equivalent to 1 mm. of lead, and by the body of the patient representing $\frac{1}{4}$–$\frac{1}{2}$ mm. of lead. Only about 2 per cent. of the direct radiations produced at 90,000 volts—the average used in fluoroscopy—will pass through this thickness of lead. Of this fraction the observer will receive less than 5 per cent., i.e. 0·1 per cent. of the rays measured at 9 in. from the anti-cathode.

Protective Aprons

The effect of the rays is cumulative, and the skin which has once been damaged is susceptible. Those who have suffered even slight damage cannot be too careful.

All workers, particularly those who have done localisation work in the war, should wear an apron when screening patients. The type of apron I use is a smock made from a single sheet of comparatively thin X-ray-proof rubber, covering both the back and the front of the body. Its protective value is $\frac{1}{4}$ mm. of lead. It has no arms and is open at the sides, where its halves are loosely held together by two chains; it is slipped on over the head, and the weight (about 6 lb.) is balanced and taken easily on the shoulders (Fig. 16). It does not drag the shoulders forward like the old type of apron which was supported by a strap round the neck and which the operator took off as soon as authority's back was turned.

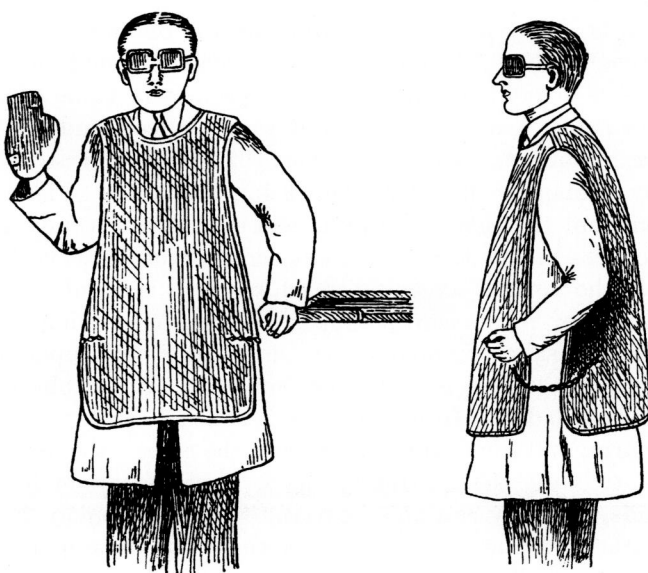

Fig. 16. Observer's smock, made of light X-ray-proof rubber. The diagram also shows the palpating glove used in manipulation (cf. Fig. 3). The goggles figured have ruby celluloid for the preparation of the observer's eyes; they are not made of protective material.

The X-ray-proof apron that hangs from the lower edge of the screen on the upright screening stand should be divided with an overlap in such a way that the observer's hand can be comfortably inserted for palpation. I find that palpation is greatly assisted if the apron is made in three strips, the central one overlapping the lateral ones, so that the palpating hand can pass between them. Usually this apron is of very thick X-ray-proof rubber, but quite thin protective rubber of $\frac{1}{2}$ mm. of lead is all that is necessary. The apron is only required to catch any stray primary or secondary radiation that might escape below the screen and would strike the observer's body. An apron of this thickness is soft and pliable and does not materially interfere with palpation. Its width should be that of the screen and it should be about a foot in depth.

The operator should make a test to see that there is no gap between the apron and the lead glass of the fluorescent screen. A beam of direct radiations through such a gap would be most dangerous, especially to the novice who has not learned to keep his illuminated area always strictly within the limits of the glass. For a similar reason protective material should also be fitted up the sides of the screen, giving a margin of safety of about 4 in. outside the lead glass to stop any direct radiation that the operator may carelessly allow to extend beyond the limits of the fluorescent screen. As the observer's face should never, in any circumstances, be exposed to the direct beam, X-ray-proof masks and goggles are entirely unnecessary. The attendant nurse should always wear an X-ray-proof apron if she cannot stand at least 6 ft. from the tube (cf. Fig. 14).

Tube Boxes

The Coolidge tube is a much more dangerous instrument than the metalix or the old gas tube, for besides the direct rays from the target an additional 5 per cent. come from the anti-cathode stem. This direct radiation and its source are readily appreciated by screen observation if the diaphragm opening is shut

Fig. 17. Pin-hole radiograph showing that radiations arise from the whole length of the anti-cathode and not only from the focal spot.

down to a quarter of an inch. This gives the effect of a pin-hole camera, and in addition to the brilliantly illuminated area there is a fainter image giving a picture of the whole stem of the anti-cathode (Fig. 17). If, therefore, a Coolidge tube is used, a box of the completely enclosed type is essential for safety. The metalix type of tube, which, like the Coolidge, is a hot-filament tube, is quite free from this particular source of danger, for all the radiation produced emanates from the focal spot of the anti-cathode. The use of this type of tube is likely to become universal, for it has the great advantage that no protective box is necessary, since the protective material is incorporated in the tube itself, thus eliminating all the bulky and weighty protection boxes that are essential with the older types of tube.

A word of warning is perhaps still necessary against certain old tube boxes that are still in use, in the manufacture of which reliance is placed on sheet iron or steel. Iron is a very poor obstructor of the rays, and it takes $\frac{3}{4}$ in. (18 mm.) to give a protection equivalent to 3 mm. lead. The usual $\frac{1}{8}$ in. (3 mm.) sheet iron only equals about 0·1 mm. lead.

Radiography during Screening

A number of radiographic exposures are usually made during a routine screen examination. The cassettes are slipped into place and the observer maintains his position during the exposure. This practice seems to be quite safe with the protection already mentioned for, although large intensities of rays are employed in the exposures, the time is only fractional. In fact, the quantity of radiation is only a very small proportion of that used in the necessarily prolonged routine of the screen examination.

Safety lies in the knowledge and realisation of dangers and, no matter how efficient the protective measures, it is the radiologist's business to look after himself and see that he is never exposed to the direct beam, always keeping it well within the limits of the protective glass of the fluorescent screen.

MEASUREMENTS OF THE DANGER
(In conjunction with W. V. Mayneord)
(A figure of 0·63 r as the daily safety limit is taken as the basis, see p. 34)

The exact conditions of screening were reproduced, but a corpse was used in place of the living subject. The measurements were made with a number of small condenser chambers, exposed simultaneously and examined immediately. They seemed to give accurate and consistent readings and confirmed the photographic estimates of the risks involved.

It can be accepted that, although some expert workers are much more rapid, the average observer spends five minutes on the actual screening of each gastric case and about ten minutes on each completed gastro-intestinal case.

(A) *The Upright Screening Stand*

The factors were as follows: time 5 min.; area illuminated 5×5 in.; K.V. 80; milliampères 5; filters 1 mm.Al. and $\frac{1}{4}$ in. three-ply wood; tube screen distance 30 in.

Under the above conditions the figures were of the order of:

(*a*) On the skin of the patient, 6·0 r.

(*b*) In the beam on the distal side of the patient, i.e. in the position of the palpating hand, 0·2 r. It would therefore need only 15 min. daily with the palpating hand in the direct beam to exceed the danger limit of 0·63 r. How long the observer's hand would be exposed in the direct ray and the way in which he used the opaque food in the stomach to hide his hand would depend on his skill. For our purpose we must assume that his hand is exposed during the whole period.

(*c*) Just outside the illuminated area the palpating hand used in the manner I advocate (p. 18) received a dose that was less than 0·01 r. It was therefore perfectly safe for an almost indefinite period.

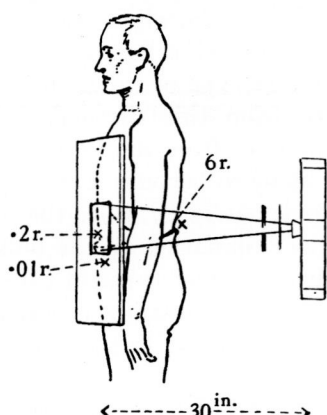

Fig. 18. In five minutes' exposure 6 r was measured on the subject's skin, 0·2 r in the position of the palpating hand in the illuminated area, and 0·01 r just outside the illuminated area.

(*d*) The usual protecting apron that hangs below the screen had been removed and in the position of the observer's abdomen the dose was smaller than 0·01r; in fact it hardly affected the condenser chambers used. Therefore, if the observer uses a small illuminated area in the middle of the screen, he is quite safe as regards exposure to his abdomen.

(*e*) Using a larger field, i.e. 12 × 15 in. illumination, there was, as expected, some slight increase in these figures, but not sufficient to affect the conclusions, except as regards the observer's abdomen. This might conceivably be exposed to a dangerous intensity. The danger is of course automatically dealt with by the apron that hangs from the fluorescent screen to protect the careless worker who allows the direct beam to overlap its limits.

(B) *Screening on the Couch*

The factors for these readings were the same but the tube-screen distance was 26 in. and the illuminated area 12 × 15 in., since large fields are frequently employed in opaque enema work.

In the position of the observer's abdomen 0·8 r was measured in five minutes.

Every worker therefore should appreciate that he stands in a definitely dangerous intensity of radiation when screening patients on the couch. The risk is mainly due to the scattered radiation that comes from the patient's body. In one screen examination of only five minutes' duration the daily safety limit of 0·63 r may be exceeded. Clearly this must be avoided, and the easiest method is to wear an apron. Tests were therefore made with a thin lead rubber apron which gives $\frac{1}{8}$ mm. lead equivalent protection. It cut this radiation down to 2 per cent. at 80 K.V.

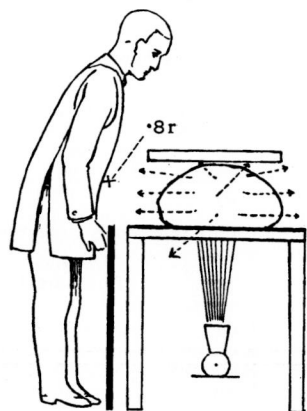

Fig. 19. In five minutes' exposure 0·8 r was measured in the position of the observer's abdomen.

and to 6 per cent. at 100 K.V. and was therefore amply sufficient to reduce the intensity far below the safety limit.

(C) *In Radiography*

The figures of the intensities employed in the radiography which is carried out in the course of screen examination were surprisingly small and corresponded closely to those of E. W. Twining of Manchester, who kindly gave me his unpublished results. When making radiographic exposures in the course of screen examinations, the intensity of scattered radiation reaching the palpating hand *outside the direct beam* was negligible, while in the position of the observer the chambers were unaffected. It is therefore absolutely safe for the observer to retain his position while films are exposed, as in fact he always does in practice. It is quite safe for him to maintain pressure with his hand, provided that he keeps it *outside* the direct beam.

It is clear therefore that the intensities of radiation to which an observer may be exposed during screen examination are small and can be easily reduced far below the danger limit. Definite danger, however, lies in carelessness and failure to study the problems and to take reasonable precautions.

According to Zuppinger[344], with the apparatus now used at the Zürich Institute the patient gets roughly the following dosage in r (550 r = 1 U.S.D.).

X-ray dose on skin of patient's back in postero-anterior position.

Distance of skin from anticathode cm.	Voltage K.V.	Current in ma.	Filtration mm.Al.	Dose per minute r.	Time taken to give one U.S.D. min.
40	60	4	$\frac{1}{2}$	12	50
	70			13	46
56	60	4	$\frac{1}{2}$	6	100
	70			7	87

The palpating hand receives the following dosage:

Distance of palpating hand from anticathode cm.	Thickness of patient's body cm.	Voltage K.V.	Current in ma.	Filtration mm.Al.	Dose per minute r.	Time taken to give one U.S.D. hours
76	20	70	4	$\frac{1}{2}$	0·004	2400
50	10				0·017	550

According to Saupe's measurements, the dosage in radiography is:

Organ	Distance from target cm.	Voltage K.V.	Current in ma.	Filtration mm.Al.	Length of exposure sec.	Dosage per exposure r.
Lung	100	45	80	1	0·15	0·08
Stomach	40	63	40	2	0·3	0·3
Kidneys	50	53	20	1	3·0	0·9
Scalp	50	60	20	1	3·0	1·2
Knee	50	53	20	1	3·0	0·8
Hand	50	40	20	1	1·0	0·3

(2) DANGERS FROM ELECTRICAL SHOCK

The evolution of X-ray apparatus from the 3 in. coil and battery of bichromate cells to the present day has brought about the gradual standardisation by the instrument-makers of much that was tentative and makeshift. The old tangle of loose wires has been replaced by rigid metal tubes and now all apparatus is being rendered entirely shockproof. Most early workers were fortunate in discovering that the discharge from a 10, 12 or 16 in. coil, although painful, was not necessarily fatal, even when taken on the head! In fact, I do not know of any fatal shocks from the high-tension side of X-ray work in the early days.

To-day it is different. Familiarity breeds contempt, but that this contempt is not justified is shown by a case recorded by Wetterstrand[336] in 1926. The X-ray apparatus was installed in a small room and a doctor and nurse were examining an ankle. While the tube was working, the doctor put out his hand to adjust it, and the nurse beside him, apparently intending to help him, put out a hand in the direction of the other end. This much the patient saw before he received a shock that rendered him insensible for a short time. When he recovered, the doctor and nurse were both lying dead beside the couch and the nurse's clothes were in flames. The apparatus itself was also on fire. This is, of course, an extreme case of ignorance, for the apparatus was furnished with a device for intimating when it was generating high voltage current. A similar accident occurred in France in 1921, when a well-known radiologist, working in a confined space, received a fatal shock from a small apparatus. A fatal case occurred in this country in 1933(349). Recently I had personal experience of a shock from a 4-valve outfit. I was just about to handle the tube, and my fingers were about 3 in. away, when a student switched on a current of 70 ma. at 90 K.V. Apart from the shock and the burns on finger and on heel where the current went to earth, I was none the worse.

With a modern apparatus I recently (1931) experienced in my own department a grave risk from the breaking of a spring which held a switch out of contact. Any shaking would form contact, and indeed it actually occurred before I noted the fault, but without any untoward result. On another occasion a fault occurred in the low-tension circuit for heating the filament, with the result that the high tension would not pass through the tube and sparked through the patient and the couch to earth. A nasty burn resulted, but there was, fortunately, no other injury. The ends of the tube should always be at a safe distance from the patient and there should be a spark-gap on the apparatus that is always set just wider than can be bridged by the voltage in use. This safety device is very frequently omitted and it should be fitted on every apparatus that is not protected by shock-proof casing.

These instances are quoted to show that no apparatus can be made fool-proof. Ignorance, and sometimes ill luck, may make the most perfect apparatus produce untoward results. There is only one safeguard, viz. a competent radiologist who understands his apparatus and is constantly alert to see that all the working risks are minimised.

Sagging high-tension leads are a source of danger. Recently, in an old department, a nurse received a shock from such a wire that rendered her unconscious for more than an hour. Fixed overhead tubes must replace all wires as high-tension leads, not only for safety but also because there is little discharge from the surface and consequently less contamination of the atmosphere.

The advent of shock-proof apparatus has completely eliminated the risks of electrical shock. There is a risk, however, that this safety may lead to careless-ness and that it may still be possible for the shock-proofing to break down.

Many unnecessary deaths have occurred from electrical shock which, in the first place, is merely shock and suspended animation. It is only in really severe cases that paralysis of the diaphragm and prolonged cessation of the heart action result. Hence, in every case of electrical shock, artificial respiration must be employed at once and persisted with for hours. Every effort should be made to rouse the patient to consciousness and, if he has not lost consciousness, to ensure its retention. So long as the patient is conscious there is probably no danger from shock. Electrical burns are, however, a different matter.

(3) DANGERS FROM GENERAL CONDITIONS

Whether the anaemias and intestinal troubles of which there are a few records are due to X radiations, or whether they result from causes such as lack of ventilation is not known, and it is very doubtful whether proof will ever be forthcoming, for the conditions in which these symptoms have developed are disappearing rapidly as X-ray departments are being given more reasonable housing. My own impression is that both factors may play a part.

Gastro-intestinal symptoms have been ascribed to X rays. In the early days of deep X-ray therapy, Röntgen sickness was marked, and in fact it is still troublesome in some departments. At first, enormous doses were given at one séance that lasted for hours. Now an even larger dose is given, but it is divided and spread over some weeks, and this complication seldom arises.

Some of the early X-ray workers experienced intestinal troubles. I had a troublesome and persistent diarrhœa that seemed to have a definite relation to periods of heavy screen examinations. It disappeared on holiday but recurred some two or three weeks after returning to work. At the time I thought it was probably due to a combination of exposure to X rays during war service with the exceedingly bad conditions of ventilation in my old department, which was housed in a basement. The trouble has gradually subsided. The very occasional attacks which I now have sometimes seem to be related to work but, as the intensity of radiations to which I could have been exposed was infinitesimal (perhaps a thousandth part of that given in an average therapy case), it seems practically certain that the cause lies in factors other than exposure to radiations. The fact that such troubles were not noted in many thousands of patients treated with heavy doses of X rays goes very far to exonerate radiations from blame and to suggest that the cause was ineffective ventilation and an atmosphere contaminated by the effects of high voltage currents.

Shortly after the war there were rumours of changes in the blood of those who worked with radiations, and deaths from aplastic anaemia were reported, but I believe that all except one of these occurred in radium workers. In this one there was the complication of a definite sinusitis. Under present-day conditions of protection, the work of assistants in an X-ray department should not be more injurious to health than that of those in any other walk of hospital life. Mottram (255), who examined in detail the blood changes in radium and X-ray workers, has recently investigated the blood conditions of thirty workers in radiological departments in general hospitals in London, and, as controls, twenty-six hospital workers in comparable employment—house surgeons, house physicians and ward sisters. He concluded that the blood of X-ray workers had not been affected by their occupation and that working conditions in these institutions provided effective protection, i.e. that in reasonably well-equipped departments workers were not exposed to radiation in sufficient intensities to be in any danger. The tenth annual report of the British Empire Cancer Campaign (347) records investigations on the blood of X-ray and radium workers, patients and normal subjects. Very great variations were found to occur in the blood-count in perfectly normal people at different times of the day, and further variations between different individuals. So great were the discrepancies that no normal standard could be established. These conclusions (described as "rather startling") destroy the evidence for blood-changes produced by radiations. The blood changes that occur in intensive X-ray treatments are of course quite definite, but these intensities are not comparable with the minute doses that may possibly be taken by the observer in the course of diagnostic work.

No useful purpose would be served by framing suggestions for the protection of assistants working in subterranean passages. The only thing to be done with departments of this type is to invite efficient inspection and, armed with the report, to demand reasonable conditions. Radiologists can take personal risks if they so desire, but neither they nor the governors of a hospital have any right to endanger the health of those who work for them.

Thanks to the service which radiology has rendered to medicine, there is now little difficulty in obtaining reasonable accommodation for an X-ray department. Moreover, a first-rate X-ray department is a good advertisement for the hospital, and visitors like to see it! There is, however, one room that is seldom seen: the dark room, and it is in this one spot—so far as my experience goes—that danger tends to persist. A small, inadequate and ill-ventilated dark room is a very definite source of danger, and I have known more than one assistant contract tuberculosis which I believe was largely, if not entirely, due to long hours in a cupboard that was given the all-too-literal name of "dark room".

B. *RISKS TO THE PATIENT*

To-day the patient who is radiographed or examined on the screen is under no risk whatever.* It was not so in the early days, when no filters were used and renal examinations, for example, involved possibly five minutes' exposure with the

* See Zuppinger's figures on p. 46.

full load that the tube would carry. Moreover, satisfactory radiographs were the exception rather than the rule, and the patient frequently had a number of exposures to each area.

A filter of 1 mm. of aluminium should be permanently fixed in the diaphragm opening of every tube box that is used for radiography or screening. This makes no difference whatever to the quality of the radiograph or screen picture. In addition, the three-ply wood of the screening stand against which the patient leans, or that of the couch on which he lies, has filtration value. This is apparently all that is necessary even for prolonged examinations.

No patient under my care has ever suffered injury, although in the early days, before a filter was permanently fixed in the path of the rays, there were serious risks. Perhaps we were fortunate in the comparative inefficiency of our tubes and other apparatus. I know of only one instance of serious injury inflicted in diagnostic technique. This was a terrible case in which a hole was burned in a patient's back, destroying skin and muscles and extending to the vertebrae. The facts were never accurately ascertained, but I strongly suspect that the patient was left lying on the couch with the tube running while the technician went away to develop a plate. It is doubtful if this appalling injury would ever have healed; certainly the patient would have been badly crippled. The suffering and mental strain, however, were more than he could stand, and he committed suicide. The case is cited to emphasise the fact that even with modern and efficiently protected apparatus accidents can occur. X rays cannot be rendered fool-proof, and are only safe in competent hands.

A number of cases have been recorded in which a burn has followed an ordinary examination. On subsequent inquiry it has been discovered that the patient, or the doctor, not being satisfied with one examination, has decided to consult another radiologist without informing him of the previous exposures. This, of course, constitutes a very definite risk, particularly if, as is likely, the first examination has been an inefficient one, conducted with indifferent apparatus and possibly by a person who is not competent. It is important to find out whether there has been a previous X-ray examination. If the patient has been exposed recently, I usually make some excuse for deferring my examination to a date three weeks after the last exposure.

The application of any irritant will make the skin unduly susceptible to irradiation. Cases have been reported in which the application of iodine as a counter-irritant has produced quite a severe reaction in a part that has received only a small dose of rays. I once saw a case in which an injury of the thumb which had been treated with iodine was X-rayed and an extremely severe and deep X-ray burn resulted.

The one important rule is that the patient should never be exposed unnecessarily, either for prolonged demonstration or for a large series of radiographs.* I have heard of a professor of anatomy who, in his keenness, subjected himself to a large number of exposures in order to obtain a cinematographic study of the movements of the large intestine. The work was abandoned because —in the words of his assistant, whose investigation this was—the professor was "used up". He must have incurred serious danger not only of extremely severe skin injury, but also of damage to the intestines and other internal organs.

Idiosyncrasy

Idiosyncrasy to the action of X rays used to be spoken of very freely and, in my view, without sufficient justification considering the evidence afforded by the X-ray treatment of ringworm, the one form of dosage which is essentially set within relatively narrow bounds, with success on the one side and disaster on the other. In a well-ordered clinic the response is little short of a mathematical certainty—there are practically no repeated exposures or cases of reaction with permanent baldness as the result. Surely, if idiosyncrasy is at all common, as used to be suggested, susceptible patients would be encountered comparatively often among the large numbers treated. Individual workers tell of thousands of cases without disaster, and suggestions of idiosyncrasy now come only from those centres where inefficiency may be suspected.

There may be variation in the individual reaction, but it seldom amounts to more than a fraction of the dose, one that can apparently be neglected in efficient ringworm work. If an over-action occurred in my practice in any ordinary treatment case, most certainly the last explanation I should give would be the idiosyncrasy of the patient. To my mind most, if not all, of the accidents that were attributed to "susceptibility" were in reality due to faulty technique, to unrecognised variations in the intensity of the rays or to the use of iodine or other irritant. With so many possible variants in the production of the rays—such as the old gas tube, and the drop or rise in the line voltage that has such a critical effect on the hot cathode tube—it is straining credulity to attribute our accidents to idiosyncrasy until we have definitely ruled out the other and far more likely causes. Years ago, MacKee (228) wrote: "If we include under idiosyncrasy acquired hypersusceptibility from known causes, then idiosyncrasy is common. If, on the other hand, we exclude from idiosyncrasy hypersusceptibility from known causes, and avoidable or unavoidable errors in technique and judgment, this idiosyncrasy is uncommon—even of rare occurrence." After eighteen years' further experience, I think X-ray workers will entirely endorse this opinion and, while recognising slight individual variations in tolerance, will regard idiosyncrasy as an extremely rare condition and may even doubt its existence.

The experiences of the last few years, in which the accurate measurement of

* An assessment of the intensities involved is given on p. 44.

the intensities of rays in international "r" units has become routine, entirely confirm the above opinions. The therapist who measures his doses with mathematical accuracy can foretell very precisely the degree of reaction that will result from any dosage. We never hear about idiosyncrasy from competent radiotherapists. The margin of error under the old colorimetric methods of measurement may have been in the region of $\pm$ 50 per cent. except in the hands of workers who were well experienced. In the circumstances the marvel is that there were not more accidents.

PART II

THE RADIOGRAPHIC EXAMINATION OF THE "NORMAL" GASTRO-INTESTINAL TRACT

CHAPTER IV

THE VALUE OF THE OPAQUE MEAL

HISTORY

The earliest record of an X-ray investigation of the gastro-intestinal tract is by Straus (249), who wrote in 1896, within a year of the discovery of X rays:

"It would be, of course, desirable in the interests of patients if we could make use of the radio-opaque property of the metals for diagnostic purposes, without subjecting them to the discomfort associated with the introduction of tubes. For this reason I have carried out experiments in the following manner: taking the gelatine capsules used for the administration of castor oil, I have filled them with reduced iron oxide and bismuth subnitrate. On screening I could make out only very indefinite shadows of these capsules on the screen. For the present I have not continued these investigations, because they appear to me to be of less practical importance than the question of changes of translucency of pathologic new formation to the Röntgen rays."

David Walsh (249), in his book published in 1897, says:

"Application of the Röntgen rays to the abdomen has not hitherto yielded results to compare with those derived from the thorax. The upper border of the liver can be well seen, and a hydatid tumour has been reported projecting from its convex surface; but the lower border is rarely to be made out. Kidneys are not visible. The stomach is sometimes faintly outlined, presumably most so when filled with gas; the intestines are to be seen at times faintly outlined."

In 1897 A. L. Benedict (249) succeeded in locating lesions of the alimentary tract with gelatine capsules of reduced iron. In 1898 W. B. Cannon (76), a physiologist at Harvard, initiated the radiological study of the intestinal movements in dogs and cats by means of large doses of bismuth sub-nitrate. His work arose out of a suggestion made by Dr H. P. Bowditch in 1896 that Röntgen rays might be used to record normal gastric movements. Cannon also, with F. H. Williams, made some observations on human beings.

The credit for the inception of the method is undoubtedly due to these workers. It is curious that their papers were overlooked by other investigators, although small doses of bismuth were later used tentatively by a number of observers—among them Dalton and Archibald Reid[107], Roux and Balthazard. The credit for initiating the use of the method on a large scale, for demonstrating that large doses of bismuth are harmless and for laying down a standard opaque meal is due to Rieder of Munich. In England A. F. Hurst, and in the United States of America A. W. Crane of Kalamazoo and Hulst of Grand Rapids were very early workers. Many other pioneers of this method have written on it, but the names that stand out most prominently in the early days are Holzknecht, Haenisch, Jollasse, Leven and Barret, Haudek, Groedel, Rosenthal, Kaestle and Case. At a pre-war meeting a long discussion on the standard opaque meal was brought to a close by Thurstan Holland, who said that he was all in favour of a standard opaque meal provided that it was the one he used! Soon after this, the bread-and-milk meal gave place to the barium mixture and the recommendations made at this meeting were forgotten.

The first radiograph of a stricture of the oesophagus was published by Thurstan Holland in 1904; it was taken after the patient had swallowed two ounces of strong bismuth mixture. Definite progress was made in 1905 when Rieder[281] suggested as a standard meal 30 g. of bismuth sub-nitrate mixed with a little milk and added to 300–400 g. of flour-gruel sweetened with milk sugar. He also advocated the use of a rectal injection of one litre of fluid containing bismuth. In 1905, also, G. E. Pfahler[249] gave an excellent account of normal and abnormal conditions in the stomach and bowel. In 1906 Holzknecht[160] wrote on the X-ray diagnosis of cancer of the stomach, using large amounts of bismuth given with food and examining by the fluoroscope.

Jollasse[249] in 1907 described the size, shape and extraordinary variations of the stomach. His meal consisted of 30 g. of bismuth in 200 g. of bread pulp. Groedel in the same year gave an account of gastroptosis, hour-glass stomach and delay in emptying. Most workers were using bismuth sub-nitrate, although some were still experimenting with the inflation of the stomach or bowel with air or carbon dioxide. The sub-nitrate of bismuth was not, however, always a reliable preparation and deaths from nitrite poisoning were reported: it was never clearly established whether these were due to changes in the drug after ingestion or to impurities. The salt earned a bad name, and was therefore generally replaced by the carbonate. Hurst, however, in 1908 objected to the carbonate on the ground that it would neutralise the free acids in the stomach and thus might alter the normal processes of digestion. Hurst[172] and Barclay[34] reported experimental work with these salts, and Hurst advocated the oxychloride of bismuth, which was satisfactory but so expensive that it never came into general use. The introduction of barium sulphate reduced the cost to a tenth, and the new salt proved quite as satisfactory as the old, although larger quantities had to be used.

In recent years the most important advance has been the intensive study of the mucous membrane. In 1924 Baastrup[25] devised a method for covering the walls of the stomach with a dry coating of bismuth after filling it with air. He also suggested a method for covering the walls with a layer of barium meal and then distending the cavity with some substance which casts no shadow under X rays. Since then Forssell[121] of Stockholm and Berg[58] of Hamburg and Åkerlund and their pupils have brought the visualisation and radiography of the mucous membrane to a fine art by careful manipulation with graded pressure (cf. p. 23).

My work on this subject began in 1906. I am horrified when I recall that each patient was examined and re-examined perhaps a dozen times, without a screening stand and almost without any protection.

Of the thirty years that have elapsed since the opaque meal method of investigation was introduced, many were so absorbed by the war and its aftermath that scientific progress was brought more or less to a standstill. There have only been about seventeen years of serious work, and yet this method of investigation has not only won its place in the forefront of diagnostic measures, but has revolutionised much of the old clinical teaching on the alimentary tract. Neither the clinician nor the patient is now content to go on year after year with treatment based on a vague diagnosis of "indigestion", "dilated stomach" or "atonic dyspepsia", without turning to the radiologist for assistance. Not that the radiologist is always right in his interpretation of what he has seen—possibly far from it—but the diagnosis of pathological conditions, particularly those that call for surgical intervention, has become extraordinarily accurate in expert hands.

FALLACIES IN METHODS OF OBSERVATION

(1) *Studies of the Abnormal*

In radiology, as in every other branch of medicine, the diagnosis of the abnormal can only be based on a sure recognition of the normal and an appreciation of the limits of normality. Radiology has suffered much from its early upbringing in a pathological environment. Only when it had already achieved maturity as a diagnostic procedure did it enter upon what should have been its nursery phase: the radiological study of indisputably normal and healthy subjects.

A. F. Hurst's early work on students should, however, never be forgotten. He was one of the very few who, amidst the difficulties of private practice, attempted to base his work on a study of the normal. There were few physiologists or physiological physicians to follow his example, and the progress has been almost entirely due to practising radiologists. In view of the difficulties that confronted the new science and its very scanty physiological foundation, the study of radiology has led to an astonishing revision of the early ideas of both form and function. Many cherished anatomical and physiological dogmas have been shattered.

For instance, when asked his conceptions of the propulsion of food through the intestinal tract, the average medical man reverts to hazy memories of the lecture rooms and visualises a peristaltic wave as a deep constriction of a tubular organ—as if a string were tied round it—which, as it travels along, obliterates the lumen of the canal, forcing the contents onwards. He might also picture writhing, pendulum and other movements that have been described in similar vivid phrases. When the radiologist watches and analyses the behaviour of shadows in the alimentary tract, he finds a very different picture.

Admittedly the opaque meal method of investigation may be subject to fallacies from the presence of an inert and insoluble salt of high atomic weight, and the radiologist's interpretation of the meaning of what he sees may not always be free from error; yet his records are at least those of natural living processes, and for this reason are less misleading than other sources of knowledge. His observations are certainly far sounder than those on which deductions were based before the use of X rays, when direct observation of normal peristalsis under normal conditions was impossible. Direct observations such as those of Beaumont in 1833 (on Alexis St Martin, who had a permanent gastric fistula as the result of a gun-shot wound) are open to criticism not only on account of the abnormality of the subject but because we now realise the enormous variations, even in a normal subject, that may arise from a multitude of causes of which we know only a few. In the light of X-ray experience, the fallacy of making deductions from one subject is obvious.

The question of whether or not the heavy salts used for the examination of the intestinal tract produce abnormal conditions is rather difficult to answer. I have met with cases in which the opaque meal has apparently led to marked consolidation and even impaction of the faeces. With the object of attempting to find out whether the barium meal had any influence on the passage of the food, I made records of eleven normal subjects. Charcoal biscuits were given and the times of the first appearance and the subsequent darkening of the stools were noted. In one or two cases normal action of the bowels was twice and in others once a day, the time of the bowel action being usually after breakfast, but in two instances it was before breakfast and in one in the middle of the day. The interesting thing about these experiments was that, although the bowels were acting perfectly normally, the charcoal was still present in the stools for two or even three days. This observation is entirely in conformity with the results obtained by Alvarez in his experiments with small glass beads (p. 178).

I then gave each of these subjects an opaque meal and made records of its passage throughout the intestine. The opaque food appeared in the stools in approximately the same time as the charcoal in each subject, and the rate of disappearance of the barium was approximately the same, with two exceptions. In one of these, the subject said that it had caused diarrhœa and the barium disappeared from the stools more rapidly; in the other, the subject said that it had caused very definite constipation and that she had had to take a purgative. These statements corresponded with the X-ray records.

It seems highly probable, therefore, that the opaque salt has no definite action in the intestine, and that its weight does not interfere with the mechanism. The two abnormalities recorded were probably due not to the action of the opaque food but to the psychical effect of an unusual meal. I think, therefore, that both the constipation and the diarrhœa that are recorded from time to time are more likely to be due to auto-suggestion than to the action of opaque food, unless it is given in quantities such as are entirely unnecessary in opaque meal examinations.

(2) *Studies under Anaesthesia*

The only peristaltic movements that can be observed through the abdominal wall are the excessive and very powerful waves associated with obstructive lesions and often with colicky pain. Under inhalation anaesthesia any definite movement of the intestines in the human subject is unusual, but under spinal anaesthesia movements are constantly seen. My impression of these is that they do not truthfully represent what takes place under normal conditions but are— largely, at any rate—the result of trauma and the abnormal condition of exposure to the air. It is not easy to see these movements in the operating theatre, but those that are seen do not look as if they would produce the effects on the intestinal contents that are observed in the X-ray department. I do not think it is wise to deduce any conception of normal movements from observations in the operating theatre.

(3) *Studies of Animals*

Observations on animals are no more reliable, as—apart from the fact that they are made with the abdominal contents exposed and subjected to trauma of varying degrees—it is quite evident that the movements in different animals may have widely different characteristics. The same criticism must be levelled against accepting as applicable to man X-ray observations of the passage of opaque foods through the intestinal tract in animals. Although much may no doubt be learned by comparison, the wide discrepancies of intestinal behaviour between animals that are relatively near to each other in the animal scale make it hardly likely that deductions from any animal can necessarily be applied to man. They may or may not be applicable. Phenomena observed in animals lead an investigator to look out for similar occurrences in man, but he is not justified in supposing that they occur in man simply because they have been noted in animals. In one institution that I visited, bran was always on the table, and guests were expected to eat it, because the experimental rats flourished on it!

(4) *Indirect Methods*

Indirect methods, introducing tambours and other devices to indicate the pressures, may also be subject to fallacy. A tambour in the lumen of a muscular tube may record one of two things, viz. the muscular action of the walls (the cause) or the result produced on the contents of the tube (the effect), and it may be difficult to disentangle the records of cause and of effect. For instance, in their graphs of the pressures in the pharynx in the act of swallowing, Kronecker and Meltzer (212) recorded the movement of the walls and the positive pressures exerted by the contraction, but their instruments were not designed to show that this muscular movement actually produced a negative pressure in the lumen, and they therefore missed the essential nature of the mechanism (cf. p. 126).

The only reasonably reliable method, therefore, is deduction from direct observation of the opaque meal in the human subject, and the radiologist will be well advised to start *de novo*, questioning everything he has learned from the anatomists and physiologists of a previous day. Much of their teaching must be unreliable, and I fear that a good deal of it is based on the "armchair" variety of work. Presumably writers felt that on psychological grounds they had to give some sort of plausible explanation of everything for the benefit (*sic!*) of the student, even though their ignorance might be deep and fundamental. We have a heritage of theories that, if incorrect, will hinder progress for many years, just as the old anatomical descriptions of the stomach delayed the true conception of the living human organ. As Alvarez has said, "It takes twenty years for a new observation to get into the text-books, but when once there, no matter how obviously wrong it may be, it takes a hundred years to die out".

Not for one moment do I wish to suggest that we know the whole story—far from it, for the information is as yet much too incomplete, especially that of the physiology. It takes a very long time to translate the meaning of the movements of the shadow contents into terms of their cause. Some of these movements—especially when there is obstruction—conform to what would be expected from the physiological description; others do not. Nature has no set patterns, either in form or in function. She varies her methods ceaselessly, and the more we see of the inner workings of her mechanics and chemistry the more we realise that they constitute a kaleidoscope of balanced form and function, the mutations of which are utterly bewildering to those who attempt to describe and tabulate them.

It is highly artificial to separate form from function, anatomy from physiology, but for convenience of text-book descriptions it is usual in one section to describe the form and position of organs and in another to give an account of their movements and function. This plan is followed here, but with the emphatic proviso that the two subjects must never be divorced in the mind of the student.

SECTION I: ANATOMY

THE ANATOMY OF THE "NORMAL" STOMACH AND THE INHERENT MOBILITY AND ADAPTABILITY OF THE ABDOMINAL VISCERA

CHAPTER V

THE STOMACH: SOME ANATOMICAL CONSIDERATIONS

It is essential to think of the alimentary tract as a whole. The water-tight compartments formerly taught to students must be forgotten, for symptoms

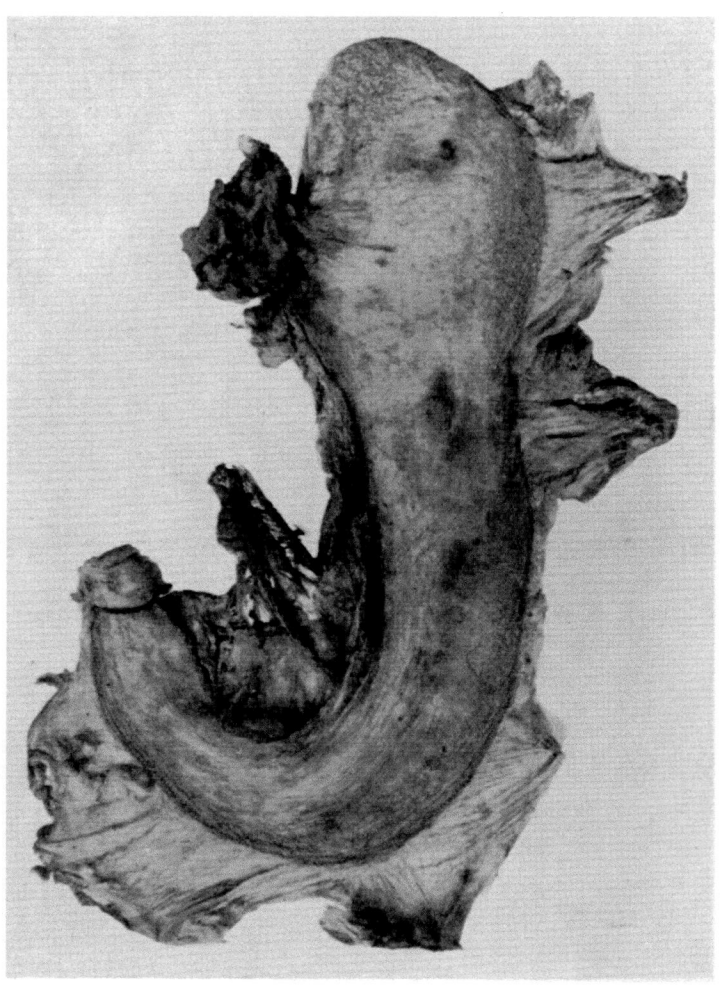

Fig. 49. Photograph of an empty normal stomach as it is believed to be during life. (Contributed by J. S. B. Stopford.)

may be referred to the stomach from any part of the tract. Moreover, there is no such thing as "normal": an alimentary tract may approximate to the average, but there is no fixed standard of normality.

The Varying Thickness of the Stomach Wall

The opaque meal shows the outline of the inner wall of the stomach, and one would expect that this would correspond fairly accurately with the outer wall when due allowance has been made for its thickness. A considerable amount of work is being done by various authorities —for example, Alvarez, McSwiney and Cole—on this subject by attaching small fragments of metal below the serous coat and observing the discrepancies between these and the opaque shadow. The early observations by this method seem to indicate that the stomach wall behaves in a somewhat unexpected manner: that it thickens up in various parts, particularly in the pyloric region, and also that it rotates in a way which suggests that there is a great deal more to learn from this method of investigation.

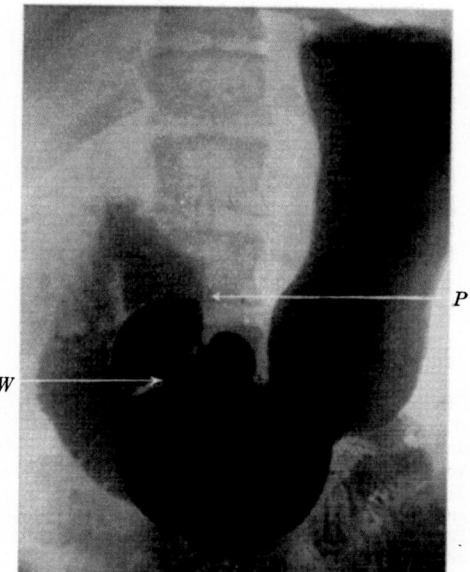

Fig. 50. Radiograph of a normal stomach. *P*, Pylorus. *W*, Peristaltic wave. (Contributed by F. Haenisch.)

The Nerve Supply

The whole tract is a continuous muscular tube which, like any other muscle, varies in shape and behaviour according to tone, and that tone is subject to many influences. The sympathetic nervous system is freely distributed to all parts of the tract. The rôle of the vagus is important, for it is not a motor nerve in the ordinary sense of the term, but an augmentor or accelerator, its final effect being to augment the existing tone or contraction of muscle (Figs. 51, 52, and 53), (M'Crea, McSwiney and Stopford (225)). According to Alvarez (11), there is now fairly general agreement that peristalsis is myogenic and not neurogenic, rhythmic contraction being an inherent property of muscle and muscle-like tissue, probably brought about by recurring cycles of chemical activity. The function of Auerbach's plexus is probably to conduct stimuli and to co-ordinate the different parts of the alimentary tract. It may also serve to control spasmodic contractions and to conduct impulses from the mucous membrane to the muscle, so that the chemical composition of the food can regulate the peristalsis.

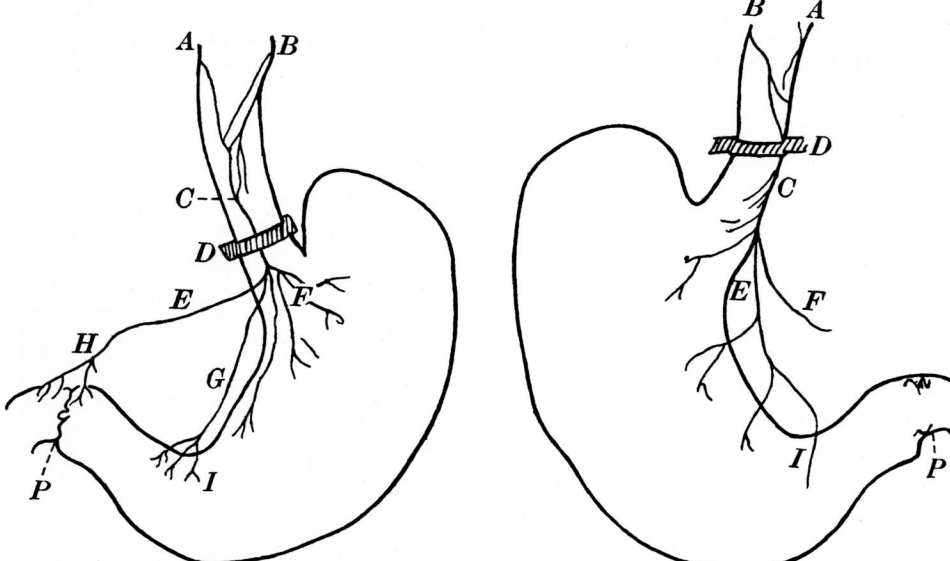

Fig. 51. Diagram made from a dissection, showing the normal formation and distribution of the anterior vagal trunk. *A*, Right vagus. *B*, Left vagus. *C*, Anterior vagal trunk. *D*, Diaphragm. *E*, Hepatic branch. *F*, Gastric branches. *G*, Principal anterior nerve of the lesser curvature. *H*, Branches to pylorus and first part of the duodenum. *I*, Incisura angularis. *P*, Pylorus.

Fig. 52. Diagram made from a dissection, illustrating the normal formation and distribution of the posterior vagal trunk. The stomach has been turned to the right, exposing the posterior surface. *A*, Right vagus. *B*, Left vagus. *C*, Posterior vagal trunk. *D*, Diaphragm. *E*, Gastric division, which lies in the coronary falx. *F*, Coeliac division. *I*, Incisura angularis. *P*, Pylorus.

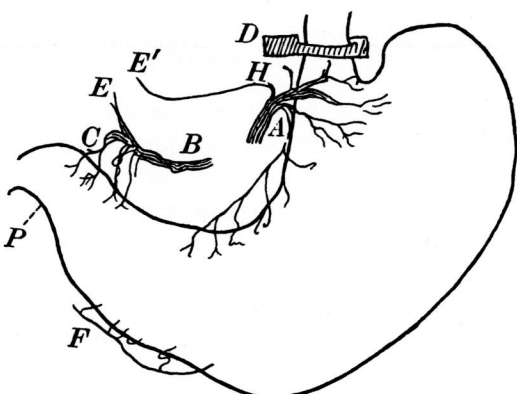

Fig. 53. Diagram to illustrate the manner of distribution of the sympathetic nerves to the stomach. *A*, Nerves accompanying and distributed with the left gastric or coronary artery (a similar arrangement exists on the posterior surface of the stomach). *B*, Nerves accompanying the hepatic artery. *C*, Branches which run a recurrent course in the right free margin of the lesser omentum and with the right gastric or pyloric artery to supply the pars pylorica and duodenum. *D*, Diaphragm. *E*, *E'*, Nerves to the liver. *F*, Twigs running with the gastro-duodenal artery and its gastro-epiploic branch. *H*, Twigs with the inferior phrenic arteries. (Reproduced from E. D'A. M'Crea.)

In the upper part of the tract two other nerves also contribute to the supply: the ninth and eleventh. Authorities still differ on the exact part innervated by each, and for all practical purposes the path taken by the fibres is less important than the nucleus of origin. It seems to be agreed that the nucleus ambiguus supplies the striated muscles, while the dorsal nucleus of the vagus supplies the unstriped muscle. The change from striated to non-striated muscle takes place about the junction of the upper and middle thirds of the oesophagus, and it is in this region, therefore, that the nerve supply changes (114, 127). This change is correlated with several interesting physiological and pathological phenomena (cf. pp. 136, 206).

The Muscular Coats of the Stomach

The stomach is entirely covered with peritoneum, and between this and the mucous membrane are the muscular coats. Throughout the whole length of the alimentary canal there are two persistent layers, namely, the outer longitudinal and the inner circular. These two are developed in different degrees in various parts of the tract. On removing the peritoneal coat by a picric acid technique devised by Forssell, the longitudinal fibres are plainly seen emerging from the oesophagus and spreading out over the stomach wall, following its contour (Fig. 54). These fibres intermingle to a certain extent with the underlying circular fibres, which are best studied by dissection from within after the mucous membrane has been removed (Fig. 55 A). These are seen to be continuous with the circular fibres of the oesophagus and to form a continuous coat encircling the stomach wall. Lying between the mucous membrane and this circular coat is an additional and incomplete but well-developed layer of muscular fibres showing powerful strands running down on either side of the lesser curvature and eventually

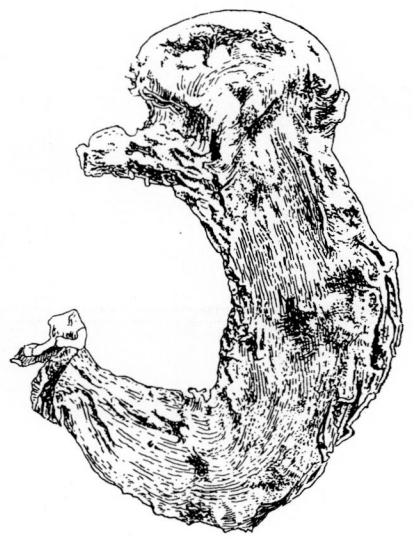

Fig. 54. Peritoneum stripped from the stomach, leaving exposed the outer longitudinal coat, the direct continuation of the longitudinal coat of the oesophagus.

spreading out in a fan to anastomose with the circular fibres. It does not encircle the oesophagus but falls down on either side of the lesser curvature, leaving a narrow strip of the underlying circular fibres exposed. The result is that this layer forms a sling from the oesophagus down either side of the lesser curvature (Fig. 55 B). These extra fibres are free for about two inches below the oesophagus and are not attached in any way to the underlying circular fibres. Developmentally, they appear to arise from an additional circular layer that originates in the fundus. These muscles have been beautifully dissected by Forssell (120) (Fig. 56), and also by G. Jefferson, from whose preparations Figs. 54 and 55 have been made. (The photographs of these dissections, however, were never published by him.)

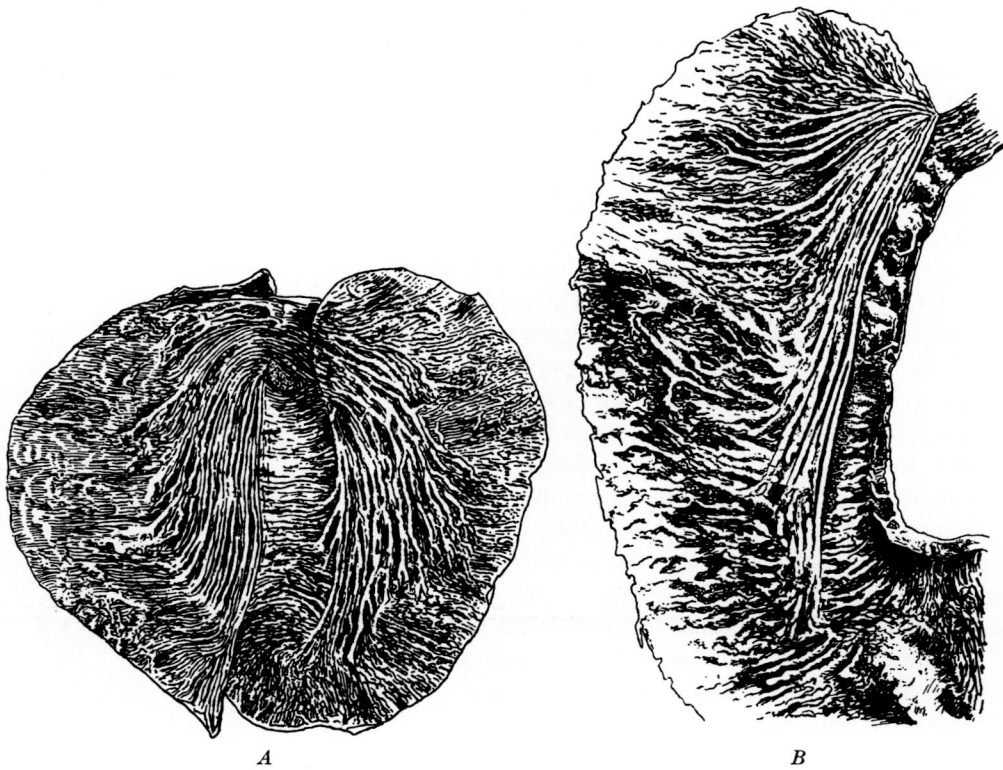

A   B

Fig. 55. *A*. Stomach opened down the greater curvature and the mucous membrane dissected off. Note the innermost coat, the oblique band running round the oesophagus and down either side of the lesser curvature and branching out fan-like. A narrow gap is left along the lesser curvature between the two sides. Jefferson has shown that in the upper 2 in. the edges of this band are quite free from the underlying muscle wall, but that lower down they spread out on either side and the fibres intermingle and fuse with the fibres of the circular coat. *B*. Fusion of the oblique and circular fibres. Note the tangle of the fibres which form the circular coat.

In attempting to explain the nature of the contraction that produces the cup-and-spill type of stomach (cf. p. 82), I thought that possibly the action of this oblique band might be the clue to the problem. If its contractions could be shown to be independent of those of the other coats, a basis would be provided for the explanation of the various forms. Moreover, independent contraction might also explain the fact that in atonic conditions of the stomach the lesser curvature retained its length, maintaining the pylorus in its usual position, although the whole of the rest of the musculature was greatly elongated. In fact the maintenance of the tone in the muscle bands about the lesser curvature, while the rest of the muscle was obviously so elongated as the result of loss of tone, could only be explained on some such supposition. In "gastroptosis", in which the lesser curvature is longer than usual, I supposed that all the muscle coats, including this oblique band and the other muscles of the lesser curvature, were elongated proportionately with the rest of the muscle wall and that tone was maintained.

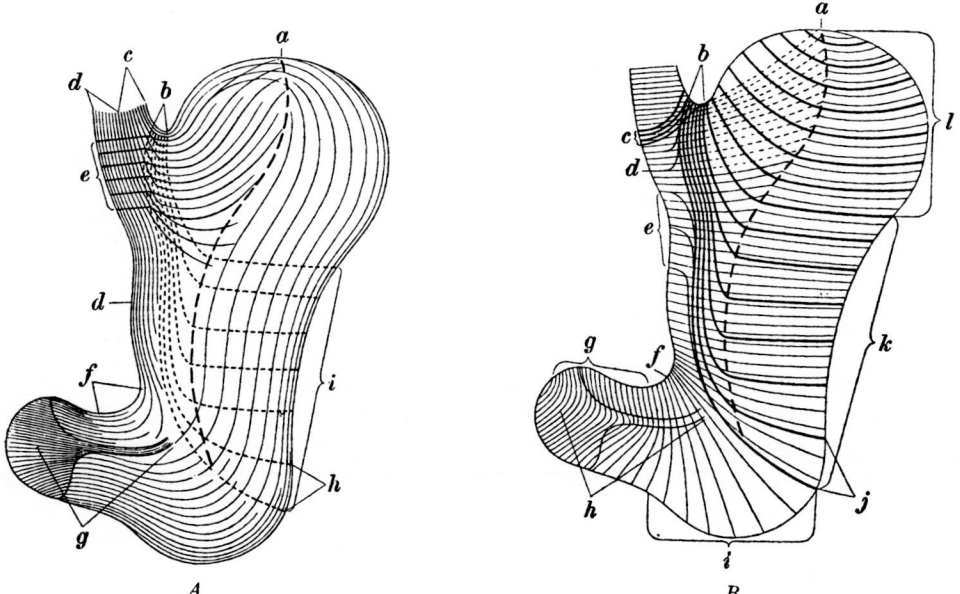

Fig. 56. *A.* Plan of the longitudinal muscles of the human stomach. The innermost layer, the oblique fibres, are shown by broken lines. *a*, Line of insertion of the oblique fibres. *b*, The oblique fibres—dotted lines. *c, d, e*, Longitudinal fibres passing from the oesophagus over the stomach. *f*, Incisura angularis. *g*, Ligamentum ventriculi. *h*, Lower oblique fibres. *i*, Oblique and circular fibres fused. *B.* Plan of the circular and oblique muscles of the human stomach. *a*, Line of insertion of the oblique fibres. *b*, Oblique fibres taking their support from the angle between the cardiac orifice and the stomach. *c, d*, A few fibres passing round the cardiac orifice. *e*, Connecting filaments of the oblique fibres. *f*, Incisura angularis. *g*, Ring muscles of the pyloric canal. *h*, Ligamentum ventriculi. *i*, Fan-shaped muscles of the sinus. *j*, Lower oblique fibres. *k*, Corpus. *l*, Fornix. (Contributed by G. Forssell.)

Some Electrical Experiments on the Stomach Muscles

I thought it would be worth while to attempt to test the reaction of various parts of the stomach wall by electrical methods and, by the courtesy of Professor E. D. Telford, a series of tests was carried out in the operating theatre on a man in whom a diagnosis of duodenal ulcer had been made, but who was otherwise in good condition (38).

A rather larger incision than usual was made and the anaesthesia was kept as light as possible as soon as the abdomen had been opened. A large indifferent electrode was placed under the patient's back and, with an olivary pointed electrode, we applied the stimulus direct to the stomach wall. At first we tried the interrupted galvanic current, but this met with no response; possibly the anaesthesia was too deep at this period. We then switched over to an interrupted sinusoidal current, and at once obtained contraction of the stomach wall (Fig. 57 a). Wherever we stimulated on the greater curvature and

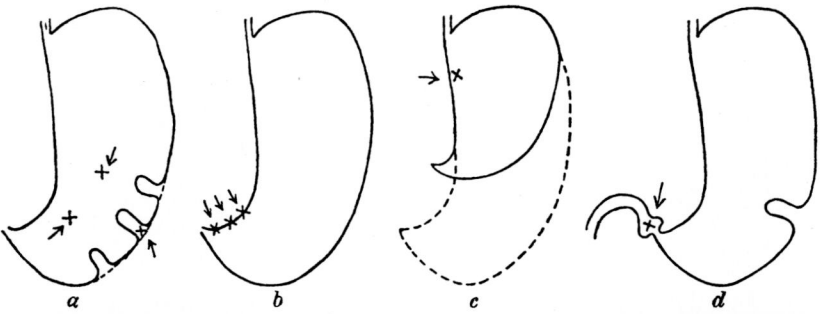

Fig. 57. Electrical experiments on the gastric muscle. Effects of direct stimulation at the points marked ×. The resulting change of outline is indicated on the diagrams.

anterior wall, a band of contraction, a typical incisura, occurred, the greater curvature being drawn in towards the lesser curvature in every instance. This appeared to be entirely due to contraction of the circular fibres drawing in the free greater curvature towards the thicker and comparatively fixed lesser curvature, as would be expected. We then applied our stimulus to the lesser curvature at various points in the lower third but obtained no contraction of gastric muscle, as far as we could see. There was, however, a very definite tendency to retching and straining; so much so that we thought the patient was coming round. However, the spasm relaxed directly the current was cut off, and did not recur when we applied the electrode at other points. The reaction seemed to be a general spasmodic contraction of the diaphragm and abdominal muscles (Fig. 57 b).

The liver was then drawn aside and the electrode applied to the lesser curvature in its upper third. The result of this was a very definite response with each stimulation: the stomach, which was bulging out of the wound, was drawn up into the abdomen, descending again slowly as soon as the current was cut off. There was apparently no suggestion of the formation of an incisura, and the reaction seemed to be due to a contraction of the oblique band acting entirely alone (Fig. 57 c).

One other point of simulation was tried, namely, the peritoneal surface of the duodenal ulcer. There was no local response whatever, but an incisura appeared in the lower third of the stomach such as would give, on the screen, the hour-glass appearance which we so often see in connection with duodenal ulcers (cf. p. 243) (Fig. 57 d).

The way in which the contractions occurred was interesting: they were not immediate, but took perhaps ten seconds to appear, attaining their maximum in another ten seconds and relaxing in about fifteen seconds. At no period of the experiments did we obtain any contraction that suggested peristaltic action.

These experiments, therefore, confirm to a very large extent the hypothesis that the oblique band can act entirely independently of the circular and longitudinal coats; and if this is correct, I think it can be said that with a long type of stomach there is elongation of the oblique band, while atony is the relaxation, lengthening and possibly stretching of the fibres of the circular and longitudinal coats, the oblique band retaining its normal length.

I believe that the chief function of the oblique band is to carry the weight of the stomach and its contents, and that the functions of the other two coats are chiefly concerned with peristalsis and with that ligamentous action of muscle which is called tonic action.

The Mucous Membrane

To Forssell (123) belongs the credit of calling attention to the part played in digestion by the movements of the mucous membrane. He showed that, whereas in the dissecting and post-mortem rooms the mucous membrane is all gathered up into disordered folds, in life it maintains a purposeful formation. In the oesophagus, for instance, the folds are arranged longitudinally; in the stomach they form a number of channels following the contour from the cardiac orifice to the pylorus (Fig. 58, A2). Forssell concluded that research on the muscularis mucosae might materially help to solve some of the problems of digestion. His work has been elaborated by Berg (58), Albrecht (8), Chaoul (95) and others. In my experience the normal mucous membrane pattern varies so much that it is unwise to define the borderland that separates the normal from the pathological. For instance, it is not unusual to find that the rugae along the greater curvature run obliquely and give a crenated outline to the shadow, while in some perfectly healthy students the pattern of the mucous membrane is disordered and quite comparable with some of the pictures that are labelled gastritis (cf. p. 270).

The Cole Collaborators seem to suggest that gastric peristalsis is a function of the mucous membrane. This hardly seems possible. In the excessive peristalsis shown in Fig. 192 the folds of the mucous membrane appear to follow

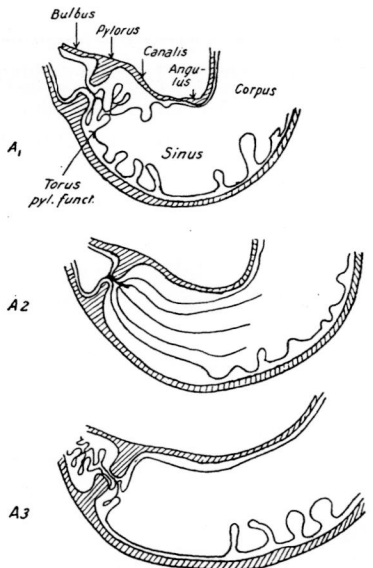

Fig. 58. Mucosa of stomach, pylorus and duodenum. (Contributed by G. Forssell.)

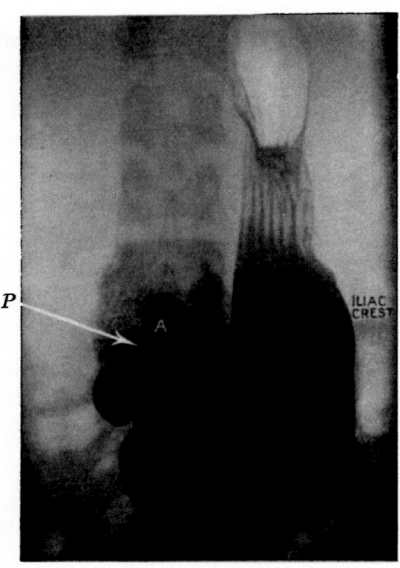

Fig. 59. Formation of the rugae in the upper part of the stomach: about eight well-defined channels. *A*, Duodenal cap. *P*, Pylorus.

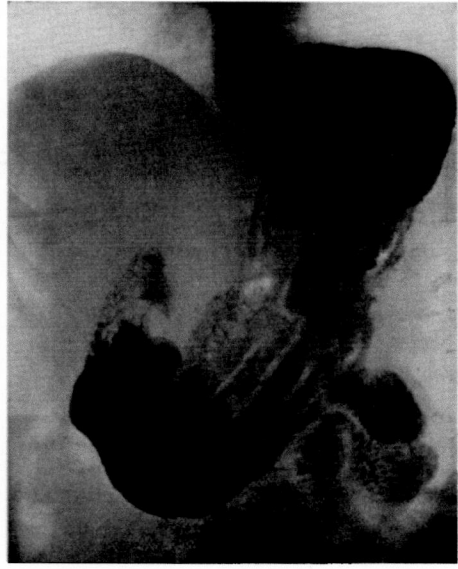

Fig. 60. Stomach lying down showing the mucous membrane pattern spread out over the vertebrae. The rugae are rather wider and straighter than usual.

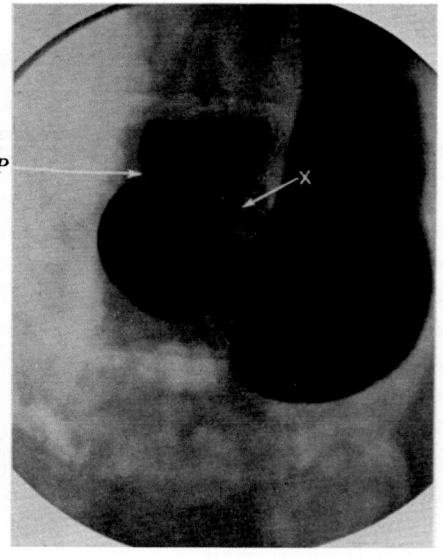

Fig. 61. Notch (×) in the shadow close to the pylorus due to a fold of the mucous membrane: "peristalsis of the muscularis mucosae." *P*, Pylorus. (Contributed by S. Gilbert Scott.)

the contour of the stomach; there is no suggestion that they are responsible for the peristaltic waves.

Near the pylorus it is not very uncommon to find a small, sharply defined notch on the greater curvature, not larger than a half pea (Fig. 61). This appearance, which is not constant, seems to be due to an aberrant ridge of mucous

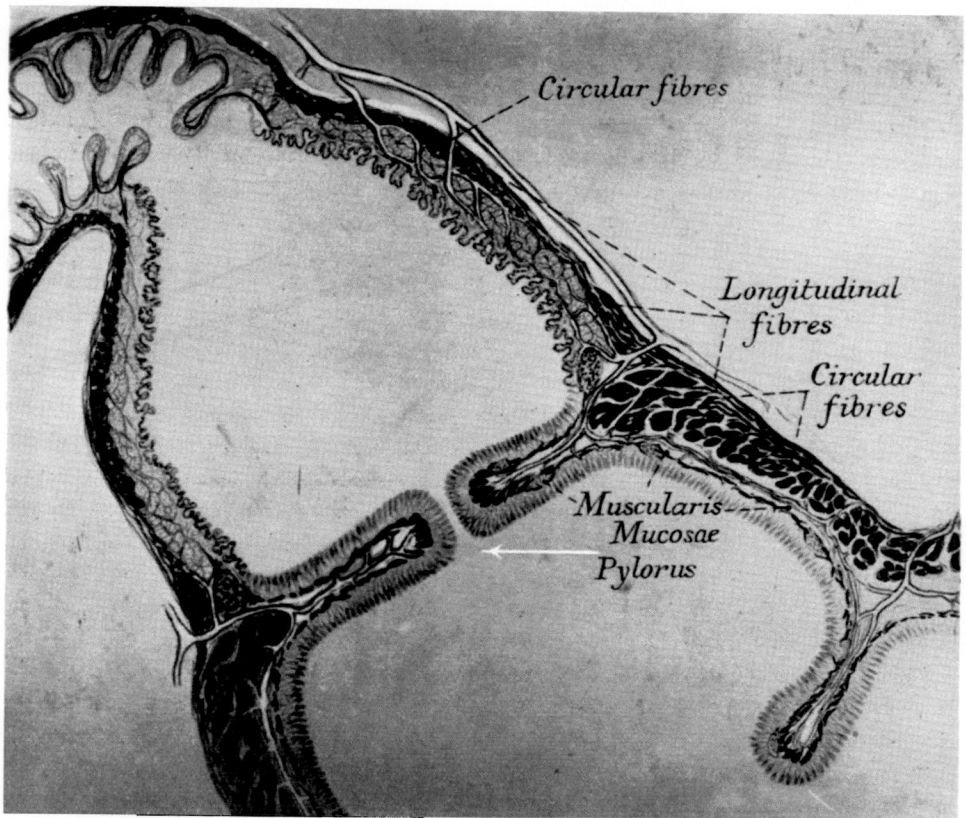

Fig. 62. Diagram of the mucous membrane and muscular wall of the pylorus and duodenum. Arrow indicates pylorus. (Contributed by L. G. Cole.)

membrane cutting into the lumen of the pyloric antrum. It may perhaps correspond to a peristaltic wave in the mucosa (cf. pp. 154 and 165).

The Pyloric Sphincter

Cole and his collaborators [103] state that the pylorus is closed by "a circular contraction of the muscularis mucosae. The pyloric valve is not controlled by any specialised sphincter derived from the circular layer of the muscularis propria. The circular fibres of the muscularis propria terminate just at the base of the pyloric valve...". Von Bergmann (62) compares the pyloric sphincter to the iris, pointing out that the muscularis mucosae is radially disposed.

The muscularis mucosae terminates sharply at the pylorus, and in the first part of the duodenum this structure and also the sub-mucous coat are absent (Fig. 62). Here the true muscular coat is also thin and incomplete, and composed almost entirely of longitudinal fibres that are continuous with those of the stomach. The circular fibres of the stomach definitely end at the pylorus and there is a gap in the continuity; there are no circular fibres in the base of the duodenal cap and, in fact, the circular fibres are not abundant till about the middle of the cap. Cole states that the junction of the cap with the small intestine is marked by the first annular fold and that at this point the muscularis mucosae and the sub-mucous coats reappear.

CHAPTER VI

THE FACTORS INFLUENCING THE FORM AND POSITION OF THE STOMACH

Nobody, to my knowledge, has attempted to reproduce radiographic tracings in conjunction with photographs of the subject so that they shall be more or less accurate representations of the organs that cause the shadows, and yet it looks so obvious and easy to produce an atlas of surface markings in this way. The difficulties and fallacies of the technique are, however, so numerous and fundamental that on more than one occasion I almost abandoned the idea in favour of line drawings.

The studies here described suggest that certain changes which must have been regarded in the past as pathological are in fact perfectly normal in response to respiratory and gravitational influences, and are found not only in ordinary subjects but also in athletes. Athletic training, even of the abdominal muscles, appears to exert little or no influence on the shape and disposition of the abdominal viscera.

Many factors may influence the descriptive anatomy of living organs as they fulfil their functions. In 1910 I (47) pointed out the effect of mental influences as shown by the behaviour of the viscera under the influence of fear, nausea and other strong emotions. Wingate Todd (312) has carried these studies farther, and has also recorded the influence of various types of food. Such factors cannot be overlooked, although they are not so readily studied as mechanical influences.

The chief mechanical factors responsible for change in shape are:
(1) The posture of the subject (the influence of gravity).
(2) The tonic action of the intrinsic muscles.
(3) The movements of the diaphragm.
(4) The distension of the organ by the bulk of the food.
(5) The weight of the food, to a small extent only.
(6) Pressure from other organs.

This chapter deals only with those factors that are directly under our control, i.e. gravity and respiration. The effect of the pressure of other organs will only be mentioned incidentally. The weight and the bulk of food are more or less indivisible, and their effect is closely bound up with that of gravity and tone. It is obvious that the movements of the abdominal organs and the modifications of their shape must at all times be a resultant of the forces at work. The effect of tone on the shape of the stomach is discussed on p. 83.

The present detailed study is confined to three normal, healthy subjects who consented to undergo the necessary tedious X-ray and photographic experiments;

but behind them is a background of observation and intermittent study of many thousands of patients. Thus, though the number described is negligible, the real significance of these cases is that they illustrate lessons which have been impressed on me by the accumulated experience of many years.

TECHNIQUE OF THE COMPOSITE PICTURES (Plate figs. 20–48)

Figs. 20–48 are grouped together on the pull-out facing p. 104.

In order to obviate as far as possible the effect of the weight of the opaque food, only a small meal—2–3 oz.—was used. It consisted of barium sulphate mixed to a cream with water, with a flavouring of sugar and cocoa.

Fluoroscopic methods were first tried. With a dermographic pencil the shadows of the diaphragm and stomach were rapidly mapped out on the abdominal wall of the subject in the screening stand or on the couch; then, the picture having been filled in at leisure with grease-paint, photographs were taken. In some postures, particularly when the patient was lying on one side, the outlines were necessarily only rapid approximations and were not satisfactory, and in any case the risks of exposure to the observer were considerable and were not justified.

An attempt was therefore made to produce a composite picture by superimposing radiographs of the organs on to photographs of the subject. The scheme was to obtain first, photographs, secondly, radiographs of the vertebral column and, thirdly, radiographs of the stomach and intestines. If correctly superimposed, these three were expected to give a reasonably accurate representation of the relationships of the organs both to the surface of the body and to vertebral levels. Experience showed that the inclusion of the whole of the vertebral column introduced too many difficulties; this was therefore abandoned, and only so much of the spine as showed in the X-ray films of the organs was included in the composite pictures.

Difficulties cropped up one after another and, for the guidance of anyone who tries to repeat this technique, I give an account of some of them. Those who remember the meticulous accuracy that was necessary in war work to make skin markings of foreign bodies a satisfactory guide to their surgical removal will realise the extent of the error to which the slightest deviation from the central ray gives rise. In this work I was taking radiographs of large areas that included organs; I was not centring on a definite point. The central beam is in the middle of the radiograph, while the surface landmarks, for repositioning on the photographs of the patient, are usually at some distance from the centre and are correspondingly liable to error.

Moreover, the position of skin markings changes according to posture. For instance, in one subject the umbilicus corresponded to the disc between the fourth and fifth lumbar vertebrae in the upright position, while in the supine position it moved up to about the third or fourth. This disparity was much increased by flexing the legs. Nor are skin markings even over the spine any more reliable. In two cases I tried this out, and in each of them the mark was a whole vertebra higher when the subject lay down on her back. There may even be a considerable displacement of the skin over the chest. I noted in a thin subject that my markings of the rib cartilages were displaced a half to three-quarters of an inch when the subject lay down.

In deep inspiration and expiration any point on the anterior abdominal wall and on the chest rises and falls considerably in relation to the vertebrae, so that, if surface markings are given, the conditions under which they are made must be stated. The photographs of subject A (Figs. 20–28) were taken in the various phases of respiration; in subjects B and C one photograph was used for all three positions. Between subject A and the others there is very little apparent difference, certainly not enough to catch the eye if it were not pointed out. As I had no facilities for placing a camera sufficiently high above the couch, I had to use the photograph of the standing subject to represent the supine posture.

Superimposing the Tracings

Attempts to superimpose reductions of actual radiographs on photographs of the subject were quite unsatisfactory, and tracings of the chief outlines were therefore employed. This method has the advantage that only the salient features are transferred into the picture.

If the same degree of reduction is applied when photographing the subject and the traced outlines of the radiograph, the one picture does not fit the other. This, of course, is due to the divergent paths of the X rays that have produced the shadow picture. A radiograph is necessarily a magnified representation of the structures that throw the shadow. Owing to the radial divergence of the X-ray beam about the central ray, this magnification is not uniform but is greatly increased towards the edge of the film. There is only one point at which this error is absent, viz. the point of incidence of the central ray. Hence, for instance, the traced outline of the diaphragm will overflow the body outline on the photograph. The same distortion is inevitable in radiographs of the vertebrae: only those shadows close to the central ray are relatively accurate. Moreover, the further a bone is from the film, the greater will be the distortion. Hence the natural curvatures of the spine caused definite inaccuracy, and the symphysis pubis is so far from the film and also from the central ray that its outline came well down the legs when I first tried to superimpose it, even when every allowance had been made (by proportionate photographic reduction) for the general enlargement. To avoid this distortion was impossible; it could only be reduced by making a number of sectional pictures and joining them together, a technique which was impracticable.

The bony outlines cannot be made to fit the subject *accurately*, and approximate correctness only can be attained. I aimed at this by measuring off corresponding points in the radiograph and on the patient. When the correct ratio was ascertained, the tracings were reduced to correspond with the size of the photographs, and printed on to them. With the camera I found the degree of reduction necessary to make these points superimpose with reasonable accuracy.

Moreover, there is another source of error. The radiographs were not all taken at the same tube-film distance. The average distances dictated by the apparatus at my disposal were 30 in. for the standing postero-anterior, 34 in. for the standing lateral, 26 in. for the supine, and 40 in. for the lateral recumbent position. The inaccuracy is relatively small, and I have ignored it. It reaches its maximum in the pictures representing the subject lying on the back (Plate figs. 24, 34, 44). In these, the fact that the tube was at a short distance and centred approximately over the pyloric region has caused such distortion at the cardiac end of the stomach (on the periphery of the film) that the diaphragm level appears to be very much higher on the vertebrae than it should be. The apparent discrepancy was so great that I had one of the subjects down again and took two more films, one centred over the pylorus and the other over the diaphragm, and satisfied myself that this appearance was due to foreshortening. (The error, incidentally, produced a picture which approximates very closely to the outlines of surface markings given in the text-books.)

The actual superimposition of the tracings on the photographs of the subject presented a number of difficulties. The one which caused the greatest trouble, and finally made meticulous accuracy impossible, was the fact that the slightest deviation from the true antero-posterior position of the subject, either in the photograph or the radiograph, at once disturbs the relationships. A fraction of rotation throws the vertebrae in the radiograph to one or other side of the middle line of the abdomen. This difficulty was especially marked with the subject lying on one side. I finally compromised on a general degree of accuracy by using the vertebral level corresponding either to the umbilicus or to a surface mark representing the diaphragm level, and making some allowance for the known distortion.

The Fallacies of the Composite Pictures

Thus, no matter how convincing the pictures may look, they are not and never can be accurate representations of the surface anatomy. They are merely approximations in which the fundamental inaccuracies are reduced as far as possible, and they indicate the main point that I wish to emphasise, i.e. the fluid nature of the anatomy of the alimentary tract.

In some instances, especially when, owing to the small quantity of opaque food used, outlines were incomplete or obliterated by other shadows, I had to insert the missing outlines from my radiological experience. These may, however, be taken as substantially correct.

When all the conditions of examination are apparently identical it does not follow that in subsequent observations the organs will always occupy the same position, even relatively to each other. For instance, in subject B, I carried out two sets of investigations on the colon (Plate figs. 38 and 39). It will be noted that the transverse colon was about two inches lower on the second occasion—possibly (or probably) because the subject was nervous about the proximity of a *viva voce* examination. The difference in the position of the splenic flexure in these two pictures is also noteworthy, but I cannot explain it. It certainly does not seem to be connected with the weight of the food.

DESCRIPTION OF THE COMPOSITE PICTURES

The three subjects of this special study were "normals" selected merely because they were available. Clearly it would be impracticable and a waste of time to apply such a detailed study in a large number of cases. No definite object would be served, and the point is sufficiently proved by the three cases taken at random but backed by a very wide experience of cases that have not been recorded in detail by this laborious method. Subject A (Plate figs. 20–28) is a well-built healthy young woman of good physique aged 27. The man, subject B (Plate figs. 30–39), is an athletic student aged 20. Although he happens to have six lumbar vertebrae, the umbilicus in the erect posture corresponds to the intervertebral space between the fourth and fifth, as in the other subjects. Subject C (Plate figs. 40–48) is an active and healthy but thin woman of 55.

The changes recorded in response to respiration and posture in the pictures of the stomach (Plate figs. 20–48) tell their own story, which is as nearly true as I can make it for the particular individuals at the particular time.

The cardiac orifice and the pylorus are the only well-defined regions of the stomach, but for descriptive purposes it is usual to speak of the cardia, the body and the pyloric antrum. The division is entirely arbitrary but is useful and necessary.

The Cardiac Orifice

The cardiac orifice is the one relatively fixed point of the abdominal alimentary tract but, owing to the attachment of the oesophagus to the diaphragm, it is necessarily subject to the diaphragmatic movement. It is usually situated at about the level and to the left side of the eleventh dorsal vertebra. Normally, apart from exertion, it moves about half an inch between inspiration and expiration, but on deep respiration it appears to move just as much as the maximum excursion of the diaphragm, perhaps three inches. This observation, however, is not at all easy to verify, as the opaque food usually slips through too soon. The level is not affected to any extent by posture.

The Pylorus

The position of the pylorus is given in the old text-books as to the left of the first lumbar vertebra. In practice it may vary within wide limits, not only according to the type of the stomach but with the posture of the subject, for the pylorus is capable of a wide range of movement. I would, however, place the average position of the pylorus, in the ordinary **J**-type of stomach in the upright posture, as at the right side of the disc between the third and fourth lumbar vertebrae. When the patient lies down, it moves upwards to somewhere near the first or second. In the small hypertonic stomach, it may even be as high as the lower border of the twelfth dorsal, while in the long stomach, as in Plate fig. 40, it lies at the right side of the fourth lumbar disc. By superimposing the radiographs, taken under varying conditions of respiration and posture,

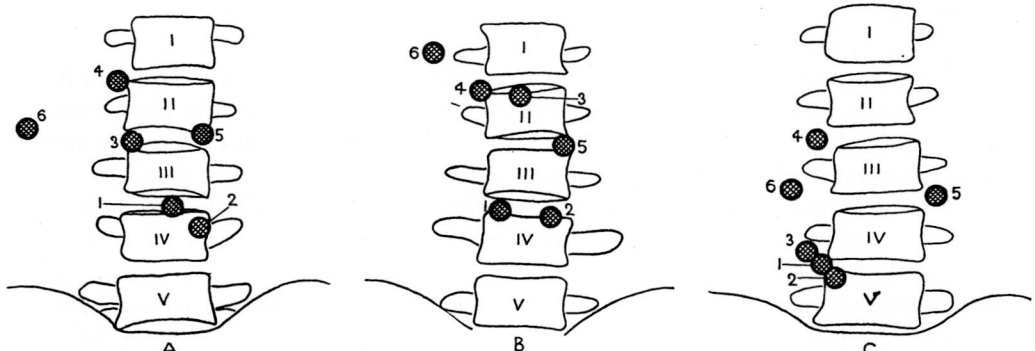

Fig. 63. Healthy woman, aged 27.   Fig. 64. Healthy man, aged 20.   Fig. 65. Healthy woman, aged 55.
(Subject A in Plate figs. 20–28.)   (Subject B in Plate figs. 30–39.)   (Subject C in Plate figs. 40–48.)

Figs. 63, 64 and 65. The position of the pylorus in various postures and in the extremes of respiration. 1, Standing at rest. 2, Standing, full inspiration. 3, Standing, full expiration. 4, Lying on the back. 5, Lying on the left side. 6, Lying on the right side.

from which Plate figs. 20–48 were made, I have tried to represent the positions in which the pylorus was found in the three subjects of my investigations (Figs. 63, 64 and 65), and to show how mobile it is. From these illustrations it appears to have a zone of possible movement perhaps 5 in. in diameter, and I do not think that this is unusual; this range could be considerably increased by manipulation (Fig. 66).

A striking feature in these three cases is the somewhat limited range of movement in the last subject, C, the elderly woman (Fig. 65). It is considerably less than in either the young man or the young woman. This is probably because the long "dropped" stomach is supported to some extent on the pelvic contents. By manipulation I have sometimes elicited an extraordinary range of movement of the pylorus in cases of this type, but in this investigation I was only posturing and was not manipulating. It is rather surprising that the range of movement of the pylorus appears to be greatest in the young athletic man.

The deduction from these observations is that the pylorus is relatively free to move within a radius of some inches; in fact, this wide range is unexpectedly found to be as great in a perfectly healthy, young, athletic subject as in the subject C, who has a relatively lax abdomen and a "dropped" stomach. Had such a wide movement been discovered in a patient with abdominal symptoms, it would have been difficult to resist claiming it as the cause. Such free mobility must, however, be accepted as quite normal.

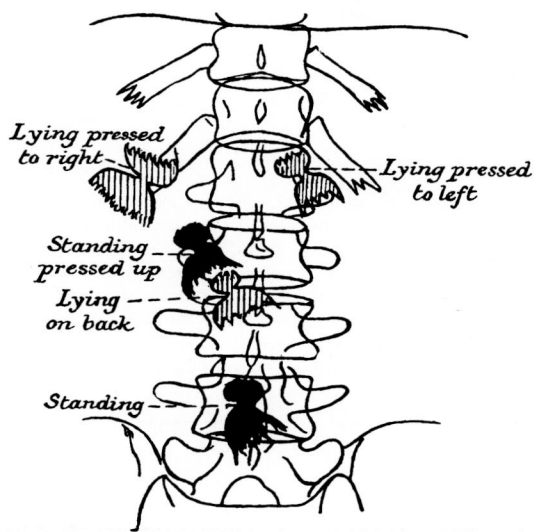

Fig. 66. Tracing from superimposed radiographs, showing the effect of pressure on the position of the pylorus. The subject was thin, and the viscera were not so mobile as they would be in a subject with more abdominal fat. (The movements of the kidney of the same subject are shown in Fig. 86, p. 96.)

THE SHAPE OF THE STOMACH (ERECT POSTURE):
MID-PHASE OF RESPIRATION
(Plate figs. 20, 30 and 40)

Naturally, if neither of the two "fixed" points between which the stomach lies is even approximately fixed, its shape is likely to vary greatly. Moreover, its size does not bear any definite relationship either to the build of the subject or to the distance between these two points.

The most common type of stomach is a **J**-shape (Fig. 67) that extends downwards to about the level of the umbilicus (the level of the iliac crests) and then turns up and across the middle line to the pylorus. There are many variations of the **J**-shape—e.g. fish-hook shape, "steerhorn" (Fig. 68), and so forth—but these variations are insignificant in comparison with the variations in length.

Early radiologists, obsessed with the prevalent and fashionable conception of visceroptosis, regarded a long stomach as abnormal, and labelled it "dropped"

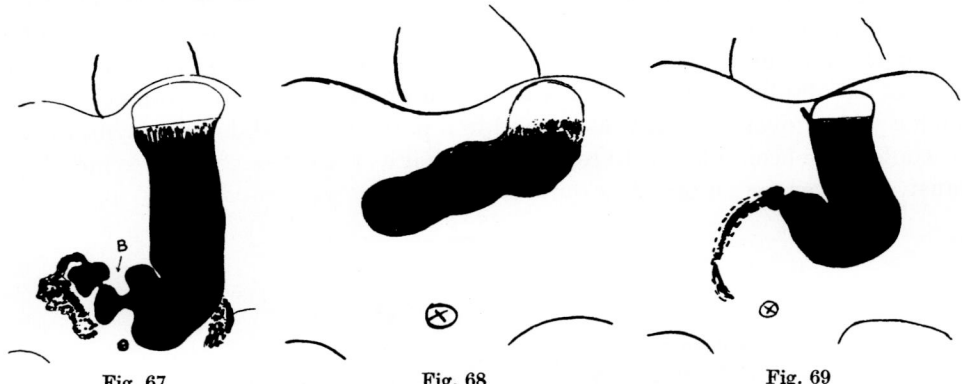

| Fig. 67 | Fig. 68 | Fig. 69 |

Fig. 67. An average J-shaped stomach, well-filled, showing peristaltic waves and well-filled duodenal cap which has just been emptied into the second part of the duodenum and been refilled. Note the small quantity of secretion collecting above the opaque food.

Fig. 68. A transversely-placed stomach, approximating to the steerhorn shape. This type is seldom seen in the female, but is common in the short stout man. The pylorus overlaps the duodenum, which passes straight backwards. To see it, a very oblique or even a lateral position would be necessary.

Fig. 69. A small stomach—often called a hypertonic stomach. The duodenum passes off more or less horizontally. The stomach happens to show no indication of peristalsis.

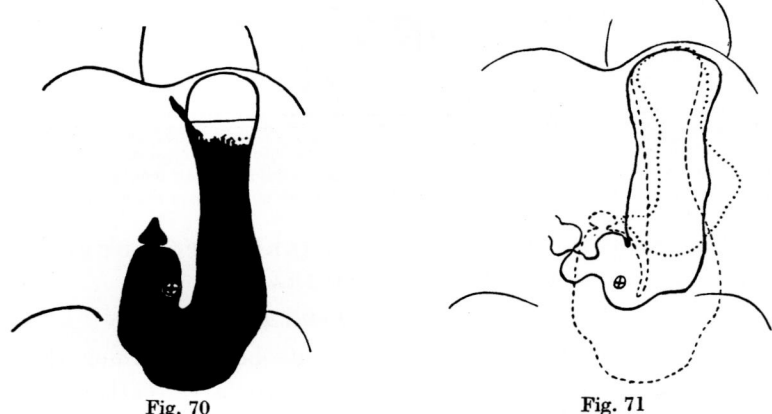

| Fig. 70 | Fig. 71 |

Fig. 70. A long stomach, such as would have been called gastroptotic. The tone is perfect. A little secretion is collecting above the opaque food. The pylorus appears to occupy its usual position.

Fig. 71. Outlines from radiographs of three types of normal stomach. Considerably smaller types are met with.

or "gastroptotic" (Figs. 70 and 77), or—if it failed to hold its contents in tubular form against the action of gravity—"atonic" (Figs. 78 and 79, p. 86). A short stomach was called "hypertonic" (Fig. 69).

The small stomach does not differ essentially from the "normal"; it is proportionately shorter and wider, and the pylorus and first part of the duodenum pass more or less transversely, or even downwards, into the second part of the duodenum. The pylorus in these cases may be on the level of the twelfth dorsal vertebra, so high that palpation is impossible because of the costal margin. This type of stomach is common in the man of short stature and prominent abdomen who habitually over-eats (Kretschmer's "pyknic" type (211)), whereas the long type is met with in tall, thin women who eat very sparely. I am confident, however, that there is no causal relationship.

The shape and disposition of the abdominal contents shown in subject C (Plate fig. 40) might be expected only in tall, thin women, yet I have seen exactly the same condition in some men students. One whom I saw recently, a man of short, sturdy, athletic build, was captain of his boat club and in training for the races. Yet his stomach and colon were almost a replica of those of subject C. Such a finding in a man of his build is doubtless unusual, but that is no argument for saying that the organs and their position are abnormal.

As there is still considerable misunderstanding of the so-called "gastroptotic" or "dropped" stomach, I shall not use either of these terms, but will simply call such organs "long" stomachs, while those formerly called hypertonic I shall call "short" stomachs. It must be remembered, however, that the form seen on one day may be quite different from that seen on the next. This is due to alterations in gastric tone (cf. p. 84). Moreover, the shape is easily altered by manipulation of the abdomen or by the pressure of intra-abdominal structures, or even by gas in the intestine. Small wonder, then, that these types are considerably modified by posture and by respiration, and that surface markings must give a false impression of organs that have no constant form.

Lateral View (Plate figs. 21, 31 and 41)

With the subject standing and the rays passing from side to side, the stomach is seen more or less in section. It takes up an angle, from above downwards and forwards, which varies with the individual, according to the prominence or flattening-out of the lumbar curvature. The average angle found in 100 consecutive subjects in the erect position was 30°, as in subject A. In subject B, with a marked lumbar curvature, however, the angle is nearer 45°, and in subject C, with the long type of stomach, there is hardly any angle at all; the viscus merely curves gently round the kidney.

This shadow outline of the stomach is not a true section, for the lower part is straddled across the vertebral column, and the "section" does not give a true idea of its antero-posterior thickness.

The Cup-and-Spill, Cascade or Drain-trap Stomach (Figs. 72–75)

In some subjects, nearly always men, the angle over the left kidney is quite sharp, perhaps 70°, so that the upper portion forms a sac or cup, while the

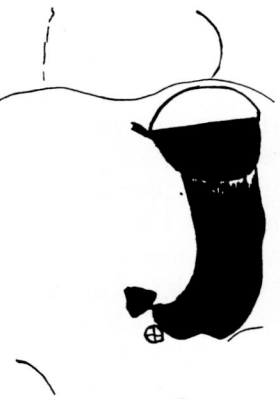

Fig. 72. Cup-and-spill stomach emptying forwards.

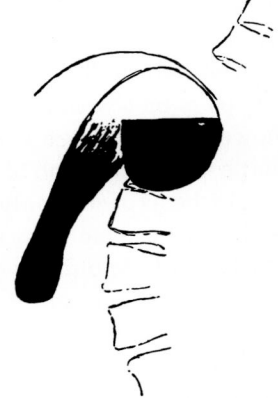

Fig. 73. Lateral view of a cup-and-spill stomach.

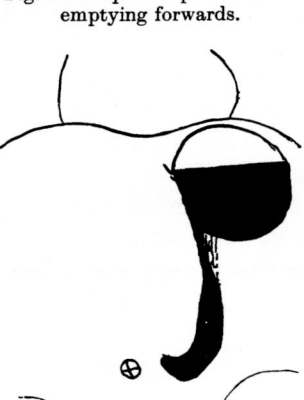

Fig. 74. Well-marked cup-and-spill stomach emptying along the line of the lesser curvature.

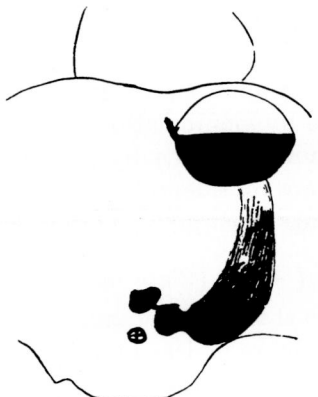

Fig. 75. Cup-and-spill stomach emptying rather to the outer side.

lower two-thirds of the organ drop practically straight down. These stomachs fill in a peculiar manner: the upper cup fills first and the food appears to spill over into the lower part—hence the name "cup-and-spill", "cascade" or "drain trap". Henri Béclère calls it "l'estomac en coupe à champagne". The food usually comes straight forward over the brim, but sometimes spills to the inner or outer side (Figs. 74 and 75). This "cup-and-spill" appearance is occasionally associated with duodenal lesions, or with a gastric ulcer high up on some part of the wall; *per se*, however, it does not appear to be abnormal but rather a variation in normal form; very often it is merely transitory. It can sometimes be produced by giving sodium bicarbonate and tartaric acid and so distending the fundus with gas.

The mechanism that produces this type is not at all clear, but can most easily be explained by assuming that the oblique band remains in its normal state of posture or tone while gas distends the fundus, stretching the thin wall above it so that the oblique band holds up the lip of the cup. Why some of these "cup-and-spill" stomachs should empty forwards and some sideways is a mechanical problem; a possible solution can be imagined by considering that the fundus of the stomach has ample room for rotation and that the cardiac orifice is the only comparatively fixed spot. The explanation is completed by carrying the hypothesis a little farther and suggesting that the two sides of the oblique band can act independently of each other, just as there is separate control of the two sides of the face. This theory, moreover, has slight support in the text-books of anatomy, which state that the nerve supply is through the terminal branches of the two pneumogastrics (with the addition of various offsets from the sympathetic), the left supplying the anterior and the right the posterior wall.

The "cup-and-spill" form may be the result of a spasmodic contraction, for it often disappears entirely on giving more food, but it is more probably due to a combination of extra-gastric factors (e.g. the lumbar curve) and spasm of the oblique fibres. Sometimes it is so pronounced that a definite hour-glass appearance is seen.

The Form in Children

In infants the stomach is comparatively spherical: it does not elongate until the erect posture is assumed, and even then only gradually takes on the adult form.

In children it is relatively short and wide in proportion to the length of the body. Whereas in the adult the stomach reaches to the umbilicus, in children it does not reach the umbilical level and assume a J-shape until near puberty. At about four years of age it usually reaches to about half-way between the xiphisternal notch and the umbilicus.

THE PART PLAYED BY GASTRIC TONE

Tonic action is difficult to explain, and there is no satisfactory definition of it. It is entirely different from active muscular contraction and has been described by Cleland as the "ligamentous action of muscle". It is the property that enables muscle to "stay put" and yet to exert force. It enables the stomach to posture or to remain stationary and yet to exert a constant, sensitively balanced and automatic pressure on its contents. It is compensatory to the influence of gravity.

Sherrington (299) says:

"The notion of tension is attached as a concomitant of shortening and supposes that with greater shortening there must run increased tension. But it has become clear that skeletal muscle in postural reflex contraction may alter the lengths of its fibres very considerably with little or no change in the tension the muscle exerts."

Speaking of the bladder, he continues:

"We may apply the term *posture* to this property...by virtue of which it solves the problem of acting as a reservoir for quantities of fluid of very varying volume from one occasion to another without allowing the intravesical pressure to attain the reflex stimulus threshold height with one particular fluid quantity only. But if we do we must attempt a definition of posture in order that the term may be clear....Active posture largely compasses the counteraction of those effects which gravitation, etc., produce in the dead body.

"Active posture may be described as those reactions in which the configuration of the body and its parts is, in spite of forces tending to disturb them, preserved by the activity of contractile tissues, these tissues then functioning statically. The rôle of muscle as an executant of movements is so striking that its office in preventing movement and displacement is somewhat overlooked. When a movement, whether active or passive, has brought about a change in the configuration of a limb—e.g. by flexing one of the joints—an important function of the musculature may be to maintain the new configuration—the posture. In doing this the muscle does not make but *prevents* movements; it then acts statically and, though in a state of contraction, it does no mechanical work, whether the tension it develops...be great or small."

In the recumbent position the action is not required to counteract gravity and largely disappears. Hence the change in gastric form when the patient lies down. The intragastric pressure is maintained constant in spite of the addition of more food, and keeps the contents in tubular form against the action of gravity, quite irrespective—within reasonable limits—of the quantity of food in the stomach; the increased capacity is obtained almost exclusively by lateral expansion (Fig. 131, p. 148). In animal experiments it is found that the intragastric pressure does not increase at all until a large volume is reached (Gianturco(132)). Tone exerts its pressure to such purpose that the whole lumen is filled by even a small quantity; a single mouthful of food is enough to "fill" the lower portion of the stomach and to keep it "full". Tone, moreover, gives the organ a relatively fixed shape and position. Hence we are not—or should not be—conscious of a full stomach when we walk or run. There seems to be some means in the stomach of adjusting it to the bulk of the contents, with the result that the intragastric pressure remains the same for any reasonable quantity of food. The rate at which the food enters is, however, apt to cause temporary disturbances in the intragastric pressure—i.e. the general tonus of the stomach has not time to readjust itself. Hence the feeling of discomfort that some patients experience from bolting their food and the clinical significance of enquiring into the way in which patients eat. This may be of far greater importance in vague cases of dyspepsia than the type of food; there was a very good physiological foundation for the practice ascribed to Mr W. E. Gladstone of chewing every mouthful forty times!

This automatically controlled power of adapting itself to varied internal and external forces so as to exert constant pressure on the contents is one of the most important functions of the gastric muscle. The intragastric pressure must necessarily be greatest at the lowest part and must be proportionately graded to the cardiac end according to the outward thrust of the column of food that it has to support. This somewhat obvious fact I have omitted in order to avoid complicating the description of a mechanism that is difficult both to understand and to describe.

Emotional disturbances, such as fear, are at once shown by a relaxation of the tone of the muscle and a consequent drop in the level of the lowest part of the outline. In the waiting period before an examination or a race, most people experience sinking sensations in the abdomen; these are due to loss of tonic action from emotional causes, with the result that the stomach becomes, for the time being, "dropped".

Many years ago I was watching an opaque meal on the screen when suddenly the lower border of the shadow dropped down from the level of the umbilicus almost into the pelvis. A door had banged and startled the patient. On another occasion when I saw the same thing the patient fainted and fell among the apparatus. In those early days of prolonged examinations and sparking apparatus, before screening stands had come into use, fainting was not uncommon, and radiologists learned to recognise this dropping of the stomach as a definite warning—a warning that had to be obeyed when apparatus was unprotected and a fall might entail serious consequences, not only to the patient but also to the flimsy supports that were the predecessors of modern elaborate and stable screening stands. Dropped stomachs used to be very frequent in X-ray departments at the first examination, but the organ was often normal in appearance when the patient, no longer apprehensive, came for further examinations.

A pleasant odour tends to increase tone, an unpleasant one to relax it. A pleasing prospect of food or drink may also have a marked effect (44). On one occasion I casually asked a man if he would like half a pint of beer, and the improvement of gastric tone was remarkable! The amount to which tone is increased seems to be proportionate to the patient's psychical reaction. Wingate Todd (312) in Cleveland examines all medical students periodically. At the end of their first year, when some of the students were warned that they might be dismissed as unfit to continue their studies, he noted a definite gastric response to

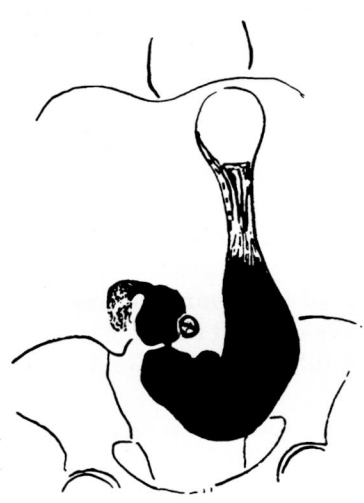

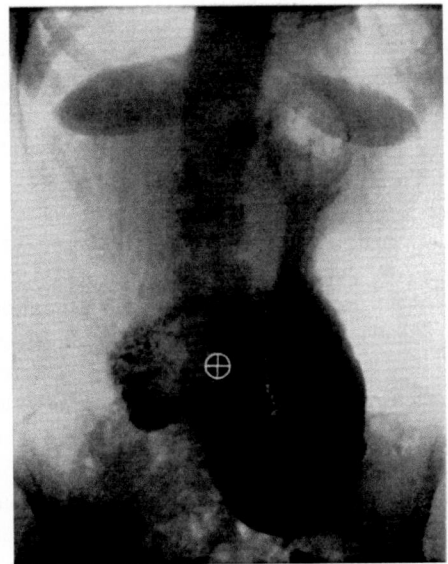

Fig. 76   Fig. 77

Fig. 76. A long stomach in which there is slight atony; the food is beginning to drag on the walls and these are probably almost, if not quite, in contact for a short distance below the air. The pylorus is low.

Fig. 77. Abnormally long stomach. Note the fragmentation beyond the duodenal cap. The circle marks the umbilicus.

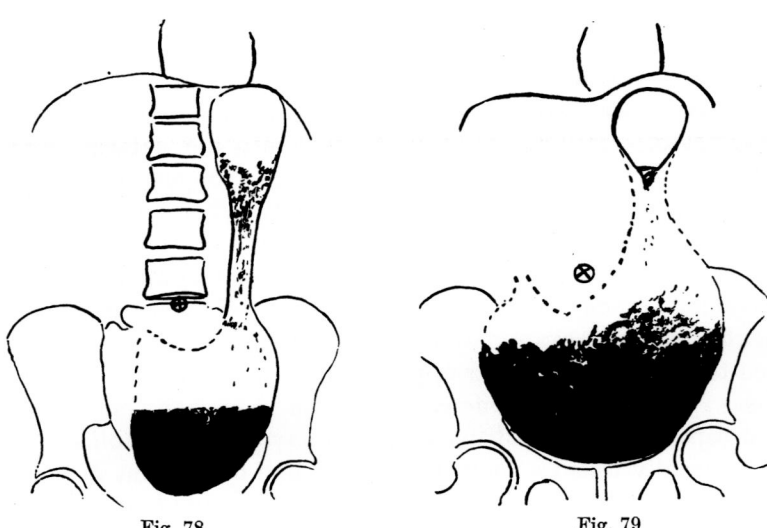

Fig. 78   Fig. 79

Fig. 78. Well-marked atony. All the opaque food has dropped to the lowest part; above this is non-opaque food or secretion. For a considerable distance below the air space the walls are in contact, probably as far as the iliac crests, and there are fragments of opaque food adhering to the walls from a meal given very shortly before the radiograph was taken. The position of the pylorus is uncertain. The case is one of pyloric obstruction with considerable residue after 24 hours.

Fig. 79. Extreme atony associated with old-standing pyloric obstruction. The greater part of the opaque food was present in the stomach after 24 hours. Note the unbroken crescentic lower outline of the food shadow. Above the opaque food is non-opaque retained food that distends the cavity almost up to the air space. The air space is pyriform and bounded below by a narrow band of fluid.

the warning: the stomach either rose or fell. Those whose stomachs dropped as the result of the threat failed to respond to the warning and were in fact dismissed, while those whose stomachs rose at the warning usually pulled themselves together and were allowed to continue.

"Atony"

When the stomach is filled, the muscular tone of the walls holds the contents in tubular form and at a fixed level (Fig. 77). If the tone is diminished from any cause, the contents tend to gravitate to the lowest part of the organ. In extreme cases the food all lies at the bottom, just as it would in a leather bag (Fig. 79). The mere fact that the opaque food drops to the bottom and does not retain a tubular appearance is not, however, sufficient ground for diagnosing atony. There may be a column of retained food or of secretion above the opaque meal, and this, although it does not appear on the screen, is keeping the walls of the stomach apart (Fig. 76). The test of atony is that the walls of the stomach are in contact above the contents, just as they would be if a heavy fluid were run

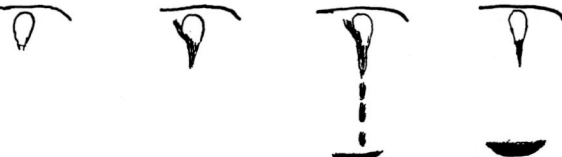

Fig. 80. Diagram illustrating the filling of an atonic stomach. The air space is pyriform, the opaque food opens out the collapsed walls and slides down between them till it meets the residual food in the lower part of the stomach. Through this it drops to the lowest part in a thick stream or in a succession of big drops or blobs.

into a flaccid leather bag. If the air space in the upper part is pyriform and has a narrow fluid line of secretion as its lower boundary, the stomach walls are very probably, if not certainly, in contact between the air space and the opaque food, and the stomach is truly "atonic" (Figs. 78, 79 and 80).

The term "dilated stomach" has been used from time immemorial to denote an atonic stomach, but seems to me misleading. To dilate means "to spread out in all directions, to enlarge". The stomach which is described clinically as "dilated" is merely one which fails to contract efficiently upon its contents and allows them to sink down to the lowest portion. The condition is certainly not one of dilatation.

My first experiment in the study of tonic action was the careful removal of a stomach shortly after death. Having suspended it by the oesophagus and along the line of attachment of the peritoneum, I filled it with an ordinary meal of bread and milk. Some bismuth-mixed food was then passed through the oesophagus and, naturally, both lots of food dropped straight to the bottom of the toneless sac, which stretched $2\frac{1}{2}$ inches under the weight. Very soon the various constituents found their level, the heavy opaque food forming the lowest, the fluid the middle layer and the air remaining at the top. This was watched on the fluorescent screen, but it was a futile experiment, and might as well have been done in any open vessel under direct observation. It did, however, emphasise the fact that the problems of the living cannot be studied in the dead subject, and that tone is essentially an attribute of the living. The dead stomach was as devoid of tonic action as a carpet bag: it had not even any elasticity; it was only stretched by the weight of the food, and had no vestige of response or recovery. In life, tone may be defective or it may be markedly deficient, but its loss never approaches the completely atonic condition that is associated with death.

Atony is not in itself a pathological condition; it is merely imperfect physiological action. It is seen, however, in varying degrees in pathological conditions and is a sign of one of two things; either that the nervous influence is below par or that the gastric muscle is fatigued (cf. p. 264). For some reason or other, gastric atony is not nearly so often seen in women as it used to be. I do not know whether changed fashions and habits of life are responsible, or whether the atonic state so often found was due to the unattractive opaque meal of former days and the dread of an unusual form of examination. The fact remains, however, that the atonic stomach, apart from associated organic lesions, is much less common than it was.

The Stomach in the Operating Theatre

The stomach which has appeared quite normal at the X-ray examination is often found at operation to be a large, flaccid, atonic sac, or vice versa. The explanation of this discrepancy is that nausea, disgust and fear bring about relaxation of tonic action, whereas in the act of retching or vomiting the stomach is contracted. Under anaesthesia the gastric muscle is fixed or stabilised in that phase of contraction or relaxation in which it happened to be when the anaesthetic affected the muscle fibres, and its appearance depends on the presence or absence of nausea or retching at that moment. Before the abdomen is opened it is never possible to foretell what its condition will be. Usually the atonic stomach of pyloric obstruction is found as a large flaccid sac, but radiographically hypertonic and normal stomachs may appear on the operating table in any form, from the tightly contracted to the large flabby. A surgeon told me that on one occasion he found a stomach so hard, firm and thick-walled that he could not perform a gastro-enterostomy. The patient died soon afterwards and the post-mortem showed a large, flaccid stomach of the "blotting paper" type.

Gastric muscle is profoundly influenced by anaesthetic agents and by the shock of opening the peritoneum, and the "operation" stomach is a very different thing from the accommodating and automatically compensating organ of the radiographic department. The occasional halting contractions seen are a mere caricature of normal peristalsis. Under spinal anaesthesia the stomach seems much more normal, so far as I have been able to study it.

GASTRIC SPASM

Visceral spasm may well be regarded as pathological and, in fact, is frequently associated with pathological conditions. Localised spasm is, however, so often noted in the stomach in apparently healthy subjects that it must find a small place in this section. As Kerley[196] says, "spasm is the bugbear of the radiologist", for it may or may not be of pathological significance, as, for instance, in the formation of the hour-glass type of stomach.

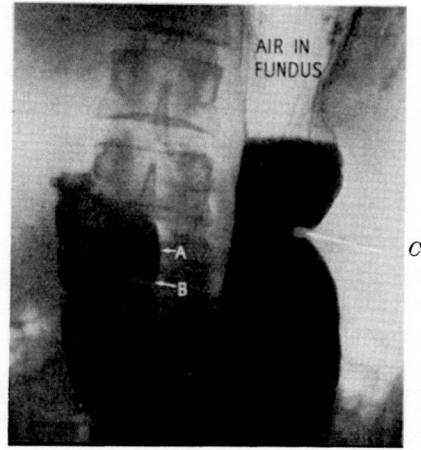 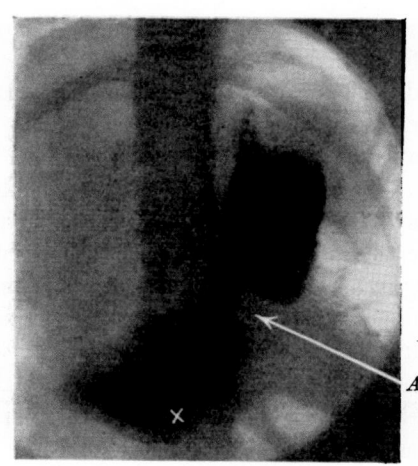

Fig. 81   Fig. 82

Fig. 81. Spasmodic contraction, C, of the greater curvature. The stomach had appeared perfectly normal on the previous day. The spasm was very persistent. Nothing was found to account for it. A, Duodenal cap. B, Pylorus.

Fig. 82. Spasmodic contraction, A, in association with a duodenal ulcer. The contraction was so extremely persistent that it was operated on in the expectation of finding a gastric ulcer with some cicatrisation. This was before the days of the recognition of an ulcer crater or the direct diagnosis of duodenal ulcer.

Not only are the two orifices of the stomach subject to spasmodic contraction, giving rise to greater or lesser temporary obstruction, but any part of the musculature may be involved. The circular fibres are apparently those most usually affected, and their contraction produces a stationary indentation on the greater curvature which simulates a wave of peristalsis (Figs. 81 and 82). Such contractions may be seen in any part of the stomach, and are usually transitory, yielding to massage and manipulation. When, however, they are seen on two separate occasions, they may be a response to some local condition of the mucous membrane; such spasm calls for very careful investigation in this region. More frequently spasm—especially pyloric spasm—is reflex, from some remote cause such as the teeth, appendix, gall bladder, kidney or even rectum (cf. p. 8).

Spasm may produce a general contraction that gives a very small type of stomach. My own experience is of interest. For some eight years I have been conscious of an occasional unmistakeable gastro-spasm. It usually occurs during a meal and the symptoms of the onset are very definite; I have to stop eating at once and stay perfectly still. It lasts only for a few minutes. There is no change of colour, sweating, or other of the usual accompaniments of vomiting. The sensation is that the stomach is completely full and that an extra mouthful would induce vomiting, and indeed this has done so once or twice. It may come on either when the stomach is empty or towards the end of a meal. Sometimes it seems to be associated with fatty foods, e.g. fried mackerel or kippers, and these, for the moment, are nauseating. More often, however, there is no nausea or distaste of the food that is being eaten, and, when the sensation has passed, the meal is continued and the incident forgotten. An Irish maid-servant gave a very apt description of the sensation: "Me stummick was sick and yet it wasn't."

The spasm may come on in the middle of the night. Occasionally I am awakened by a sense of impending vomiting, accompanied by an extremely profuse salivation, saliva literally pouring out of the mouth. Retching occasionally occurs, but there is seldom anything in the stomach other than the saliva that has been swallowed before waking. It is probable that this spasm is reflex and I suspect that it is associated with the colon, for diarrhoea and loose offensive stools are sometimes noted for a few days afterwards. Very occasionally the sensation has persisted for a few days and an X-ray examination has shown that while the symptoms are present the stomach is contracted down to an absurdly small size: a narrow J-shaped tube through which the food pours straight into the duodenum. Probably also the food is held up to some extent in the oesophagus at the cardiac orifice, judging by the sensation, but I did not

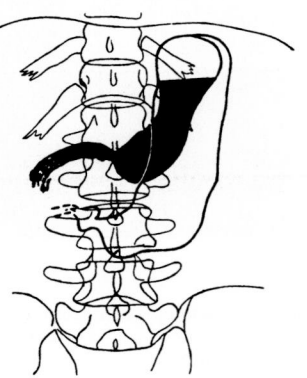

Fig. 83. General gastric spasm. The stomach was considerably smaller and narrower on the first occasion on which it was examined during spasm, but no radiograph was taken. The outlined stomach is from a film a month later after a holiday.

see this when I examined myself. Fig. 83 is from tracings of the stomach made when the symptoms were subsiding. A previous examination when symptoms were more severe showed a considerably smaller and narrower stomach, but no radiograph was taken.

THE EFFECTS OF POSTURE ON THE STOMACH

Recumbent-Supine Position, antero-posterior view (Plate figs. 24, 34 and 44)

A healthy, well-toned stomach shows far less alteration in shape from changes in posture than one in which tone is defective: in fact, in the very early days, Hulst said that that stomach was most normal which was least affected by change in posture.

When the subject lies on his back the chief alteration is a narrowing and emptying of the pyloric end and a widening out of the cardiac end. The food slides by gravity into the cardiac end, leaving the pyloric antrum either empty or occupied by the air that, in the erect posture, fills the fundus. The length of the organ, from the fundus to the lowest part, is also diminished, and the pyloric end slides up on the posterior wall of the abdomen. The variation is best appreciated by comparing Plate figs. 20, 30 and 40 with Plate figs. 24, 34 and 44, and also by noting the records of the position of the pylorus in Figs. 63, 64 and 65.

Recumbent-Supine Position, lateral view (Plate figs. 25, 35 and 45)

In the recumbent posture, with the rays passing from side to side, the food is seen in the cardiac end—the pyloric antrum is empty. The way in which the air from the fundus can distend the pyloric end should be noted. In each of these cases there was a fair quantity of air in the stomach when the examinations were made. It was the percussion of this air that gave such an unreliable guide to the size of the organ in pre-X-ray days.

It is of interest to compare these pictures with the corresponding ones (Plate figs. 21, 31 and 41) taken in the erect position, and to note the way in which the spinal curves flatten out when the subject lies on the back, a change which is largely responsible for the shape that the organ assumes. The greater the lumbar curve, the greater the tendency for the cardiac end to fall backwards and drag the pyloric end up over the kidney and pancreas.

Recumbent Position, lying on the left side (Plate figs. 26, 36 and 46)

When the subject lies on the left side the stomach sags down into the left flank, dragging with it the pylorus and duodenum. The greater curvature is moulded to the contour of the left flank, while the lesser curvature sweeps down from the cardiac orifice and up again to whatever position the pylorus has assumed. This is not, of course, a routine position in gastric examinations and I have not studied it often, but I once observed a subject in whom the pylorus was actually over the left kidney when he lay in this position. Contrary to expectation, the displacement of the pylorus in this posture in the tall, thin woman, subject C (Fig. 65), was less than in the two young subjects (Figs. 63 and 64). (The relatively slight variations in this subject for posture and respiration are rather surprising.) I am satisfied that the weight of the opaque food does not account for the distortion of the shape of the stomach, and that the present figures are almost identical with those that would have been produced had it been possible to radiograph ordinary food instead of an opaque meal.

Recumbent Position, lying on the right side (Plate figs. 27, 37 and 47)

When the subject lies on the right side the pyloric end comes right across the middle line, in such a way that it seems as if the duodenum must be kinked. Yet this is the accepted position for aiding digestion, and obviously there can be no kinking; the duodenum must adjust itself to the position. The cardiac end of the stomach is pulled out from the dome of the diaphragm, but what takes its place I do not know.

THE EFFECTS OF RESPIRATION ON THE STOMACH

Deep Inspiration (Plate figs. 22, 32 and 42)

On deep inspiration the lower border of the stomach does not descend to anything like the same extent as the cardia. This is due to a "concertina" type of action in the stomach muscle, presumably controlled by muscle tone, which tends to counteract the effect of the excursion of the diaphragm. In the J-shaped stomach this action, possibly assisted to some extent by the angle at which the stomach lies, compensates almost completely for the downward movement of the diaphragm in inspiration. It is also probably of considerable importance in assisting the food to pass on.

Where, however, the tone of the gastric muscle is diminished, the degree of movement of the lower part of the shadow in response to respiration is almost, if not quite, as great as that of the diaphragm. This movement may even serve as a rough gauge to measure the degree of atony of the stomach. But the very long stomach, as in Plate fig. 42, shows practically no movement on deep inspiration, for it is already resting on the pelvic contents. The greatest degree of downward movement in response to inspiration is in stomachs that present a relatively slight degree of atony, i.e. where the concertina action is impaired but where the lowest part is still well above the pelvic floor.

A curious and unexplained feature in Plate fig. 42 is the fact that the fundus appears to leave the diaphragm, whereas in deep expiration, with the diaphragm high up in the chest, the fundus occupies its usual position under the dome (Plate fig. 43)—the exact opposite of what might reasonably be expected. This may be due to pressure of the spleen in between the stomach and the diaphragm, for the same feature is noted with the subject at rest supine (Plate fig. 44). There is some support for this suggestion from the lateral supine picture (Plate fig. 45), in which the fundus does not seem to lie so far back in the abdomen.

It will be noted that the fundus leaves the diaphragm to a greater or lesser extent in all three subjects when they lie on the right side (Plate figs. 27, 37 and 47), and perhaps the explanation is the same.

Forced Expiration (Plate figs. 23, 33 and 43)

The pictures of the stomach on forced expiration show a striking upward excursion of the whole organ. After seeing the effectual way in which the concertina action compensates for the movement of deep inspiration, one might expect to find a corresponding relaxation of the gastric muscle in expiration which would stabilise the position of the lower part of the stomach, but I have found little evidence for this and, more often than not, the stomach seems to rise as a whole with the forced expiratory excursion of the diaphragm. Whether this is due to the absence of relaxation of the stomach wall or to the action of the abdominal muscles in the forced expiratory effort I do not know, but in ordinary unforced respiration there is only a slight degree of this upward displacement.

The change of shape of the stomach in deep expiration approximates closely to that seen in the supine recumbent posture (Plate figs. 24, 34 and 44). The effect of forced expiration on the viscera is not uniform, and depends on the type of respiration. The changes are more marked in subjects in whom the abdominal type of respiration predominates.

Models of the Stomach

Some years ago I [37] made models of the stomach to show the more important of its varying forms as revealed by X rays. Photographs of these models are shown in Fig. 84. Another method that has been developed by Hasselwander [147] of Erlangen is to make models from stereoscopic films of the stomach and other organs with an adaptation of the Wheatstone stereoscope, using prisms instead of mirrors. The observer can see through the prisms to a mass of plasticine placed behind, and this is shaped to the form of the stereoscopic image. A system of lighting gives the balance of illumination between the stereoscopic image and the phantom, which is moulded in exact reproduction of what is seen in the stereoscope. To employ this method, an exceptionally well developed sense of stereoscopic vision is necessary, but the results amply justify the pains that are necessary in making these interesting and instructive models (Fig. 85).

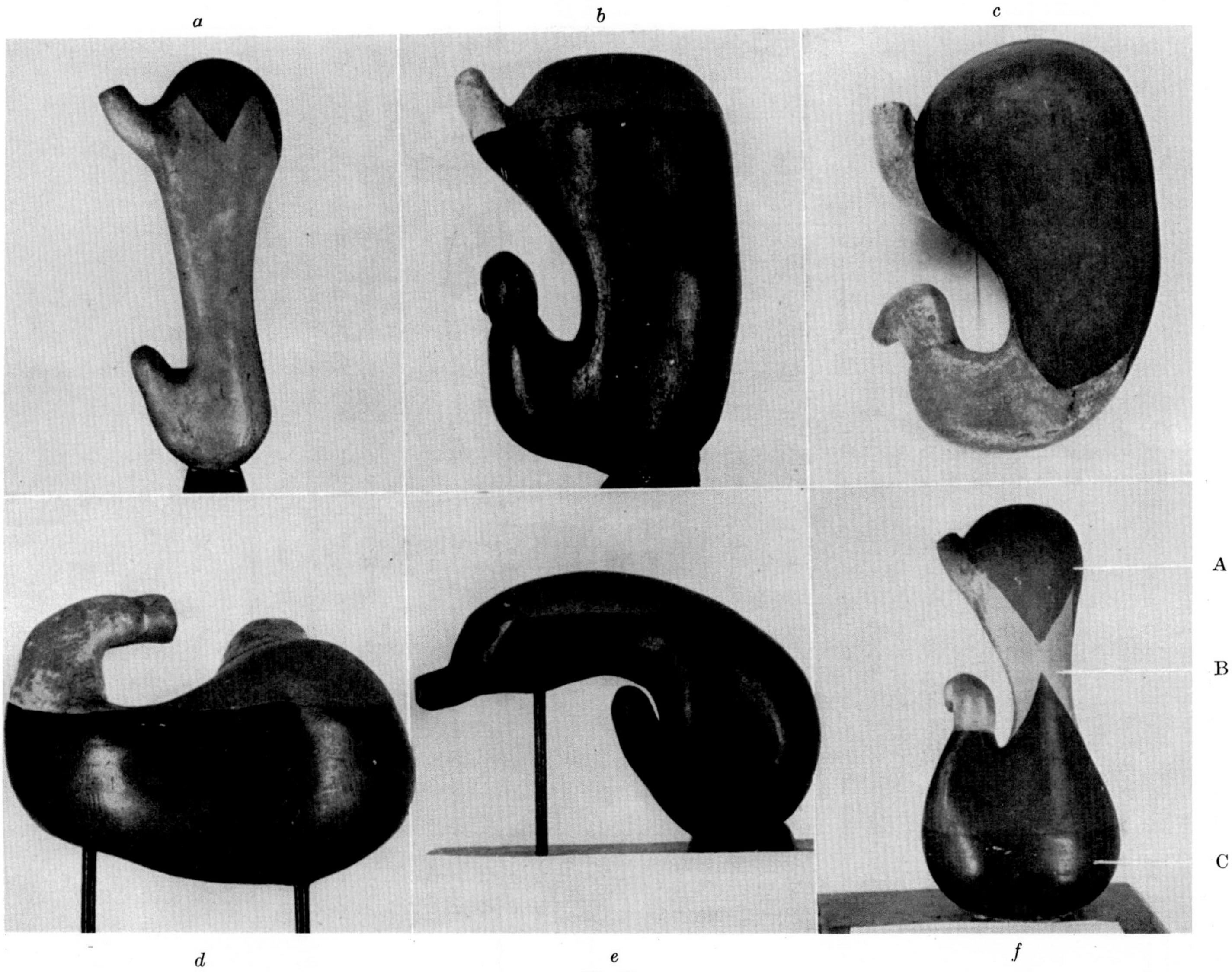

a   *b*   *c*

                                                                    A

                                                                    B

d   *e*   *f*   C

Fig. 84.

Fig. 84. Models of the "normal" stomach constructed from radiographic observation.

a. Normal empty stomach. Upright position. Dark area represents air in the fundus. It is pyriform in shape and fades off at the lower end. This is suggested by the wedges of shading extending down on the anterior, posterior and lateral aspects.

b. Normal stomach (full—about ¾ pint). Light area represents the air in the fundus. Dark area represents the opaque food. The model is not mounted quite correctly—the lesser curvature should be almost straight.

c. Normal stomach. Subject lying on the back. The air (dark area) is spread out over the fundus chiefly, and the food gravitates to and distends the cardiac end. The pyloric portion is empty and is spread out across the vertebral column.

d. Normal stomach. Subject lying on the left side. The air (medium shade) lies along the lesser curvature—sometimes a pocket of air is occluded in the pyloric end. The pylorus is usually to the left of the middle line. The greater curvature lies along, and is supported by, the left wall of the abdomen. The indentation caused by the spleen is often seen.

e. Normal stomach. Subject lying on the right side. The air (light area) lies along the greater curvature, which is drawn out from the dome of the diaphragm and away from the lateral abdominal wall; as a rule it lies near the nipple line, but even in a healthy organ fully three-quarters of the stomach is to the right of the middle line. The pyloric portion is markedly distended as compared with the upright position (*b*). The pylorus is inclined backwards and to the left, almost giving a "kink"

f. Marked atonic (dilated stomach). Note the pyriform shape of the air space (A); the dragged out and collapsed walls in the middle and the retained ordinary food (B) that tapers up into the collapsed portion of the stomach. The opaque food (C) lies at the lowest part, giving a crescentic outline. The pylorus lies in its normal position, and the lesser curvature is not increased in length. The lower part of the stomach is six inches below the pylorus in this case. Such a condition may be the result of obstruction at the pylorus or duodenum, or it may be a condition *per se,* which gives rise to delay in emptying because the peristalsis of the stomach is not sufficiently powerful to raise the food to the pylorus. The weight of the opaque food exaggerates the appearance of the atony.

See *Journ. Anat.* 1920, LIV, 260.

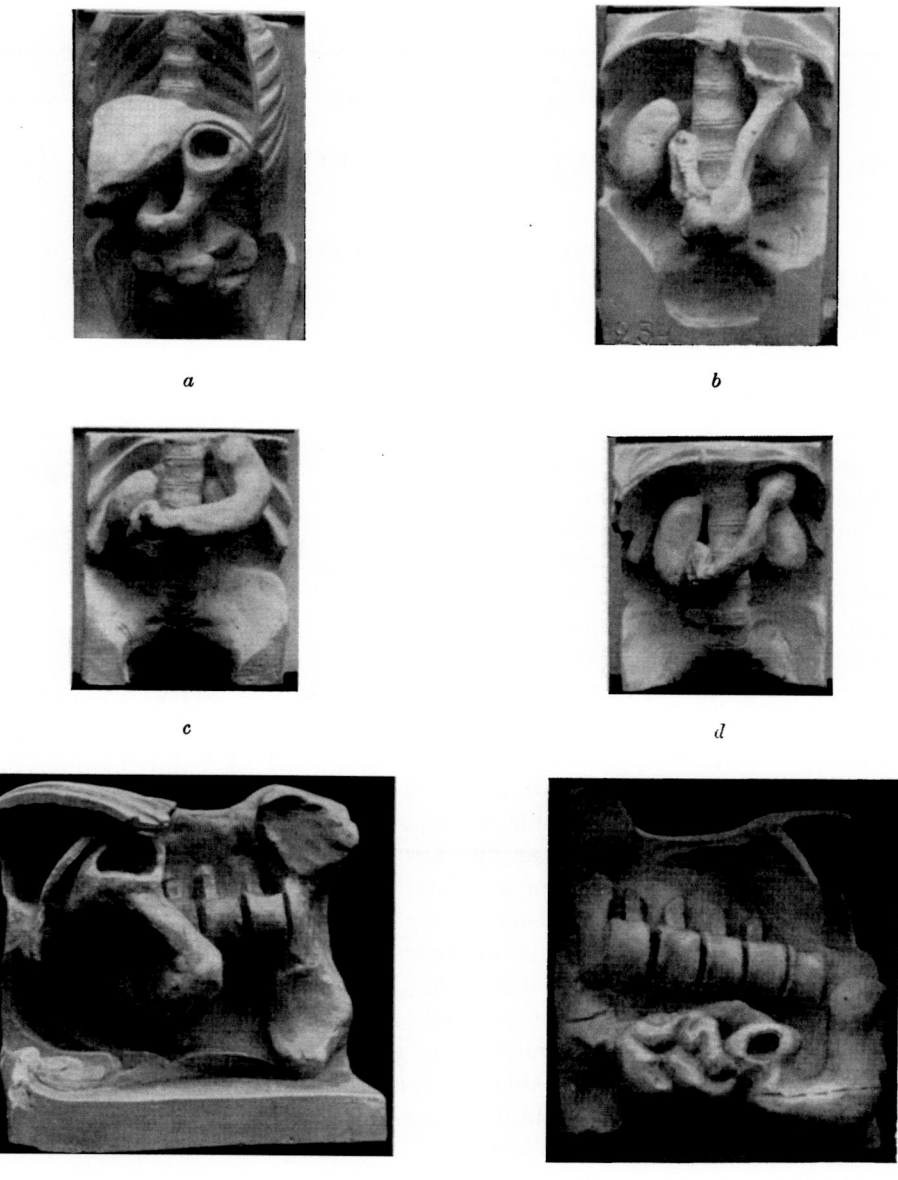

Fig. 85. Photographs of models of the stomach made by direct reconstruction from stereoscopic radiographs by Professor Hasselwander of Erlangen.

a and b. Reconstruction of "normal" and "long" stomachs in the erect posture.
c and d. Reconstruction of two stomachs in the recumbent position.
e. Reconstruction of the stomach with the subject lying on the left side.
f. Reconstruction of the stomach with the subject lying on the right side.

CHAPTER VII

EFFECTS OF POSTURE AND RESPIRATION ON OTHER VISCERA

THE LARGE INTESTINE

Caecum and Appendix

The position in which the radiologist finds the caecum varies within rather wide limits. It is obviously capable of very extensive displacement in response to posture, respiration and manipulation. In Fig. 86 I have plotted out the positions of the caecal end of the appendix in the supine position in thirty unselected cases. Although wide variations are indicated, the majority lie approximately round about McBurney's point: the junction of the middle and outer thirds of a line drawn from the anterior superior spine to the umbilicus. In the upright position, however, the appendix lies, on an average, two or three inches below this point. I have not the material available to plot out the position on a chart, as the appendix is comparatively seldom seen and radiographed in the erect posture, owing to the overlapping of the caecal and other shadows, and also because it lies so low

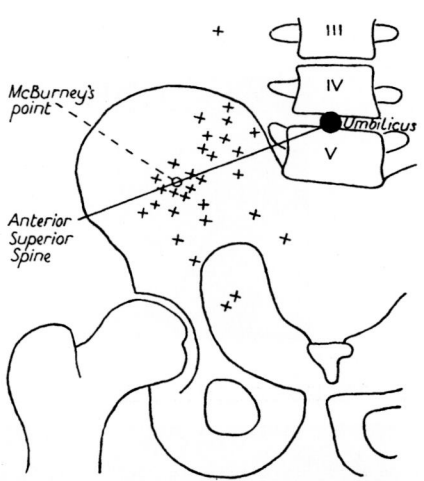

Fig. 86. The site of the caecal end of the appendix traced from 30 unselected radiographs. These were all taken in the supine position and, in many, compression has been employed to free the appendix from other shadows.

down that the organs cannot be reached and separated by palpation. Even in the recumbent posture manipulation is generally necessary to separate the appendix from the other food shadows, and the pressure of a pad or spoon is nearly always needed to maintain its position while the radiograph is taken. Hence the positions marked on the chart may not give a true indication of the actual normal position in the supine posture, but they do give some indication of the mobility of the caecum under ordinary conditions. In my tracing, the positions in which the caecal end of the appendix was found are covered by a circle seven inches in diameter centred on McBurney's point. The caecum that fails to rise out of the pelvis in the Trendelenburg or a similar position is usually anchored down by old adhesions.

Colon (Plate figs. 28, 29, 38, 39 and 48)

The filled large intestine, seen radioscopically, is a more or less uniform tubular organ with regular haustral segmentations, suggesting a string of chestnuts. Whether they are caused by contractions of the muscularis propria or of the muscularis mucosae I do not know. The solid appearance of the contents is due to the tonic contraction of the walls and not necessarily to the solid nature of the faeces. The fluid nature of the contents is evident directly a mass movement occurs: the haustra disappear and the contents respond like a fluid to the action of the bowel wall. There is no evidence of any sphincter between the caecum and the ascending colon; in fact, the radiologist develops the habit of thinking of the caecum and ascending colon as one organ. Whenever any tendency to distension and "sloppiness" is seen, it seems to involve the caecum and ascending colon as far as the hepatic flexure.

The whole of the large intestine, including the caecum and sigmoid, moves with forced respiration, and the flexures have as great, if not a greater range of movement than the diaphragm. Generally speaking, however, the further away a viscus is from the diaphragm the less the movement in response to respiration. In some cases I failed to observe any movement, even on forced jerky respiration, and concluded that its absence was accounted for by adhesions. Rotky and Herrnheiser (153) examined a large number of cases to determine the position of the colon in health and in ptosis, but did not arrive at any definite conclusions; they stated that there must be certain limits, but that even so there would be many exceptions.

Posture affects the whole of the large intestine, and Plate figs. 28, 29, 38, 39 and 48 illustrate its effect. Wide differences are recorded, even in these few unselected cases and, indeed, the variations both in normal position and in the range of movement of the flexures due to posture are very striking, quite apart from the added excursion that is due to respiration. Forced and jerky movements of the abdominal muscles cause the colon and other abdominal viscera to move in a manner that can hardly be described as anything less than acrobatic (cf. p. 103).

The usual position of the *hepatic flexure* in the standing posture is an inch or a little more above the iliac crest, while it generally rises some two or three inches higher when the subject lies down. The flexure looks like an acute angle, but this appearance is, of course, due to foreshortening (cf. p. 112).

In the majority of cases the *splenic flexure* is found high up under the dome of the diaphragm, in the position indicated in the anatomy books, but in about one-third of the students examined it is considerably lower. Occasionally it only just rises above the iliac crest in the erect posture. It often contains a collection of air and is as closely related to the diaphragm as is the fundus of the stomach, moving freely with it.

The position of the *transverse colon* is very variable. In the two women of my series it happens to be low down in the pelvis, and on the whole I think it is lower in the female than in the male, but not uncommonly the same low position is seen in men who are in perfect health and in training for sports. In fact, muscular development does not appear to be a controlling factor at all. The varieties of transverse colon encountered are innumerable. In most cases its general direction is at an angle of 40° up to the splenic region, and it forms a festooned loop, often with a subsidiary festoon that drops down almost, if not quite, into the pelvis. It is all very freely movable. The position in the upright posture depends on the length of the transverse meso-colon and of the stomach, for the colon hangs from it by the transverse meso-colon. Hence, if the stomach becomes atonic and drops, the colon likewise drops. Occasionally the transverse colon is found crossing the stomach. This is generally the result of ascites or abdominal tumours, the gas in the colon floating it up in front of the stomach, where it may become anchored.

The concept of coloptosis is one that might well have been abandoned before it was thrust upon a confiding public, for it has given rise to endless misinterpretations of normal phenomena, and the hypothetical condition it denotes has been blamed for symptoms which it would not have been at all likely to produce, even if it had actually existed. It is surely unnecessary to labour a point which is obvious to anyone who sees a reasonable number of normal healthy subjects and studies them with an open mind. It is regrettable that radiologists had no opportunity of investigating the normal and its possibilities before they were plunged into the study of abnormal subjects.

The descending colon drops straight from the splenic flexure to the iliac crest, and at this point is said to become fixed, losing its mesentery and being merely covered by the peritoneum. In actual practice, however, the supposed absence of a mesentery seems to make very little difference to mobility. In a certain proportion of cases the descending colon has a long mesentery; it drops down over this relatively fixed point and there may be a tendency to kinking.

A noteworthy point about the radiological anatomy of the sigmoid is the close relationship that the loaded caecum and the sigmoid may bear to each other: sometimes they seem to be actually in contact.

THE PANCREAS

The pancreas is probably the least mobile of organs, but it cannot be seen radiographically. Dr A. F. Hurst, however, wrote to me personally (28. iv. 32): "I firmly believed with you that the pancreas must be immobile. About three years ago I had a patient with a large ulcer on the lesser curvature which looked as if it was eroding the pancreas. As, however, it moved a little on respiration and actually dropped about two inches on assuming the erect position, I decided that it could not involve the pancreas but must be passing into the gastrohepatic omentum. At operation, however, it was found firmly adherent to the pancreas, which formed the base of the ulcer. It is clear, therefore, that the pancreas, like the duodenum, can drop behind the peritoneum."

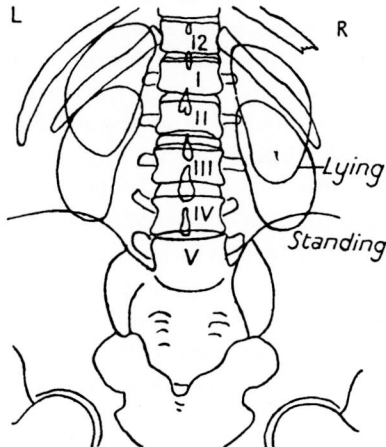

Fig. 87. A healthy man, aged 46.

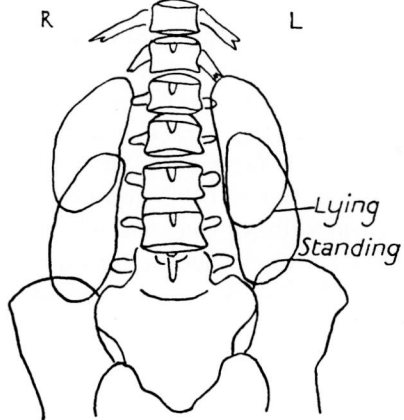

Fig. 88. A healthy woman, aged 37.
(Same subject as Fig. 66.)

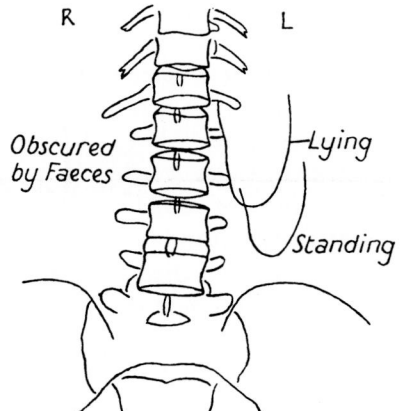

Fig. 89. A healthy woman, aged 27. (Same subject as Figs. 94–103 and Plate figs. 20–28.)

Figs. 87, 88 and 89. Superimposed tracings of radiographs showing the position of the kidney with the subject standing and lying supine. The mid-phase of respiration was used in each case.

THE KIDNEYS

The kidneys are not readily seen on the fluorescent screen, but their outline is visible on radiographs. Until recent years they could not be seen unless some device for compression and fixation against respiratory and other movements was used; consequently they always appeared higher than they should normally be. Compression is now no longer needed, and we find that an excursion of an inch or more in a direction downwards and outwards, parallel with the edge of the psoas, is normal. I asked a friend to radiograph a normal subject and expose films both in the standing and the recumbent postures under identical conditions of respiration. He selected a workman of average build about 46 years of age. A tracing of the bony parts showed that both films had been taken in exactly the same position, except for the posture. On this tracing the kidney outlines, which were clearly seen in both films, were filled in, and the result is shown in Fig. 87. The difference in position of the kidneys, due entirely to posture, is far greater than I ever expected. Accordingly I made similar observations on two other subjects (Figs. 88 and 89), and found a degree of movement of the kidneys that was slightly more in one and slightly less in the other than that shown in the first subject. These subjects were healthy young women of small build. So far as I can see, however, the kidneys are less subject to movement from respiration than from posture; nor do they appear to be displaced by violent movements of the abdominal muscles to nearly the same degree as the stomach and intestines.

THE LIVER

The liver is subject to the full range of the diaphragmatic movement, and is also affected by gravity. Some ten or twelve years ago, when pneumoperitoneum was being explored as a diagnostic radiographic method, the whole outline of the liver was well shown, and the displacements that occurred without any untoward results were remarkable. In the only instance of which I have records, I found that in the standing posture it slid down almost to the iliac crest, while when the patient lay on the left side it slid round until more than half of it was across the middle line. Fig. 90 shows line tracings from the actual radiographs of this case, which was, of course, regarded as very exceptional. (In this instance the outlines of the liver were visualised by the injection of air per rectum—a procedure seldom employed

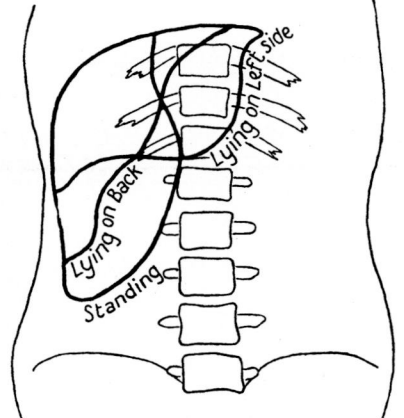

Fig. 90. Line tracings from radiographs of a case in which the liver was regarded as exceptionally mobile, seen standing, lying supine and lying on the left side.

but one which is sometimes very valuable in the investigation of conditions in the abdomen outside the intestinal tract. It is now being used by a few workers in the investigation of the mucosa of the large intestine.)

Free movement of the liver is said to be associated with Glénard's disease, but I have noted fairly extensive movement in quite healthy subjects. It is a remarkable fact that in the radiography of the gall-bladder for diagnostic purposes its position is found to vary within very wide limits. On the average, it approximates to the orthodox anatomical position, but it is sometimes found considerably higher and quite often far lower than would have been thought possible. The gall-bladder may actually overlap the shadow of the crest of the ilium, and shadows of gall-stones have been found even in the true pelvis! (cf. p. 334). Moody and van Nuys [245] showed that the liver in perfectly normal subjects could vary considerably in length, some types having their lower border as far down as 5 cm. below the iliac crest. This long type is more common in women than in men.

THE SPLEEN

The spleen is not seen on an X-ray film in ordinary circumstances, and I have made no observations of its movements. It must, however, move with the diaphragm, and clinically it is often palpable and can be easily displaced. Moreover, a spleen which is palpable with the patient standing is sometimes not felt when he lies down. While the lower border of the spleen is usually found opposite the upper half of the third lumbar vertebra, Moody and van Nuys [245] showed that spleens reaching to the lower half of the fourth lumbar vertebra were quite normal and commoner in men than in women.

A technique for visualising the spleen and liver has been devised, but I have no experience of it. It consists in the intravenous injection of 25 per cent. solution of thorium dioxide (thorium: atomic weight 234·4). This salt is said to have an affinity for reticulo-endothelial cells, and is taken up so freely by the liver and spleen that a satisfactory radiogram can be obtained. With this technique it should be easy to obtain records of the movements under normal conditions. Editorial articles in *The British Journal of Radiology* [345] refer to original work in this field.

Oka [261] has pointed out that thorium dioxide gives radio-opaque shadows of liver and spleen if a 10 per cent. solution of it is given mixed with glucose in 8 to 10 doses. The patients are apt to suffer from fever and diarrhoea afterwards. Radt [277] has improved the technique by using a salt of thorium called tordiol which is deposited in the reticulo-endothelial cells of the liver and spleen in fine granules. The whole structure of the organ is thus rendered somewhat opaque to X rays and any gaps or areas of altered structure are shown up by contrast as less opaque. Some workers have expressed distrust of the method because they feel that large quantities of a radio-active salt remaining in the body for an indefinite period are bound to have some effect, which will probably be a bad one. In my opinion the risks of leaving a radio-active material in the tissues are considerable, and the technique is probably unjustifiable except in the presence of malignant disease.

TRANSPOSITION OF VISCERA

There is little to be said about this condition except that the abdominal viscera, and nearly always the mediastinal contents also, are transposed. It is rare and is usually recognised at a glance. There is, however, a condition in which the colon only appears to be transposed. Golob (136) distinguishes this from transposition under the name of "congenital non-rotation of the colon". If the normal rotation fails altogether, the large intestine lies behind the small. If arrested later, the colon lies to the left of the small intestine; at a still later stage, to the left but with the ileo-caecal region about the mid-line. Arrest of growth after this leaves the caecum under the liver, or only partially descended to the iliac fossa. Golob says that these conditions may be symptomless for years, but that, being the point of least resistance, they may give rise to trouble. (Cf. Hunter's work (166).)

Rosselet and Mengis (286) describe a case of congenital abnormality of the stomach in a woman of fifty who enjoyed good health but had suffered a good deal from indigestion as a child. Her only complaint was of flatulence. The barium, having passed the diaphragm, continued through an elongated oesophagus to a cardia which was situated on the back of the stomach about 20 cm. below the diaphragm. The duodenal cap was placed high up, 5 mm. above the cardia and about 3 cm. to the left of the mid-line. They ascribed this anomaly to the failure of rotation of the stomach depending on an absence of activity in the duodenal papilla.

Boulton Myles recently showed a case in which there was displacement producing an apparent filling defect of the greater curvature of the stomach. On investigation he found the appendix in the left flank, to the outer side of the greater curvature. He then carefully traced out the course of the colon with an enema and, although it was much distorted, the greater part of the colon appeared to be transposed, and the right iliac fossa was empty. Similar cases have been described by Waugh under the title of "Congenital Malformations of the Mesentery" (331). The patients were investigated by giving a barium meal and a barium enema simultaneously. Dr Courtney Gage, his collaborator in the radiographic investigation of these cases, has seen eight instances.

In one instance of complete transposition, I was faced with a problem that still awaits solution. The symptoms were those of a definite appendix lesion and an operation was intended. It was only at a subsequent X-ray examination that the transposition was noted and the appendix found on the opposite side to the symptoms! There was definite ileal stasis and everything pointed to an appendix lesion except the site of the pain, where there was no suggestion of anything wrong. Was it possible that, although the viscera were transposed, the nerve supply pursued its normal course on the right side? The problem is not solved, for the patient recovered without operation and is still perfectly well. Out of curiosity I examined him again some years later and found no indication of ileal stasis or adhesions in the appendix region.

A DEMONSTRATION OF MOBILITY

It is easy to give students dramatic demonstrations of the great mobility of the stomach and other abdominal contents. I arrange for one of the class to have his colon filled by an opaque meal. With the aid of a looking-glass he notes

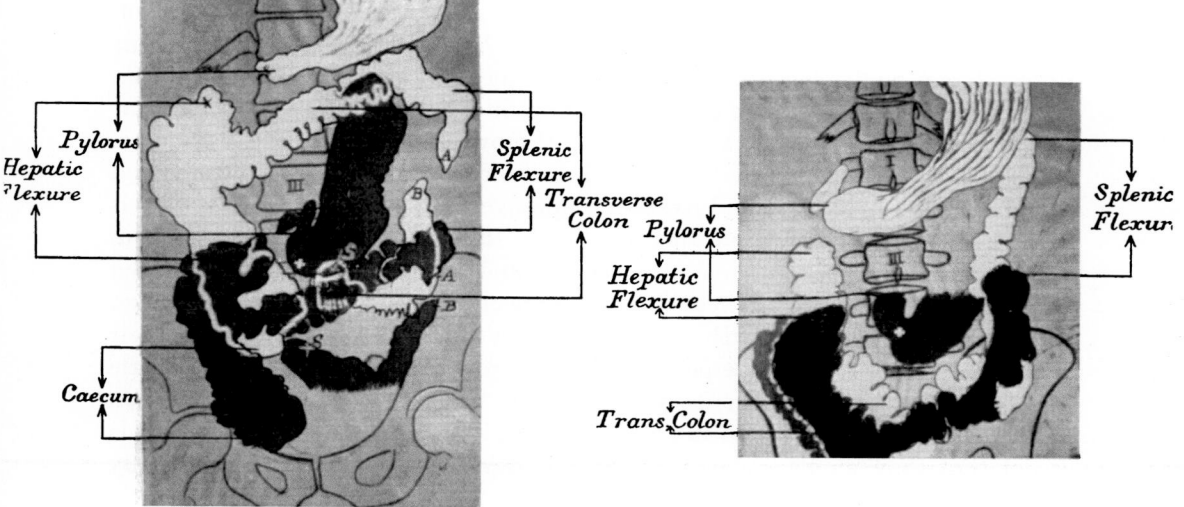

Fig. 91   Fig. 92

Figs. 91 and 92. Composite tracings from radiographs of two healthy subjects, showing the extremes of movement due to the combined effects of posture and respiration. The dark shadows of the viscera are traced from radiographs taken with the subjects standing and in the *extreme phase of inspiration*. The light shadows of the viscera are traced from radiographs taken with the subjects lying supine and in the *extreme phase of expiration*. Moreover, the abdominal muscles are retracted, causing a considerable movement in addition to that obtained by respiration alone. The extraordinarily wide range of movements indicated is somewhat exaggerated by the radiographic technique owing to the divergence of the X-ray beam (cf. p. 75).

Fig. 91. From a medical student of rather tall, slim build. The excursion of the lower border of the stomach as measured on the abdominal wall was recorded as 9 in. In the radiographs, however, there was not quite such a big disparity, as the subject could not hold the stomach in the position into which he was able to jerk it by the action of his abdominal muscles (he was watching the effect of his movements with a looking-glass).

Fig. 92. A woman of 27. (The same subject as in Plate figs. 20–28 and Figs. 94–103). Note that, although the flexures of the colon show marked movement, yet the transverse colon hardly moves at all. Obviously it is anchored down into the pelvis by some adhesions. The transverse meso-colon must be unusually long to allow of such free upward movement of the stomach.

the effect of deep respiration on the shadows of the stomach and colon. This, combined with the amusement of the class, usually makes him laugh, and his laughter causes vigorous jerky movements of the abdominal muscles, to which the organs respond. The greatest and most mirth-provoking movements are, however, produced when—as suggested by Dr R. S. Paterson—the subject voluntarily retracts and protrudes his abdomen. In response to this movement, the organs look almost as though they had no attachments at all, and their range of movement is considerably greater than that of the diaphragm. The hepatic flexure straightens out and rises several inches, and the stomach and transverse colon show an excursion of as much as nine inches! That the lower border of the stomach should be capable of such an excursion seems absurd, but this is the actual measurement recorded in a subject lying on a couch (cf. Figs. 91 and 92). The whole abdomen behaves like a rubber bag, the contents of which can be displaced into any part by squeezing the sides. It well merits the description of "a jumble of slithery things in a hole".* Even a caecum that is low in the pelvis will show some range of movement in these circumstances.

I am inclined to think that some such technique as this might be developed for the detection of abnormal fixation. Moreover, it looks as if exercise of this kind would be more effective therapeutically than any form of manipulation, for the whole of the colon, even the caecum and the sigmoid flexure, is moved in a way that could not be effected by massage or manipulation of the abdomen.

Laughter not only makes the organs move, but also excites peristalsis in their walls. It will often stimulate peristalsis in a resting stomach, and fill the pyloric canal and duodenum. Its effects would seem to explain its close association with good digestion and plentiful adipose tissue! And the moral for thin people is not that they should eat more, but that they should laugh more, especially at and after meals!

* H. B. Fell.

CHAPTER VIII

THE MOBILITY AND ADAPTABILITY OF THE VISCERA

In every range of intellectual life, whether in science, art, religion or politics, men seek a formula, a form, a concrete outline on which to build the structure of their beliefs and knowledge. In medicine this tendency is no less marked than elsewhere, and in my view it has many dangers, for, as foundations for our ideas of health and disease, such forms are often veritable quicksands. This is particularly true of the anatomy of the alimentary tract. I shall endeavour to show how utterly fallacious is the conception of fixity conveyed to the student by descriptions based on the study of the dead body.

One often hears it said how very alike two people are. Is it not rather a matter for endless wonder that, among the millions of faces that we see, it is so seldom that two bear a resemblance to one another? Or how different hands are, even to the skin markings, the finger prints that bear the unfailing and unchanging stamp of individuality throughout life? Wherever we look in the outward form, we find that each human creature, although formed after a pattern, bears the stamp of the craftsman and of the individual creation, and this is believed to be imparted at the very union of the ovum and spermatozoon, or maybe it is inherent in each separate ovum and spermatozoon. And if, in the outward things that are patent to all, the individuality of each living thing is impressed, is it not likely that the same wide elasticity in design and function will be found in the viscera?

It is exceedingly difficult for those who have been brought up on the formulae of descriptive anatomy, with its conception of fixed and definite relationships, to visualise and appreciate the essential mobility, both relative and actual, of the abdominal viscera. Undoubtedly this descriptive outlook is a handicap that still persistently hinders me: a dead weight of tradition that, despite my radiological observation of actual facts, still makes me think in the terms of traditional anatomy. Unfortunately, there seems to be no alternative to the descriptive methods of tradition. All the time the radiologist feels that there is something quite wrong, for the descriptions he attempts are always inadequate to convey a satisfactory idea of the living anatomy he sees on the fluorescent screen; it is as though he were attempting to describe a work of art in the units and formulae of mechanics, physics and chemistry.

The conception of living anatomy is one of mobility, of complete absence of fixed points. It was with a view to emphasising the essential mobility and adaptability of the abdominal viscera, a fact which radiologists see illustrated every day, that the foregoing series of investigations was made. The bearing of the observations on abdominal surgery seems even yet to be inadequately appreciated, and perhaps this small study will do something to prick the last bubble of "fixation" and similar operations. The one thing to be avoided is the production of fixed points, for these must interfere with and hamper Nature's mechanism. The normal abdominal viscera have no fixed shapes and no fixed positions, and every description of them must be qualified by a statement of the conditions existing at the time of observation. Moreover, profound change may be caused not only by mechanical forces but also by mental influences.

The traditional ideas of the form and relationship of the internal organs have necessarily been derived from the cadaver, which has passed through rigor mortis and been hardened at a time when every organ was lying flaccid, toneless, dead and in the supine position; or else from living bodies, also in the supine position, under the abnormal condition of deep anaesthesia. The picture they compose is very different from the "jumble of slithery things in a hole" seen by the radiologist, and it is curious that this jumble should present such a relatively constant pattern in the dissecting room. With the opaque meal it is possible to study living, conscious subjects in almost any desired position, and it is obvious that the results thus obtained must approximate more closely to the real conditions of life than the observations on which text-book descriptions are based. The previous chapters, founded on a paper recently published [40], present a series of observations and illustrations representing the changes of form produced by respiratory movements and gravity. The surface markings shown in Plate figs. 20–48 (p. 104), although they do not pretend to be accurate, demonstrate the extraordinary mobility of the organs.

PREVIOUS WORK

The literature on the subject of displacement and mobility of the abdominal viscera is profuse. Nowhere, however, have I noted the point that forms the text of this chapter, viz. that fixation of the viscera in definite positions in relation to the abdominal wall and to each other is foreign to Nature. The following is a brief outline of the salient historical points.

The early anatomists believed that the abdominal viscera had definitely fixed forms, positions and relationships, and considered any departure therefrom to be abnormal. Thus, Franciscus de Pedemontium [267] described a dislocated kidney in 1589, and Antonius de Haën [146] published, in 1747, several plates showing such abnormalities as an undescended caecum and a transverse colon looping down below the umbilicus. In 1761 Morgagni [247], who laid the foundations of modern pathological anatomy, described twenty autopsies in which he had found the stomach and colon abnormally low, and states that he had observed the same in many other cases. He believed that this disposition of the viscera was far more common than was usually supposed, and suggested that these abnormalities might be congenital.

In 1825 Matthew Baillie (26) described a movable kidney in a healthy woman, and in the following year Aberle (1) published four autopsies in which the kidney, palpable during life, was found unduly mobile post mortem. Meckel (234), writing in 1816, was the first to observe that the stomach frequently, and especially in women, occupied a vertical position instead of the classical horizontal one.

As Bedingfield (56) remarks in his admirable critical analysis, there was utter confusion for many years on the subject of gastroptosis and allied conditions, and the position was not clarified by the French writers who, using the stomach tube, assumed that a low position of the stomach indicated atony or dilatation.

The name of Glénard (134) is closely associated with the condition of ptosis and abdominal looseness, by reason of a series of papers that he published from 1886 to 1899, his main work being *Les ptoses viscérales*, published in Paris in 1899. Glénard was the first to connect the condition of prolapse of the abdominal viscera with certain local and general symptoms, and this symptom complex has since borne the name of Glénard's disease. He regarded the descent of the colon as an important feature and used the terms "visceroptosis" and "enteroptosis" synonymously. At first he gave mechanical explanations for the descent of the viscera, but later on he shifted his ground and held that the abdominal wall was not the chief factor. He then suggested that the cause of enteroptosis was a reduction of intestinal volume dependent on perverted liver function, leading to deficient gas content in the bowel.

Invalidism associated with flabbiness of the abdominal wall and lack of resistance in the epigastrium has been dealt with by many writers, particularly in this country by Treves (315), and by Clifford Allbutt (9) in his lectures *On Visceral Neuroses* (London, 1884). A deluge of literature, perhaps as many as a thousand communications, appeared in the early years of the twentieth century and up to 1912 (see Bedingfield (56)).

Previous X-ray Observations

In the early days of X-ray observation, "gastroptosis" was an accepted fact, and many views were expressed on the X-ray appearances. Leven and Barret (217) maintained in 1903 that when the stomach was dropped the cardiac end was drawn away from the diaphragm. Schlesinger (291, 292) (1910) also thought that the lengthening of the stomach drew down the cardia, but later on Béclère and Meriel (55) (1912) demonstrated that the cardia did not leave its position under the dome of the diaphragm.

In 1908 Cerné and Delaforge (94) defined gastroptosis as a deformity in which the "grand cul-de-sac de l'estomac" disappeared coincidentally with some dropping of the lower border. Groedel (143) (1910) held that the low position of the pylorus was the most important point in the diagnosis of gastroptosis, while Holzknecht (160) in 1906 considered that gastroptosis was present when the pylorus was not the lowest part of the stomach, and Kaestle (189) (1913) regarded a high pylorus with a low greater curvature as the criterion. Hurst (173) in 1915 defined gastroptosis thus: "When the stomach is not only abnormally low in the erect position, but the greater curvature reaches below the umbilicus in the horizontal position." He also laid down that there are two general forms of the normal: the cow's horn and the fish-hook or J-shaped stomach.

In order to reach a definite conception of the normal stomach, Mills (238, 239, 240) and Ansell (22) in America carried out extensive observations on students and others, but apparently worked on a preconceived idea that each individual could be fitted into a certain type—hypersthenic, sthenic, hyposthenic or asthenic—and that for each type there was a more or less constant gastric form. From observations on 2500 patients with gastric disturbances, Mills drew the important conclusion that there was no *causal relationship between the form and position of the stomach and the digestive symptoms*. He also noted that the passage of the food through the tract did not appear to be influenced by the position of the viscera and the tone of the gut.

In 1922 I (46) wrote that gastroptosis, *per se*, was apparently of no significance, but that when the duodenum remained in its normal high position a drag was produced on the attachments which might give rise to symptoms suggestive of duodenal trouble. Atony, moreover, did not cause drag on the duodenum, because the lesser curvature was not lengthened. It produced symptoms, however, because the pylorus was very high compared with the lowest part of the stomach, so that its position caused difficulty in emptying. I maintained that the tonic action stabilised the stomach, held it in posture and counteracted the diaphragmatic movement and gravitational effects.

The most extensive study of the normal stomach is that of Moody (1923 and 1926) who, with Nuys and Chamberlain (243, 244), examined 600 healthy American students in the upright posture. Later, they studied their subjects both in the vertical and recumbent positions, finding greater variation in the female than in the male. The pylorus lay anywhere from the upper border of the first lumbar vertebra to a point 5 cm. below the inter-iliac line. This accurate and painstaking study was continued by Moody (242) in London on 100 English students with results not appreciably different from those found in the United States. *He definitely concluded that the stomach, caecum and colon were able to function normally irrespective of their positions.*

Among other workers who have come to the same conclusions are K. Faber (116) and Campbell and Conybeare (74). On the clinical side Conran (104) showed that the low stomach is quite compatible with perfect health, and that symptoms could not be associated with any particular gastric form.

In 1909 I (28) pointed out that tone is independent of the position of the stomach and of its peristaltic activity, regarding atony as defective physiological action rather than as a pathological condition. Hurst (169), who also held this view, concluded that the terms "hypertonic" and "atonic" were misleading, since manometer experiments showed no change in the intragastric pressures as compared with the normal. He showed that the tone of the muscle adapts itself automatically to the volume of the contents and that the pressure remains constant. Experiments on both the hypertonic and the dropped stomach also gave the same result, and he considered that the only satisfactory explanation was to accept these different forms as anatomical variations in type.

Chamberlain (243) observed that an athlete, by training the abdominal muscles to an abnormal degree, produced no appreciable alteration in the disposition of the viscera, and Mackeith, Spurrell, Warner and Westlake (229) in 1922 reported an important case of congenital deficiency of the anterior wall of the abdomen in which they found the stomach normal in tone and occupying a position slightly higher, if anything, than normal in spite of this defect, thus proving that the position of the stomach is not necessarily dependent on the support of the abdominal wall.

Many theories have been advanced to explain how the organs are maintained in position in the abdomen and why in some cases "displacements" apparently give rise to symptoms. Keith (193) in 1903 held that the diaphragm was the chief factor in maintaining the position of the viscera, being so delicately poised that any alteration had a marked effect on the abdominal contents. He also analysed the relative displacements of the viscera in cases of anomaly of the diaphragm. Later on he came to regard the transversalis muscle as the most important factor in regulating the piston action of the diaphragm and thus holding the viscera in position. He held that the function of the mesentery was to limit movement and not to act as a support, a conception which harmonises with Alvarez's contention that the viscera "float" in the abdomen.

Although most writers regard the abdominal wall as of the greatest importance, Agnes Vietor (318) argued that the fundamental cause of visceroptosis was a failure of normal development which was usually associated with a retracted lower thorax; this resulted in an alteration of the size and shape of the abdominal cavity and was accompanied by defective fixation of the viscera.

The possibility of kinking of the intestine as a cause of symptoms was very prominent for a time. It was suggested that these kinks were often due to the low position of the viscera, but Hurst (168), Mixter (241), Schwarz (294), Carman (80), and many others, besides myself, were unanimous in stating that, apart from adhesions, they had never found such a condition obstructing the onward passage of the food. The mobile caecum and proximal colon have been regarded as the cause of symptoms by Hausmann (150) (1904), Waugh (331), Morley (250), Carslaw (83), and others, but Flint (118, 119) and Carson (84) were sceptical of this explanation. Alvarez says: "I think I would as willingly ascribe symptoms to a large navel, to a hooked nose, or to flaring ears, as to a mobile caecum or a redundant sigmoid flexure." I entirely agree.

ABDOMINAL BELTS AND FIXATION OPERATIONS

Glénard's work led to a fashion for abdominal belts, on the assumption that the mere mobility or displacement of the viscera was the cause of symptoms, and that the belt would support them. In 1896 Duret (111) suggested a technique for shortening the stomach, and gastropexy became a favourite operation, especially under Rovsing (287). Since then there has been a gradual decline in the popularity of this and similar operations. The vogue for abdominal belts to support "dropped" stomachs has also to a large extent passed. It is well known to radiologists that these belts very rarely, if ever, raise the viscera as they are supposed to do. Nevertheless, as their beneficial effect is undoubted, some other explanation of their action is necessary. The influence of suggestion and of rest is difficult to gauge, but certain experiments* hint that the belts may act by pressing on the abdominal veins and so helping to maintain an adequate return of blood to the heart and to raise the arterial blood-pressure. So far as I am aware, no clinical observations on the effect of abdominal belts upon blood-pressure have been made.

It is a fact that I do not remember having examined any patient in whom the supporting pads effected the purpose for which they were designed; they invariably pressed on the *middle* of the long stomach, ensuring that the dropped lower part should remain low down in the pelvis! If we regard an atonic stomach as a flaccid bag, covered with peritoneum, the function of which is to allow the abdominal contents to move freely over each other, how could we imagine that any reasonable and bearable pressure could prevent the stomach from slipping down? The benefit is certainly not brought about in the manner intended, and it is therefore a corollary that the symptoms which were relieved cannot have been due to the dropped condition of the organs.

The Failure of Fixation Operations

In the early days I saw a number of cases in which operations for slinging up the dropped stomach had been performed and, so far as my recollection goes, my examinations showed that the stomach had always adjusted itself and returned to its former appearance, provided that the patient had been fortunate enough to escape adhesions that caused displacements and restrictions of move-

* See Appendix IV.

ment that were not intended. The animal, vegetable and mineral kingdoms were searched for materials that would be effective in anchoring not only the stomach but all the abdominal viscera and, whenever the opportunity of subsequent examination occurred, it was found that these materials had failed in their purpose and that the only effective way of "anchoring" was by producing adhesions. Yet it was never suspected that the very looseness which was blamed might be Nature's attempt at repair and that what we were striving after was ill-conceived: Nature, if not hampered by the results of inflammatory processes, is nearly always capable of dealing with and making the necessary allowances for any displacements. Twenty years ago Case(90) wrote: "It is the fixed adherent bowel, rather than the mobile bowel, which is the seat of stasis and the source of symptoms." In fact, if it is necessary for her design, Nature actually produces adhesions to assist her own mechanics, as for instance in the so-called Jackson's membrane. We now know that a large range of mobility and variation of relationship is normal, and we can therefore say with certainty that the old operations for shortening and fixing the stomach and for replacing and fixing the once fashionable "mobile proximal colon" were based on false premises. The fallacy is well pilloried in the witty aphorism of a German gynae-cologist: "*Wer viel pexiert, viel pecciert.*" We realise that the ptosed stomachs of a few years back were nothing but rather long normal specimens and that a very wide range of form and mobility in the viscera is usual and probably essential for the natural functioning of all the abdominal organs.

FLUID ANATOMY

It is probable that many radiologists have conceived the idea of revising the anatomy of the abdomen in the light of X-ray observation so as to give a satisfactory idea of the "living stomach" and other organs, but their books still remain unwritten.

Some time ago I(37) made a series of plaster casts of what I then considered "the normal stomach" (see Fig. 84, p. 94). They are still of assistance in giving the student a grasp of the general contour of the organ that throws the shadow picture on the fluorescent screen. But these models have the defect that must be associated with every attempt to crystallise ideas of the "normal stomach"; the terms of orthodox anatomy are not applicable to descriptions of the conditions of life; the symbols of our formulae are unrelated to the actual facts. They may be correct for the dead subject but they are quite inapplicable to the subject with which the clinician has to deal.

Descriptive terms and diagrams can at best only indicate a given phase of form or relationship, and surface markings that give a mental picture of fixed positions cannot be satisfactorily applied to the essential changefulness of living conditions. True, in the living subject in a given posture each organ has something of a relative position in regard to other organs, and is usually found in this position, but the difference between orthodox anatomy and actual conditions is something like that between an ordinary photograph, which gives a fixed and unchanging picture, and a cinematographic record, which is a succession of photographs portraying the movement and change that are essential living factors. Even a cinematographic film would be an imperfect record, for a true conception of the living organ would take into account a dozen other factors, such as the influence of the mind on the body, to which the changes in form and function of the abdominal organs are merely the response. The death-mask of Napoleon gives little clue to the living face of the man as he watched and directed his armies, or to those inscrutable eyes, the colour of which none could describe after he had gone.

Further, we should not look upon the stomach or any of the abdominal viscera as entities that can be studied individually and separately, any more than one sentence out of its context can give an idea of the whole chapter. The anatomy of a living organ—and, for that matter, its function also—is an expression of many influences both in the organ itself and elsewhere. We are, in fact, justified in regarding the stomach as one of the most responsive organs in the body, for we know that it may react to almost every emotion and sensation that man is capable of experiencing (Barclay [33] and Todd [312]). I may seem to exaggerate the importance of this outlook, but surely it is far less cramping to the understanding of the living, moving, responsive anatomy and physiology of the abdomen than that to which we have been accustomed.

In recent years I have had occasion to examine many healthy students, and have been increasingly impressed with the need of regarding the anatomy of the abdominal viscera as fluid. There is no set and standardised pattern; divergences from the average are common. Some of them are extreme, yet the subjects have been healthy. There is much food for thought for clinicians in these observations; had I been examining these subjects with a view to discovering the aetiology of some complaint, I could not have resisted the temptation to claim such divergences from the average as the obvious cause of their symptoms.

To take an example: a radiologist investigating a case of constipation finds—as I did recently in a healthy student—a caecum deep down in the pelvis with an ascending colon of more than double the usual length extending up into the dome of the diaphragm (Fig. 93), and the hepatic flexure in a mysterious position *behind* the liver, housed in the peritoneal pocket, a potential space that runs up behind the liver as far as the bare area! Absurd to suppose it possible for the food to pass on without obstruction in such a confined space and, even if this were admitted possible, the intestine must be "kinked" as it entered or left this space and found its way out round the posterior lower edge of the liver and up to

what appeared to be a normally placed splenic flexure! Could the radiologist
resist putting such an obvious two-and-two
together, and could any surgeon have
doubted the propriety and expediency of
adjusting such a gross and definite source of
the trouble? Yet the condition was present
in a student who did not suffer from constipation and was perfectly normal in
every respect. Lately I have found that
my own entirely satisfactory hepatic flexure also occupies this position! A similar
anomaly was noted by a friend of mine,
but it had gone before he could take a
radiogram. There is little doubt that all
the older workers—radiologists, physicians
and surgeons alike—nurtured in the tradi-
tions of descriptive anatomy and ignorant
of the extraordinary elasticity of Nature's
mechanics, have often been misled by
their desire to find simple mechanical
explanations of symptoms.

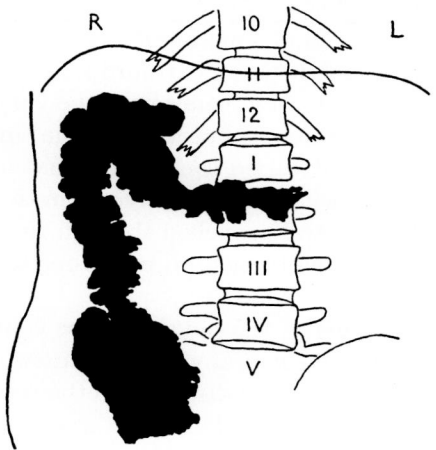

Fig. 93. Abnormal ascending colon and hepatic flexure. The caecum is deep in the pelvis, the ascending colon is unusually long and extends up to an hepatic flexure that lies behind the liver and close under the dome of the dia-phragm.

NATURE'S MECHANICS

We are slow to learn the reason for the mobility that we see, but it is obvious.
We cannot judge and criticise Nature's mechanics by the standards and formulae
of the workshop and laboratory, for whereas we rely on fixed points, Nature
insists on complete freedom of movement. Even the fundamentals of human
and laboratory mechanics have little in common. The alimentary tract is a
wonderfully efficient apparatus, and so very unlike the familiar mechanisms of
the machine-shop or of the laboratory that comparisons are impossible and
should not be attempted. There is no base plate, framework or fixed point to
act as a fulcrum, no revolving or reciprocating part; there is no known formula
on which the human machine works. It is a band of moving, co-ordinated tubular
muscle that is subject not to one but to many directing impulses. It is lined by
an absorbing and secreting mucous membrane. The whole tube is influenced, in
part or entirely, not only by the contents but also by all sorts of forces and
influences of mental, physical, chemical and mechanical origin.

The world of mechanism can produce no comparable phenomenon wherein the
distribution of the load varies all the time and there is no fixed method of producing the desired result. Nature can always produce the same effect in several
different ways, balancing up the varied forces she has at her disposal. To enable

her to do her work she demands freedom of movement with alternating periods of activity and rest.

The "fluid" mechanics of the mobile and adaptable organs within the abdomen constitute an extraordinarily efficient method designed by Nature not only to allow for and counteract the varying loads that result from change of posture and movement, but at the same time to accommodate large or small quantities of food of varied consistency that have to be reduced to a fine state of division, mixed with the digestive secretions, assimilated into the lymph and blood streams and propelled through the length of the alimentary tract, leaving only the residue to pass on to the rectum. The distribution of the load varies all the time.

Formerly, the physician was content to explain symptoms in terms of which neither he nor anyone else knew the meaning. The patient suffered from a "humour"; the disease was the result of "diathesis", and so forth. Yet I often wonder whether less harm was not done by this obviously speculative outlook than by the present-day practice of couching all descriptions in the precise terms of a science that is often incomplete and may or may not be applicable to living man. Of a million cells each takes its co-ordinate part and performs its function, perhaps even independently to some extent, and over all is the presiding power of life itself, about which we have not as yet the first glimmerings of knowledge. This is no reason why we should not attempt to explain what we see as far as we can, always provided that we realise the limits of our knowledge and do not indulge in flights of fancy into the unknown, elaborating plausible explanations that are capable neither of proof nor disproof and which, like so much of the knowledge we have inherited, may hang as a smoke screen to hamper the progress of those who follow after.

CHAPTER IX

THE DIAPHRAGM

The position of the diaphragm exercises an important influence upon the disposition of the abdominal contents. In the anatomical text-books the levels cited rest on a basis of observation on dead subjects.

The Normal "At Rest" Position

The normal "at rest" position or neutral level of the diaphragm is the position in which a subject naturally holds it when asked to stop breathing for a few seconds. The following table, compiled for me by Dr J. B. Higgins, shows this position as defined in various works of anatomy, followed by the figures obtained from X-ray observation in the upright position:

	Right dome	Left dome	Cardiac orifice	Pylorus
Quain's *Anatomy*	8th D.V.	9th D.V.	10th D.V.	12th D.V.
Text-book of Anatomy, Cunningham	8th D.V.	9th D.V.	11th D.V.	
Text-book of Anatomy, Gray	8th D.V.	8–9th D.V.	10th D.V.	1st L.V.
Manual of Anatomy, Buchanan	8th D.V.	9th D.V.	11th D.V.	1st L.V.
Practical Anatomy, Fagge	—	—	11th D.V.	1st L.V.
Practical Anatomy, Cunningham	7th D.V. (on forced respiration)	8th D.V.	10th D.V.	—
Surface Markings, Rawlings	7–8th D.V.	8th D.V.	11th D.V.	1st L.V.
Symington's *Atlas*	10th D.V.	10–11th D.V.	11th D.V.	1st, 2nd L.V.
Wingate Todd's *Clinical Anatomy*	9–10th D.V.	—	11th D.V.	2nd, 3rd L.V.
Author's Observations	11th D.V.	11th D.V.	12th D.V.	3rd L.V. lower border

These figures show not only the variations in the data given by the anatomist, but also the difference between the anatomy of the dead and the anatomy of the living as revealed by X rays. The figures in Todd's *Clinical Anatomy* were largely taken from X-ray findings, but the others were derived from post-mortem observations: the diaphragm and viscera had all slipped up in the body when muscle tone ceased at death. The corpses that I have X-rayed showed the diaphragm at the level given in the text-books. If the subjects had been preserved in the upright position there might have been an equal disparity in the opposite direction, for the action of gravity might have drawn the diaphragm and all the viscera into the abdomen.

I have found as the result of numerous observations that the average normal "at rest" position of the diaphragm is the upper margin of the eleventh dorsal vertebra. The manubrio-xiphoid junction corresponds fairly accurately with the general level of the top of the diaphragm in the neutral phase.

The "at rest" position may be altered by illness. I once investigated it in a subject whose extreme positions I had recorded fifteen months before (Figs.

98–103). Although all the conditions were identical with those of the previous examination and the excursion of the diaphragm was unimpaired, I found the normal position of rest within half an inch of full inspiration, an inch below where it had been at the previous examination (Fig. 94). A similar investigation after illness in another subject gave a like result, i.e. the reserve of inspiration was apparently diminished. The only explanation of the discrepancy was a slight attack of influenza, with occasional spasmodic cough, from which the subject had just recovered, in one case, and a recent operation in the other. Presumably it was due to some impairment of the tone of the abdominal muscles; had it been due to alteration in tonic action of the diaphragm that muscle would appear on a higher level than normal. If this observation is confirmed the sign may be very important in assessing the reserve vital capacity of the lungs, especially in such conditions as silicosis when the question of compensation arises.

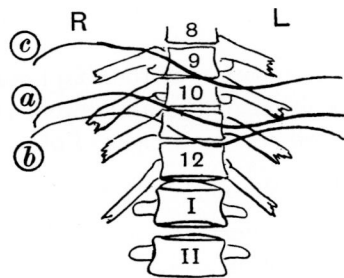

Fig. 94. Tracings of the outline of the diaphragm: *a*, at rest; *b*, in full inspiration; *c*, in full expiration. Note that the position at rest is not midway between the two extremes, as it usually is, but much nearer the position of full inspiration. (Same subject as Figs. 95–103, and also subject A, Figs. 20–28, Plate I.)

Unfortunately, however, there seems to be difficulty in obtaining satisfactory records even in normal subjects, for in the average student examined, the diaphragm is forced above the natural limit of expiration by retraction of the abdominal muscles in efforts to expel the air from the chest. My records of students show that, on the whole, the at rest position is nearer the limit of inspiration, but this may, as suggested, be the effect of abdominal retraction.

The Costo-Phrenic Angle (Figs. 95, 96 and 97)

The costo-phrenic angle is the lowest limit of the excursion of the lung into the angle of the pleural cavity that forms a potential space between the diaphragm and the chest wall. In full inspiration it usually extends right down to the costal attachments of the diaphragm. In the figures of the lateral aspect the diaphragm appears to come well down below its attachment to the xiphisternum, which, as an anatomist pointed out to me, is impossible. What the figures actually show is the costo-phrenic angle to either side of the middle line, i.e. that part of the diaphragm which is attached to rib cartilages. In the median section there must be some structure like the frenum of the tongue running up to the xiphisternal attachment, but it is not easily seen radiographically. The outlines in all the antero-posterior views represent the highest level of the dome; the lines run away down the side to the costo-phrenic angle.

The position of the costo-phrenic angle appears to vary widely with the individual, but its excursion seems as a rule to be rather more extensive than the photographs of this subject suggest. The way in which the diaphragm

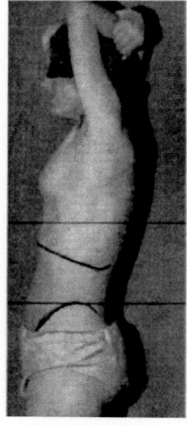 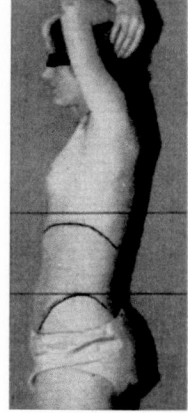 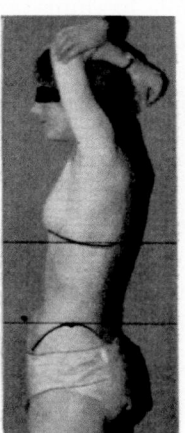

Fig. 95. In full inspiration.   Fig. 96. At rest.   Fig. 97. In full expiration.

Figs. 95–97. Photographs of a subject after the limit of the left costo-phrenic angle has been marked under X-ray guidance. N.B. The conditions under which the X-ray observations were made were repeated in taking the photographs.

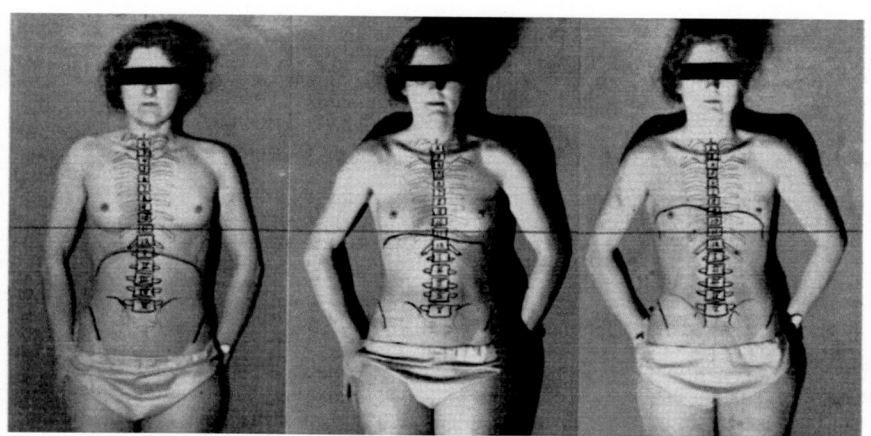

Fig. 98. Standing, in full   Fig. 99. Standing, at rest.   Fig. 100. Standing, in full
inspiration.   expiration.

Figs. 98–100. Photographs of a subject on whom the diaphragm shadow has been marked.
(Same subject as in Fig. 89.)

extends so much lower behind than in front, carrying the pleural cavity—the costo-phrenic angle—much farther down than one expects in all phases of respiration, is an anatomical point of clinical importance. Figs. 101–103 and 95–97 show this fact clearly. Since this angle is the site of the collection of the first fluid in a pleurisy with effusion and of resulting adhesions, its importance in the radioscopic examination of the chest is very great. The method of obtaining these photographs is described on p. 123.

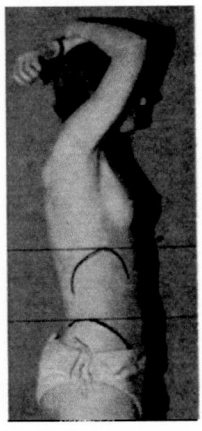 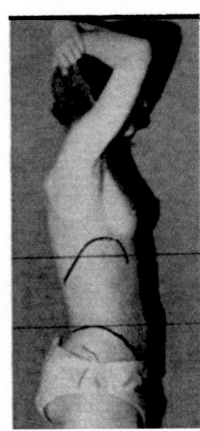 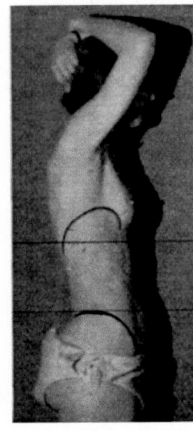

Fig. 101. Lateral outline of diaphragm, standing, in full inspiration.

Fig. 102. Lateral outline of diaphragm, standing, at rest.

Fig. 103. Lateral outline of diaphragm, standing, in full expiration.

Figs. 101–103. Photographs of a subject on whom the diaphragm shadow has been marked. N.B. The line of the diaphragm appears to come lower in front than its attachment to the xiphisternum. The line of the diaphragm represents what is seen, and this is the lowest part, i.e. to the side of the middle line where the diaphragm is attached to the costal cartilage.

THE LEVELS IN RESPIRATION

The right side of the diaphragm is always recognised to be about half an inch higher than the left, but this relationship is not constant, for on deep expiration the difference may be accentuated to the extent of almost one inch. On deep inspiration, however, there is a tendency in the opposite direction, and there is very little, if any, difference between the levels of corresponding points on the two sides (Figs. 104 and 105).

In quiet respiration the usual excursion of the diaphragm is about half an inch on both sides; on forced respiration an excursion of three inches is usual and in some students as much as four inches is sometimes seen. Individuals vary widely in the extent to which they use the diaphragm in forced breathing, and even athletes, when asked to breathe deeply, quite often comply by chest expansion only. The best way of inducing a subject to use his diaphragm over its full range is to give him a looking-glass so that he can watch its movements.

The excursion of the diaphragm on forced respiration is approximately as follows: on the right side from the upper border of the ninth or tenth dorsal vertebra to the twelfth dorsal vertebra, and on the left from the tenth dorsal vertebra to the twelfth dorsal vertebra or even lower.

Figs. 98–103 show the positions of the diaphragm in a normal athletic female aged 27, in the standing position, as seen from the front and the right side. Figs. 104 and 105, tracings from radiographs of another subject, show that on forced respiration there are definite changes, which are not symmetrical. On the left it is an even dome on forced expiration, and it maintains approximately this shape on forced inspiration, except that it is hung by its attachments at the left crus. On the right, the dome shape of the expiratory phase is replaced on

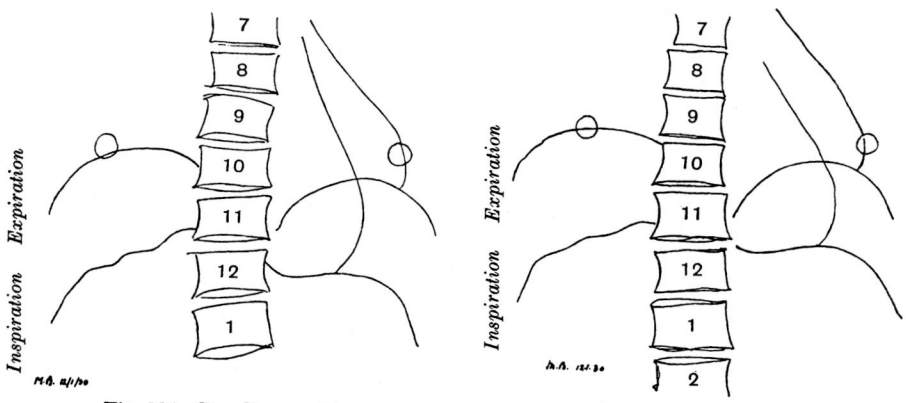

Fig. 104. Standing position. Fig. 105. Supine position.

Figs. 104 and 105. Superimposed tracings of radiographs and heart outlines, showing the diaphragm levels in the extremes of respiration.

deep inspiration by what is almost an inclined plane. The crural attachments appear to be definitely higher by about one vertebra on the right side than on the left. The irregular wavy outline of the right side of the diaphragm in deep inspiration, shown in both tracings, is not, I believe, pathological and is very frequently seen. I do not know of any satisfactory explanation.

The effect of posture

In the eighteenth edition of Gray's *Anatomy* (1926, p. 442) it is stated that "Skiagraphy shows that the height of the Diaphragma in the thorax varies considerably with the position of the body. It stands highest when the body is horizontal and the patient on his back, and in this position it performs the largest respiratory excursions with normal breathing. When the body is erect the dome of the Diaphragma falls, and its respiratory movements become smaller. The dome falls still lower when the sitting posture is assumed, and in this position its respiratory excursions are smallest".

Moreover, it has been suggested that massive collapse of the lung might be explained by a theory which is based on the assumption that the diaphragm is normally at a much higher level in the recumbent position than in the upright, thus causing compression of the lungs. One exponent of this theory has said: "When the posture of the patient was changed from the upright to the supine, there was immediately an elevation of the diaphragm;...probably...the expansion of the lower lobe was dependent not so much on the movement of the diaphragm as upon the position of the diaphragm in the chest. If the diaphragm were high up in the chest, the lower lobe would not expand, even though the diaphragm continued to move."

My own observations on normal healthy students do not confirm these statements. I have often marked the level during a demonstration, and have seldom

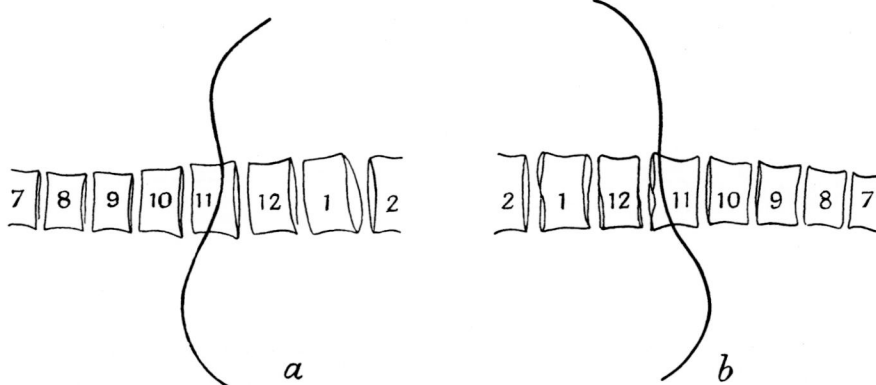

Fig. 106. Diagrams to show the way in which the diaphragm swings as if pivoted on a central point when the subject lies (a) on the right, (b) on the left side.

found that it varied more than half an inch between the standing and the supine positions, though I have never found it lower in the supine than in the vertical position. The apparent difference can generally be attributed to inaccurate skin marking or to the displacement caused by the student drawing up his knees when he lies down. Incidentally, as noted elsewhere, skin markings are very unreliable. A skin mark, even over the spine, will change in relation to the vertebrae very considerably between the upright and horizontal positions.

The position of the diaphragm in all stages of respiration is practically the same in the supine as in the erect position. If anything, there is a very slightly increased excursion in the recumbent position, but the difference is certainly not great enough to possess any clinical or pathological significance. The capacity of the chest in the ordinary healthy man is therefore practically the same in the vertical and supine positions.

Lateral Recumbent Position

When a healthy subject lies on one side or the other the general position of the diaphragm does not seem to alter much, but even in perfectly healthy athletic students it swings or pivots about a central point, so that the lower side goes up into the chest and the upper side becomes correspondingly lower (Fig. 106). There is no marked difference between the general level in the upright and the recumbent positions, but when the subject lies on one side or the other the diaphragm seems to swing according to the intra-abdominal and intra-thoracic pressures exerted by gravity. The right dome of the diaphragm seems to swing more freely up into the chest when the subject is on the right side than does the left dome when he is on the left side. At first I thought that these wide movements in lateral recumbency would only be seen in conditions of ill-health, but as a matter of fact they are universal among perfectly healthy people, as will be seen in Plate figs. 26, 27, 36, 37, 46 and 47, where the tilting of the diaphragm is well but not accurately shown.

In the prone position the pressure on the abdomen is transmitted to the diaphragm and pushes it up into the chest, almost to the position of full expiration. (Subjectively we all know the effect of lying flat on the face, especially after a full meal.)

The Tonic Control of the Diaphragm

In Gray's *Anatomy* (18th ed., p. 442) the control of the position of the diaphragm is attributed to three factors: "(1) the elastic retraction of the lung-tissue, tending to pull it upwards; (2) the pressure exerted on its under surface by the viscera: this naturally tends to be a negative pressure, or downward suction, when the patient sits or stands, and positive, or an upward pressure, when he lies; (3) the intra-abdominal tension due to the abdominal muscles." No mention of the tonic action is made, and yet this appears to me to be the one deciding and all-important factor. The position of the diaphragm is obviously controlled by some mechanism—which we call "tone"—that compensates for the effect of gravity and maintains the same general level whether the subject stands or lies down. Presumably this mechanism is the tonic action of the diaphragm muscle.

Fig. 107 shows a series of tracings of the diaphragm at rest in an athletic woman of about 35 years of age in the standing, recumbent and "hanging upside down" positions. The outlines of certain vertebrae and the diaphragm and heart have been traced from the films and superimposed. It was certainly a surprise to find that the shadow of the outline of the diaphragm in the standing and in the "hanging upside down" positions corresponded exactly, while the outline in the recumbent position was slightly higher. This series of observations has only been made once—for obvious reasons it is not an easy one to make—and I do not claim that it has universal application. Indeed, I should not be surprised to find quite a different result in non-athletic subjects, particularly in those who are in poor health and whose muscular tone is diminished. The excursion of the diaphragm in forced respiration in the upright and "hanging upside down" positions is shown in Fig. 108.

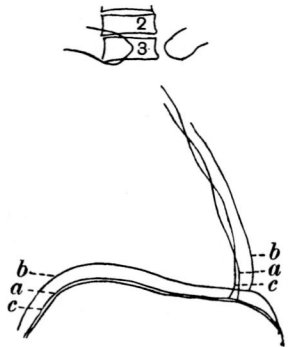

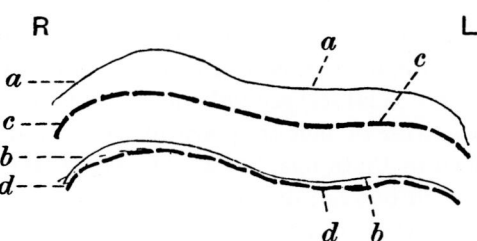

Fig. 107. Tracings showing the effect of posture on the diaphragm. Superimposed tracings from radiographs of a subject: *a*, standing; *b*, lying; *c*, hanging upside down. Mid-phase of respiration in each case.

Fig. 108. Effect of posture on the diaphragm. Tracings of the diaphragm level in full inspiration and expiration with the subject standing and hanging upside down: *a*, full expiration, standing; *b*, full inspiration, standing; *c*, full expiration, hanging upside down; *d*, full inspiration, hanging upside down.

Independent Control of the Two Sides

I have recently found a number of students who exhibited quite definite independent voluntary control of the two sides. Prof. J. M. Woodburn Morison told me of a "strong man" who had developed this ability to such an extent that he had complete independent control over a phenomenally large range of movement of both the chest wall and the two sides of the diaphragm. At the word of command, he could expand the right side of the chest and fix the right diaphragm while the left chest wall was fixed and the left diaphragm made a big excursion. Conversely, he could fix the right chest wall and move the right side of the diaphragm. In this way the intra-thoracic pressures were so balanced that there was no displacement of the mediastinum by these abnormal movements. The subject had developed this type of respiration as a trick, having learned his ability to do it during an attack of pleurisy. He imagined that he was only controlling his chest expansion, and did not know of the compensatory diaphragmatic movement. It was after I had narrated this case to a class that some of the students showed that they also would almost certainly be able to develop as complete a control. With a little practice they were able to move the left leaf and keep the right fairly still, the balance of pressure being equalised by greater chest expansion on the side on which the diaphragm did not move so freely.

THE TECHNIQUE OF INVESTIGATION OF THE DIAPHRAGM

If the vertebral levels, the skin markings and the diaphragm levels are to be correct the beam must be accurately centred on the normal or "at rest" position of the diaphragm. When the X-ray tube is centred exactly on the level of the diaphragm, it gives its exact relationship to the levels of the vertebrae, but as X rays are divergent and not parallel, the error in full inspiration and expiration with a fixed tube is appreciable. It depends on the distance of the tube and the diaphragm from the screen or film, and can only be eliminated by moving the tube up and down orthodiagraphically with the diaphragm. On making an orthodiagraphic check I found a total error of half an inch; i.e. the excursion of 3 inches on the screen represented $2\frac{1}{2}$ inches' actual movement (the tube being 30 inches away and the top of the dome of the diaphragm being roughly $4\frac{1}{2}$ inches from the fluorescent screen or film). The tube being fixed, the error is proportional to the distance from the screen image of the part of the diaphragm that casts the shadow but, as the vertebrae are also distal from the film, the relative observed positions of the diaphragm and vertebrae are not markedly inaccurate.

Figs. 95–103 were made as follows: The subject was placed in the upright screening stand and the tube accurately centred on the middle of the diaphragm. Distortion was therefore eliminated at the centre, but not at the edges, as no orthodiascope was available. The result is that the outer margins of the diaphragm appear to slope down more acutely than they should. The outline of the diaphragm was rapidly marked with a skin pencil on the subject and then photographed. This series of operations was repeated for each position and for each phase of respiration, under exactly the same conditions.

The vertebral outlines of the subject were superimposed on the photograph by the means adopted for the composite gastric pictures. I abandoned the idea of skin-marking the three positions of the diaphragm on one single photograph of the subject, as the movement of the anterior chest wall and of the skin introduced too big an error.

SECTION II: PHYSIOLOGY

THE MOVEMENT OF FOOD FROM MOUTH TO ANUS

CHAPTER X

THE NORMAL MECHANISM OF SWALLOWING

The classical description of the mechanism of the act of deglutition was given in 1817 by Magendie, who described the three stages in the passage of food through the mouth, pharynx and oesophagus. He believed that the principal coefficients of the motor power were the constrictor muscles of the pharynx, but it was afterwards shown by Kronecker and Meltzer (212) (1883) that the swallowing reflex is a complex co-ordinated mechanism, depending mainly on the mylohyoid and hypoglossal muscles.

Extraordinarily little research seems to have been carried out on the mechanism of swallowing. The work of Kronecker and Meltzer is copied from one text-book to another together with the graphs of the pressures they recorded, and no later work appears to have found its way into the text-books, although several papers have been published.

As long ago as 1911 Schreiber (293) suggested the possibility of negative pressures, but his work has apparently been overlooked by everyone except Laurell (215). Yet we have only to watch the infant at the breast to note that our earliest nourishment is obtained by suction. Speaking to a veterinary surgeon on the subject, I found that he accepted as a commonplace that horses and other animals swallow by suction to a large extent and almost exclusively so when they drink. In 1923 Payne and Poulton (265), by means of linen-covered rubber balloons filled with water, measured the pressures produced by peristaltic waves in the human oesophagus, and in a general way confirmed Kronecker and Meltzer's results. They found that, after swallowing, a wave of contraction descended the oesophagus, preceded by a small wave of relaxation. The latter produced a fall in pressure of 0·5 to 1 cm. of water, and the former produced a large rise of pressure amounting in some cases to 30 or 40 cm. They found negative pressures in the middle and lower end of the oesophagus, 12 and 16 cm. from the cardia; these they ascribe to the negative pressure of the thorax. Mosher (254), in conjunction with Macmillan, made some radiological studies, but these were mainly concerned with the action of the tongue and did not differ materially from the descriptions in the text-books.

It is curious that Schreiber's important observation escaped attention. Unfortunately his work, like that of so many others, was done on abnormal subjects, and—necessarily—under abnormal conditions, since it is evident that the mechanism of swallowing can be considerably varied to meet different conditions; our sensations tell us that any unusual circumstances call for a modification of the usual process. If a balloon is introduced into the pharynx the effect is that of a large bolus which, being attached outside the mouth, cannot be passed down by the natural forces. Hence it produces a condition of "obstruction" which calls up the reserve muscular force which is only brought into action in cases of difficulty or obstruction, when the normal force is insufficient to accomplish the passage of the bolus. In every case of obstruction that I have observed, the mechanism has been quite abnormal and suggestive of a muscular propulsive act of the peristaltic type. It is this abnormal process that has been recorded by all workers with the balloon method.

Boldireff[65] criticised the balloon method of investigation of hollow and empty intestines on the ground that the balloon itself is sufficient to excite abnormal movements, and A. J. Carlson is inclined to agree with him; but Payne and Poulton maintain that with their technique this criticism does not hold, on the ground that a balloon may rest in the oesophagus or duodenum without exciting any movement at all after it has been in situ for a few minutes. Personally, I cannot see the force of this argument, for we all know that relaxation may and does occur when foreign bodies are lodged in the oesophagus; after a time they may cease to cause symptoms. The type of peristalsis in such a condition depends on whether the presence of the foreign body has or has not become accepted and tolerated by the viscus. If it is accepted and does not cause any obstruction, it is quite likely that the mechanism will be "normal", but if the viscus decides that this foreign body is a thing that should be passed on, there will be an entirely abnormal and forceful effort to dislodge it and allow the food to pass freely. In other words, the type of movement or pressure recorded by a balloon in a viscus will be governed by mere chance, and the longer the balloon is in situ the greater the chance of recording conditions that may be normal. But there is never any guarantee that the conditions recorded are normal.

Hugo Laurell[215] recently published a study of the mechanism of swallowing in cases of pharyngeal pouch, where the pouch itself acts as an obstruction, and he regards the peristalsis which he has seen in these cases as the natural and normal mechanism. The conditions are, however, quite abnormal.

The same arguments apply equally to the use of bougies, but a thin, smooth, soft tube is much more likely to lie unrecognised in a viscus, particularly in the very highly sensitive pharynx, than a relatively large balloon of the irregular and expanding shape that would easily suggest to the sensations a bolus which has become arrested. I hold that, while any mechanism for recording pressures in the pharynx introduces some abnormal factor, the least offender is a thin nasal catheter. Prof. Anrep, in the experiments described later, used a thin, soft rubber catheter with a sufficiently wide bore to give accurate readings on a very sensitive recording apparatus; this method has practically no lag or inertia and does not seem to elicit forced and artificial swallowing. I have not tried fine ureteric catheters, but I imagine that they would tend to get blocked and would offer resistance, so that the instrument would lack sensitiveness.

Gravity

In spite of the knowledge that it was possible to swallow in the inverted position, gravity has always been assumed to play a very large part. Numerous observations have been made on its influence. Palugyay (263) stated in 1922 that the progress of food through the oesophagus could be more satisfactorily studied in the Trendelenburg position because it was then seven times slower than normal, but in his later work he admits that there is no difference in the time. Hurst and Schreiber both observed the effect of gravity on the passage of food through the cardiac orifice and found that cachets and opaque food were hindered if not altogether prevented from passing into the stomach with the patient inverted.

Dr Mukherji, one of our students, observed, however, that ordinary postures made little difference to the act of swallowing. We therefore timed with a stop-watch the passage of a fairly thick, sticky bolus from the mouth to the cardiac orifice; there seemed to be no appreciable difference between the rate of passage in the lying and in the upright position, the average being four to five seconds. In one subject the horizontal time was actually shorter than the vertical. We did not, however, invert the patient or take records with the head at a lower level than the cardiac orifice. It seems fairly clear, therefore, that with the foods we employed gravity does not play any important part in propelling the bolus down the upper part of the oesophagus.

Current Views

Ever since the opaque meal method was introduced, radiologists have watched patients swallowing food and accepted what they saw as the radiological expression of the things which they, as students, had been taught of the mechanics of swallowing. Leaving out the details of the muscles used, the following summary from Starling's *Physiology* (1920) gives an outline of the explanation of swallowing that has, up to now, found common acceptance:

A sudden elevation of the tongue throws the bolus back through the anterior pillars of the fauces. The passage of the food through the pharynx is rapid, and accompanied by closure of the two openings of the air passages. The nasal cavity is cut off by raising the soft palate and approximating the posterior pillars of the fauces. The larynx is shut off largely by approximation of the arytenoid cartilages, so that the laryngeal opening assumes the form of a triradiate fissure. At the same time both false and true vocal cords come together, while the movement of the dorsum of the tongue backward enables the closed laryngeal orifice to lie directly under the back part of the tongue. The food is passed down by the direct action of certain muscles.

Starling does not mention the epiglottis. His diagram shows it as a lid over the larynx, and this position is common to all the diagrams I have seen which purport to show the mechanism of swallowing, but Anderson Stuart (306) exploded this hypothesis in 1892 by his work on a subject in whom, owing to an operation, direct observation was possible; he showed that in this subject the epiglottis remained vertical in the act of swallowing. The figure of the parts

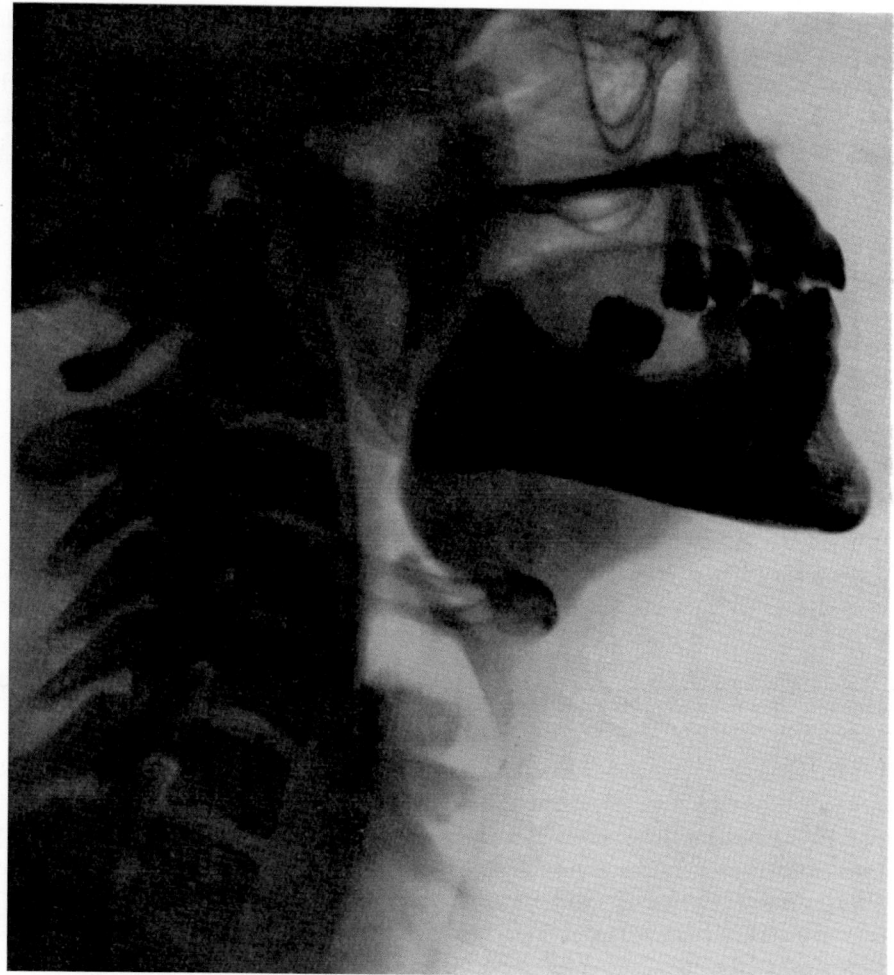

Fig. 109. Radiograph showing the normal outlines of the pharynx.

reproduced in Gray's *Anatomy* (18th ed. 1926) is, however, apparently correct as checked by means of radiographs (Fig. 109 and 110).

The diagrams reproduced in many of the text-books are obviously at fault and profess to show positions and mechanisms that are certainly wrong; when the radiologist analyses what he sees, he cannot escape the conclusion that most of these ideas need drastic revision. Unfortunately the rapidity of the passage of the food and the fact that the whole complex sequence of movements is completed in a fraction of time make direct observations difficult. Even when thick food is swallowed, the sequence of events is so rapid that the shadow only takes perhaps one-eighth of a second to pass from the soft palate region to behind the larynx. If specially thick foods are used in order to retard the action, the swallowing becomes forced, abnormal and propulsive, and it may take two or more gulps to pass the food on. A fluid, on the other hand, is useless, for it passes far too rapidly for visual observation. It is essential,

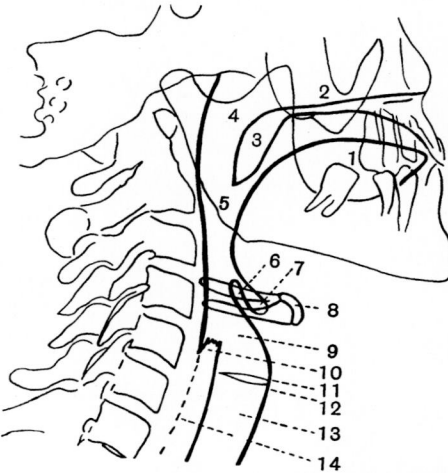

Fig. 110. Tracing from Fig. 109. 1, Tongue. 2, Hard palate. 3, Soft palate. 4, Nasopharynx. 5, Pharynx. 6, Epiglottis. 7, Vallecula. 8, Hyoid. 9, Laryngeal vestibule. 10, Laryngeal pharynx. 11, False vocal cords. 12, True vocal cords. 13, Trachea. 14, Course of the oesophagus.

therefore, to use a bolus of opaque food as thick as is compatible with easy normal swallowing, that is, about the consistency of well-masticated food.

For this investigation many radiographic records have been made in the shortest intervals of time practicable without specially elaborate apparatus; but it is obvious that really efficient cinematographic radiography which, owing to the efforts of Russell Reynolds, Janker, Gottheiner and others is now within sight, will be of enormous value in confirming visual observations and allowing leisured study of the successive phases which, in the circumstances, have been worked out largely from screen observations and deductive evidence.

A Subjective Study of Swallowing

Many attempts have been made to catch the various phases of the mechanism of swallowing. The more it is watched, the more complex the mechanism seems to be. Not only are wide individual variations possible, but each subject can probably vary the mechanism according to his needs. For instance, the mechanism employed to deal with a large, difficult bolus appears to be definitely propulsive and essentially different from the ordinary act. It is necessary, therefore, to attempt to analyse the average normal process.

Everyone knows that he can vary the normal process of getting the food past the back of the tongue, but when once swallowing has started he has no further control; the involuntary and automatic functions take complete charge. He knows that he can swallow lying on his back or on his face, if he adapts the mechanism to the posture, and he can even swallow in the inverted position. He knows also that the mouth must be shut in order to swallow. If, however, he can fit his tongue to the roof of his mouth, he can swallow with the lips and teeth parted. In swallowing he is aware of a certain sequence: the mouth is closed; the tongue feels contracted and the tip comes against the palate. The bolus of food lies in the hollow of the tongue and is lightly compressed against the hard palate. The nasal cavity is felt to be suddenly and automatically cut off, and often the change of pressure in the Eustachian tubes is noted. Simultaneously the larynx is drawn up about half an inch. Almost precisely at this moment the tongue comes into action more forcibly against the palate, throwing the food backward into the pharynx; this is probably the stage at which food is pushed into the naso-pharynx in cases of paralysis of the soft palate.

A definite sensation of suction is experienced on the attempt to swallow a plug of nasal mucus which has stuck just too far below the naso-pharynx to be dislodged by sniffling and just too high to be swallowed easily. Each attempt to swallow it, however vigorous, seems to have the same effect; apparently only a certain amount of force can be exerted on a plug that lies in this position. The muscular action of the forced swallow, when analysed, proves to be an attempt to dislodge the plug by suction, which cannot be increased beyond a certain point.

The process seen radiographically

When the act of swallowing is watched on the screen several very definite events are noticed and are by no means what would be expected from the classical descriptions:

(1) The whole larynx rises.

(2) Suddenly the pharyngeal space is obliterated, just for a fraction of a second, *before* the food slips over the back of the tongue.

(3) The pharyngeal space usually appears again and into it comes the swallowed opaque mass. There it is, apparently just thrown back into this cavity by the action of the tongue, and it seems to shoot as though through space, at a tremendous speed, as if the cavity had no walls. In fact, it appears not only to shoot through this space but actually to go on dropping for some

distance down the oesophagus, although one would presume this to be a narrow collapsed tube of muscle, a potential space. That food should shoot like this through a narrow tube seems absurd; yet the bolus is usually seen to travel with only slightly diminishing speed to about the level of the clavicle, and not until this point does it appear to be entubed, sticking to the walls and proceeding in a manner more like what would be expected of such material progressing through a muscular tube.

The bolus as it travels gives the impression of being sucked rather than pushed down. We all know the appearance of a bolus of food when it is being forced through a coil of small intestine; we see the evidence of the muscular action behind the bolus, the *vis a tergo* moulding it as it pushes it along. There is evidence of definite muscular action behind the mass as it is propelled from the mouth. In the pharynx and upper part of the oesophagus, on the contrary, there is normally no evidence of *vis a tergo*, yet the rapidity with which the food passes down is most extraordinary. The same type of food dropped or squirted into a wide glass or rubber tube would stick and slide down very slowly. The mass looks like a large drop (see Fig. 115 and Plate figs. 116*b* and 117*b*) with a rounded lower border and a long drawn-out tail, like that of a comet, as though it were being drawn down by gravity or other inductive force.

The Pharynx

What happens in the pharynx? Obviously, all three openings into it must be closed before the natural act of swallowing can take place. Radioscopically it is quite clear that the pharynx is completely emptied of air—becomes a potential space—just for a fraction of a second before the swallow (Fig. 112); yet this space seems to reappear during the phase in which all its openings remain closed (Fig. 113). The appearance is comparable to what takes place in the cylinder of a four-stroke internal combustion engine. As the piston rises, pushing out the exhaust gases, it obliterates the space, and then, with the exhaust valve closed, it descends and produces a vacuum into which, when the inlet valve is opened, the explosive mixture is sucked. All the conditions for producing negative pressure are present. Moreover, the way in which the food enters and passes through the pharynx confirms the appearance of a vacuum that is sucking the food down; gravity plays little part, for exactly the same phenomena are seen when the patient is recumbent.

To study the closed phase of the pharynx, which is very short (one-twentieth to one-tenth of a second), numerous sets of serial pictures have been taken, each film being exposed for about one-twentieth of a second and each set of three exposed within one and a half to two seconds. A number of deductions have been made; some of them were expected and others were not.

From the work of Anderson Stuart I expected that the epiglottis must be

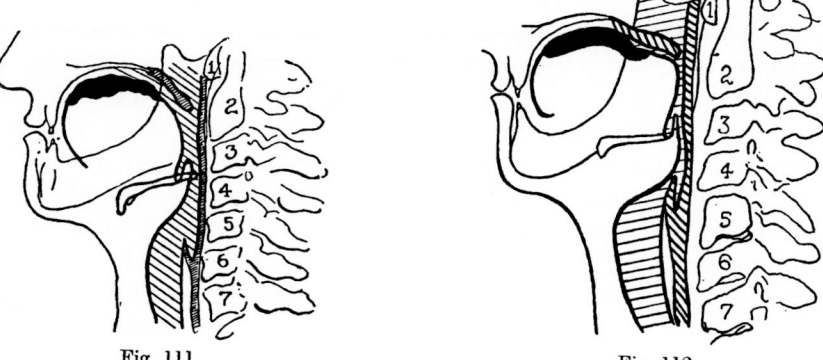

Fig. 111   Fig. 112

Fig. 111. Before swallowing; bolus lies in curve of tongue. The figure shows the beginning of the act of swallowing. The bolus is compressed and the soft palate thrown against the posterior wall. The larynx is rising with the hyoid and the pharynx is narrowed.

Fig. 112. Bolus compressed, nose closed off, larynx raised, pharynx and upper larynx obliterated.

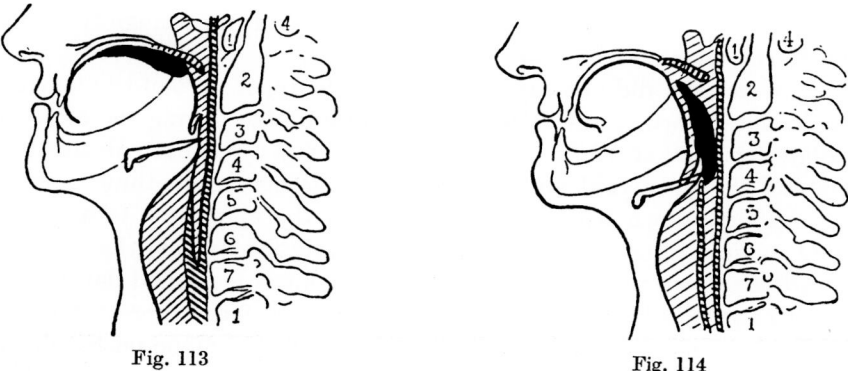

Fig. 113   Fig. 114

Fig. 113. Pharynx opening up, laryngeal pharynx drawn up to epiglottic position. Oesophagus is an open tube and upper larynx is open again.

Fig. 114. Pharynx open; laryngeal pharynx is in epiglottic position and food drops over epiglottis into open oesophagus. Food caught on the epiglottis is deflected down aryteno-epiglottic folds.

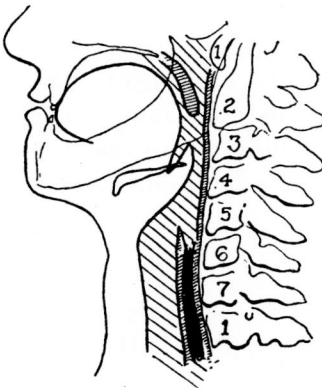

Fig. 115

Fig. 115. Laryngeal pharynx and oesophagus drop with contents back to normal position. Bolus looks like a big drop in space.

vertical and lie flat against the posterior wall of the pharynx during the phase when the pharynx is a potential space. This I confirmed by observing a fleck of barium lodged in the vallecula. From its movement I was able to make certain that the position of the epiglottis in this closed stage of swallowing was flush against the posterior wall of the pharynx (Fig. 114). When the food passes down and the pharynx opens, the epiglottis protrudes into the space and stands out rather like a rock under a waterfall. Ordinary food probably goes over without touching it, but some of the thick sticky food I used seemed to divide on it and be caught in the vallecula or diverted to both sides, passing round and down into the oesophagus in one or both of the ridge channels formed by the aryteno-epiglottic folds. The epiglottis does not appear to take any vital part in the act of swallowing or in the closing-off of the larynx. The sticky opaque food that often lodges in the vallecula can be watched in the postero-anterior position during swallowing. Usually it is squeezed out by a second act of swallowing and passes over the top of the epiglottis in the middle line, but it sometimes escapes down the line of the aryteno-epiglottic folds into the pyriform sinuses and so into the oesophagus.

An observation I did not expect was that the upper part of the larynx—the vestibule right down to the false cords—is obliterated during the closed phase (see Plate figs. 120 and 122). This is a definite fact, yet anatomically I cannot understand it. The hyoid and thyroid rise together. Something comes from above and slips down between the hyoid and the epiglottis, forming a well-rounded shadow across the top of the larynx and obliterating the whole laryngeal vestibule down to the false cords. The epiglottis is pushed flat against the posterior pharyngeal wall. This descending shadow must represent either the back of the tongue or structures which the back of the tongue pushes down into this position. There is no suggestion that the posterior pharyngeal wall comes forward at all, or any other sign that indicates a constrictor action of its muscles. The pressure of the back of the tongue flattens the pharynx and epiglottis against the posterior pharyngeal wall and obliterates the cavity. As the hyoid rises, it embraces the tongue; the tongue is "swallowed" by the hyoid and pressed by it against the pharynx and the upper part of the larynx, obliterating the vestibule as far as the false vocal cords. That is, the laryngeal vestibule and the pharynx are obliterated by compression and not by constriction from the so-called constrictors. Laurell states that the pharynx widens laterally in deglutition. This seems to be a fact, and to add considerable support to my theory of the mechanism.

The Laryngeal Pharynx

At the same time that both the pharynx and the laryngeal vestibule are obliterated something else is happening: the laryngeal pharynx, together with

PLATE II

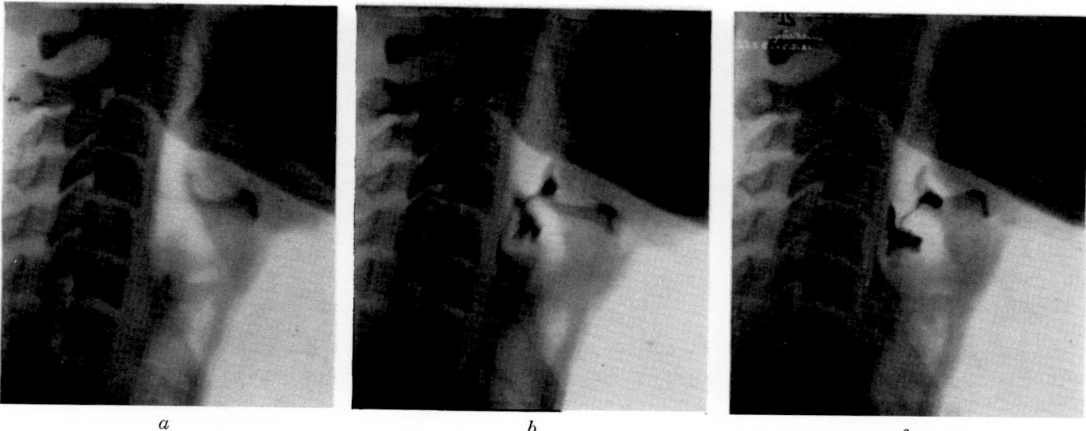

a   b   c

Fig. 116. *a*. Swallowing is just starting, but the bolus has not left the back of the tongue. *b*. About ½ sec. later. The bolus has passed right down and is seen as a large drop just disappearing. Traces are left in the vallecula, aryteno-epiglottic folds and sinus pyriformis. *c*. The food has completely disappeared except for traces left as in *b*.

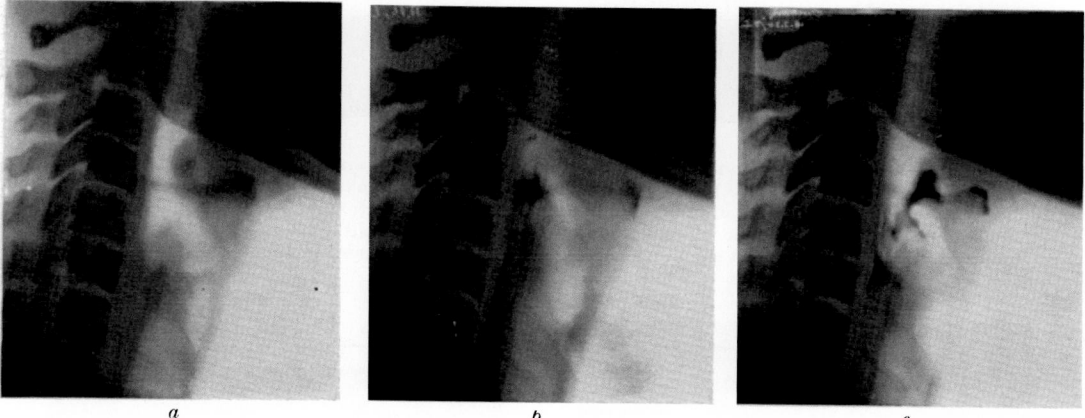

a   b   c

Fig. 117. *a*. Swallowing has not yet started. *b*. About ½ sec. later. The bolus is disappearing like a large drop, leaving traces in the oesophagus which suggest that it is a complete open tube behind the larynx, i.e. from the epiglottis downwards. *c*. The bolus has passed on, leaving traces. Note particularly the behaviour of the heavy shadow on the level of the hyoid in *b* as compared with *c*, which strongly suggests that, in the phase shown in *b*, the laryngeal pharynx rises up to the level of the epiglottis and is in contact with it.

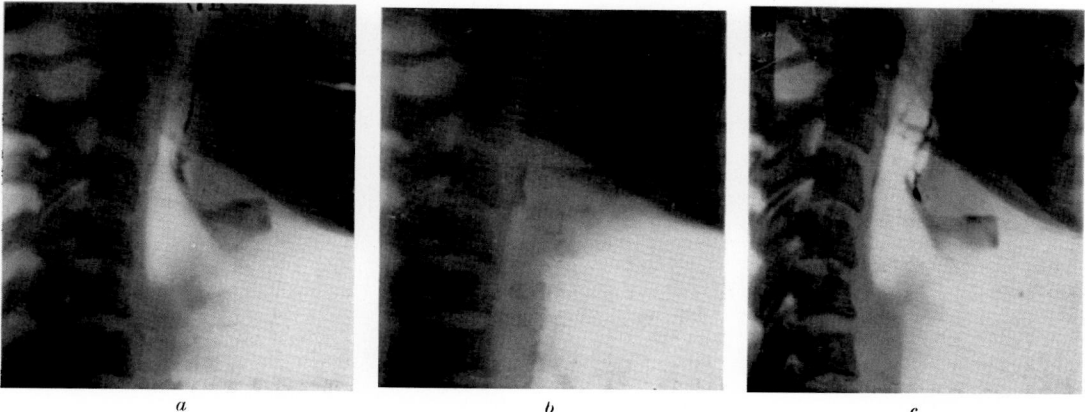

a   b   c

Fig. 118. Traces of food are left on the back of the tongue and in the vallecula. *a*. The subject is just about to swallow. *b*. The closed phase of the pharynx. Note the way in which the larynx rises with the hyoid, and that the traces of food are pressed against the posterior pharyngeal wall. Observe particularly the position of the shadow in the vallecula, which indicates that the epiglottis lies flat up against the posterior wall. *c*. The swallowing act was not effective and the trace of food has not been dislodged from the vallecula.

Figs. 116, 117, 118. Three sets of serial radiographs. Each set taken with intervals of ½ to ¾ sec. between each radiograph. The exposures were about $\frac{1}{20}$ sec.

PLATE III

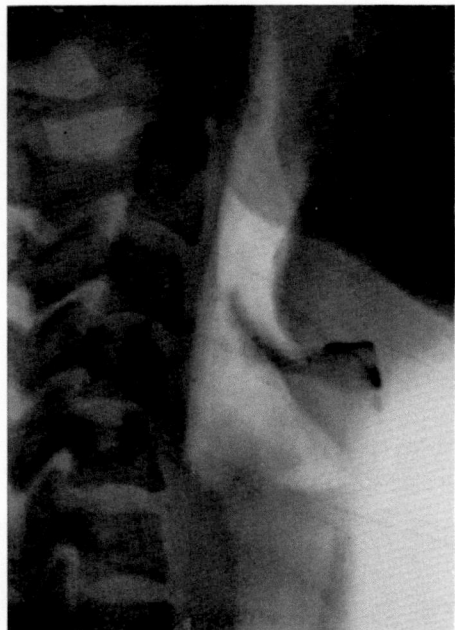
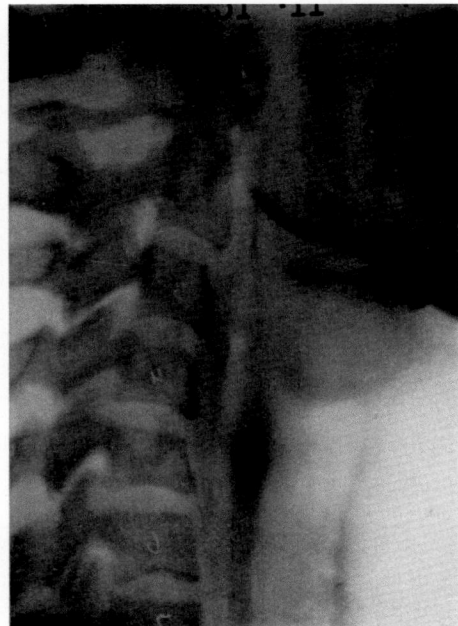

Fig. 119   Fig. 120

Figs. 119, 120. The comparison between the open and the momentarily obliterated pharynx. (Two radiographs out of another series.) The larynx is pulled up, the hyoid is on the level of the lower edge of the maxilla. Below the hyoid is a rounded shadow obliterating the pharynx (except for a streak of air running down into the oesophagus). The whole of the laryngeal vestibule is obliterated down to the false vocal cords. (I have not yet found a subject who could hold this closed phase, and have only succeeded in obtaining radiographs of it on a very few occasions.)

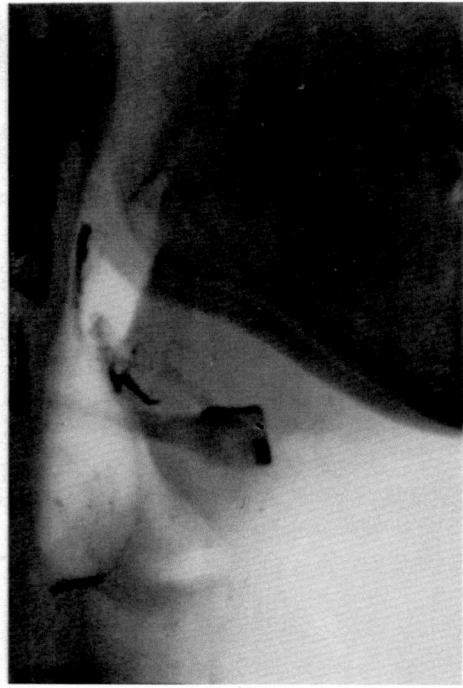
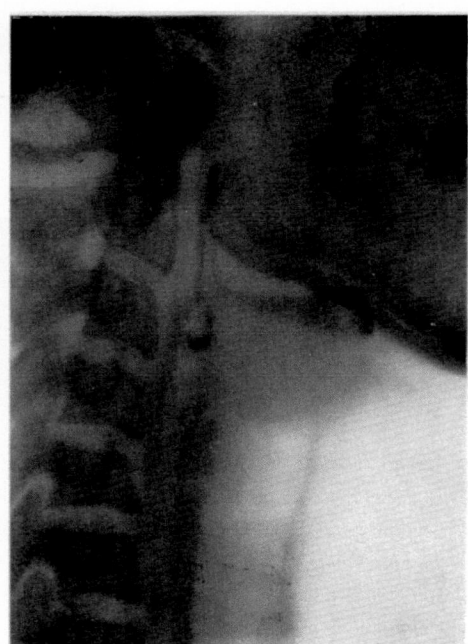

Fig. 121   Fig. 122

Figs. 121, 122. The same comparison as in Figs. 119, 120, but with fragments of food. (Two radiographs from another series.) The epiglottis is pressed back against the posterior wall but does not rise so much as the larynx and is apparently pressed back into this position by the base of the tongue; on the other hand, the fragments of food on the posterior wall of the pharynx rise very considerably, suggesting that this wall performs a considerable upward movement.

the mouth of the oesophagus, appears to be pulled up behind the obliterated laryngeal vestibule until it actually comes into contact with the aryteno-epiglottic folds and epiglottis, completely covering the laryngeal opening. The laryngeal vestibule is therefore in this brief phase not only obliterated and closed off by the tongue, but apparently also covered by the laryngeal pharynx, drawn up like a curtain behind it. It is not easy to see how, anatomically, this can happen, but the mucous membrane of the laryngeal pharynx is very loosely attached and, in the dead specimen, is covered with abundant and redundant folds, which may well be provided in order to allow very free movement. The curtain that shuts off the mouth of the larynx may therefore be formed by the mucous membrane of the laryngeal pharynx. Whether there is in addition, as described in text-books, some shaping or narrowing of the laryngeal margin by movements of the arytenoid and other cartilages, I have no means of determining, but I do know that the laryngeal pharynx forms a complete tubular channel behind the laryngeal opening. The entubed appearance of the food passing behind the laryngeal opening is seldom recorded in radiographs but is discernible in Plate fig. 122. Pancoast [264], who has made a careful investigation of the mechanism of swallowing, holds that the epiglottis, and not the back of the tongue, closes off the air-passages. With this I agree, but it is the back of the tongue that pushes the epiglottis backwards while the larynx is raised to meet it.

In a number of the films showing the obliterated pharynx phase, a streak of residual air is noted in the laryngeal pharynx and oesophagus. This appearance seems to indicate that when the laryngeal pharynx is pulled up to this epiglottic position it becomes an open-mouthed receptacle like a Christmas stocking, so that the food, as it leaves the back of the tongue, just drops into it. It looks, therefore, as though the mouth of the larynx were covered by the mucous membrane of the laryngeal pharynx at the moment when the whole larynx rises at the beginning of swallowing.

On the screen another surprising thing is seen: the laryngeal vestibule appears to open up as the hyoid comes down, before the food passes, and yet the food does not enter it (Plate figs. 116b and 117b). Our sensations, and the fact that the food "goes the right way", tell us that the larynx must in fact be still closed, but the manner in which it is closed off is most unexpected. My interpretation of the appearances is that the laryngeal pharynx waits up in its epiglottic position for the bolus to be popped in, just as the nestling bird holds up its open beak to the mother. It is not until this has happened that the laryngeal pharynx drops down to its normal position behind the larynx, as the nestling sinks back with the worm into the nest. A number of the film records strongly suggest, even if they do not actually prove, that this surmise is correct. It is certainly not easy to see why the laryngeal vestibule should be obliterated before the act of swallowing and yet open up again before the food passes over the mouth of the larynx. The only suggestion I can make is that its closure is connected with the raising of the unsupported mucous membrane of the laryngeal pharynx to the epiglottic position. The mucous folds appear to be the only structure available to form the curtain that obviously covers the laryngeal aperture while the food goes past, and possibly this preliminary closure of the laryngeal vestibule is designed to ensure the apposition of the mucous membrane curtain to the epiglottis. This, however, is pure hypothesis and is merely put forward as a possible explanation.

The general character of the superficial cells of the mucous membrane in this region gives some support to these theories. The respiratory passages are lined with ciliated columnar cells, whereas the mouth, pharynx and oesophagus are covered with stratified epithelium to stand wear and pressure. Only the upper portion of the posterior surface of the epiglottis and the upper part of the aryteno-epiglottic folds are covered with stratified epithelium, and these portions also have taste buds, suggesting that, in the act of swallowing, the upper part of the epiglottis and the adjoining folds are exposed to the food stream while the lower part is protected, presumably in the manner I have suggested.

The Anatomical Segment concerned with Swallowing

The act of swallowing begins with the tongue, but where does it end? I suggest that this complex co-ordinated act extends through a segment the lower limit of which is the junction of the upper and middle thirds of the oesophagus. Several indications point in this direction: the rapid progress of the bolus is slowed down as it reaches the level of the clavicle, and evidence of peristalsis is sometimes seen at this point; above the level of the clavicle, except in abnormal conditions, peristalsis is not seen. The anatomical structure changes in this region from striated voluntary muscle to non-striated involuntary muscle; the muscularis mucosae, which is almost absent above, becomes prominent, and the nerve supply changes. The fact of this change was deduced from the behaviour of the opaque food in certain cases of paralysis (Barclay[44]), and was only later found to be correlated with the dual nerve supply arising from the two separate nuclei in the medulla (cf. p. 65). Incidentally, this is the point at which nearly all coins or middle-sized foreign bodies lodge in the oesophagus. These facts fit in with the observations to support the view that a bolus travels with one co-ordinated impulse from the back of the tongue to the level of the clavicle.

Obviously swallowing is not the simple, almost peristaltic movement that it was once considered. The initial impulse that pushes the food out of the mouth plays a small part, but it does not explain why and how the bolus traverses the pharynx and the first few inches of the oesophagus with such extreme rapidity, and one is driven to accept the explanation of negative pressure as the main force at work. In some of the subjects examined there has been greater radiographic suggestion of suction than in others, and the records of actual pressures measured in these cases have confirmed the visual observations. Apparently, also, the negative pressure is markedly increased if the swallower commences the act by sucking the teeth, and, in fact, James and Hastings (183) have demonstrated that negative pressure is usual in the mouth when it is closed.

Experimental Proof of the Negative Pressure

The foregoing obervations call for much explanation, both physiological and anatomical. No attempt has as yet been made on the anatomical side. On the physiological side, however, Prof. Anrep, then of the Cambridge University

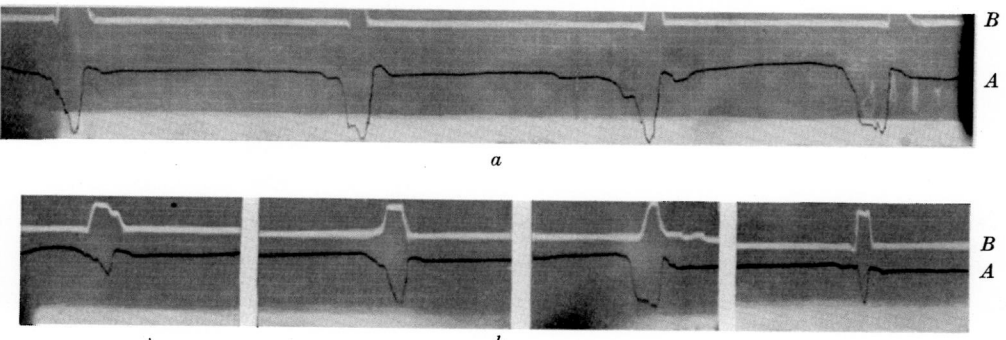

Fig. 123. *a, b.* Typical graphs, obtained by Prof. Anrep. *A,* showing the negative pressures in the pharynx and upper oesophagus. In certain instances a simultaneous graph, *B,* was obtained of the movements of the thyroid cartilage. The vertical lines indicate $\frac{1}{25}$ sec. The graphs read from right to left.

Physiological Laboratory, made some observations for me. We found that the suggested phase of negative pressure definitely occurs (Fig. 123), varying with different subjects and with the type of food. When materials such as bread

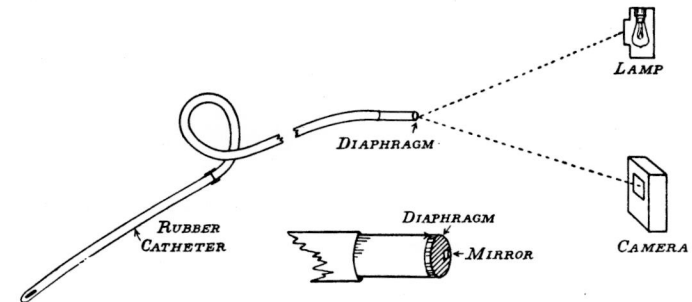

Fig. 124. Apparatus used for recording pharyngeal and oesophageal pressures. (Prof. Anrep.)

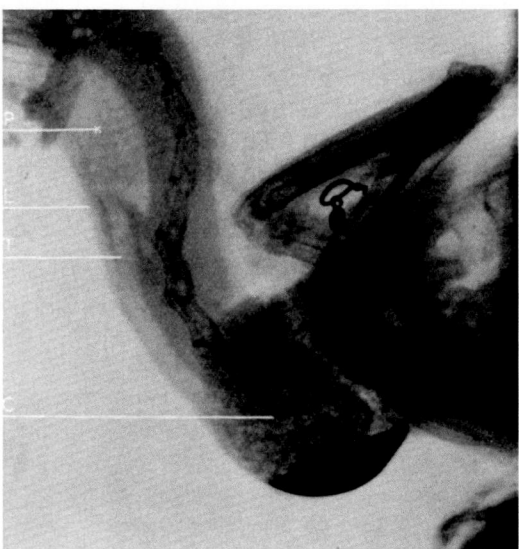

Fig. 125. The hen at rest. Note the large pharyngeal cavity, *P*, and the position of the larynx, *L*. The trachea, *T*, is seen passing down through the shadow of the crop, *C*, which is full of ordinary food, with some opaque food in the lower part. The wire is an identification tag on the wing.

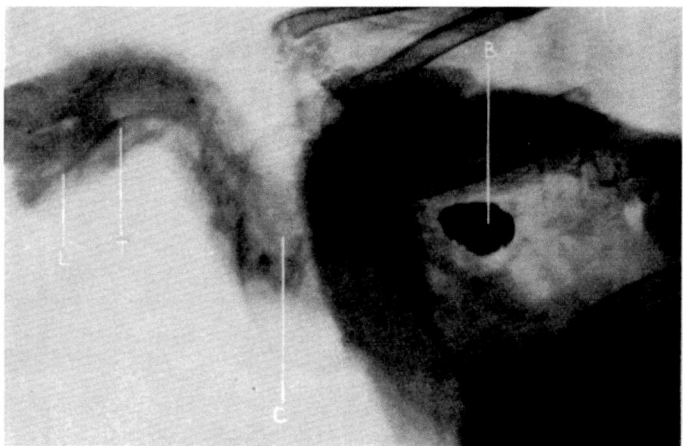

Fig. 126. The hen reaching forward to swallow. The pharynx is completely obliterated, and the larynx, *L*, takes up a position right underneath the tongue. Note the arched trachea, *T*, as compared with the last figure. The crop, *C*, is distended with air, and a large bolus, *B*, is passing on towards the gizzard.

are swallowed, this negative pressure is somewhere about 16 to 18 inches of water. The records were made by introducing a thin soft rubber catheter through the subject's nose into the pharynx and oesophagus, controlling its position by X-ray observations. The outside end of the catheter was connected with a membrane manometer, the segmental capsule of which carried a mirror which projected a beam of light into a paper film camera (Fig. 124). The vibration frequency of the manometer was 55 per second and its magnification such that the beam of light was deflected 10 mm. by a change of pressure of 12 cm. of water. In some of the experiments the subjects performed "empty swallowing", i.e. swallowing saliva only; in others they swallowed bread or water. In most of the experiments the eye of the catheter was left open; in a few cases it was covered with a thin rubber balloon which was *very* slightly inflated after introduction. If the balloon was more inflated, the direct action of the muscular wall upon it was recorded as positive pressures, such as were observed by Kronecker and Meltzer. Moreover, the subject felt the catheter gripped by the muscular action and pushed out through his nose, presumably by the lifting of the larynx and the associated movements. Prof. Anrep has written to me that he is continuing the work on the pressures concerned in swallowing and that, so far, his observations confirm our previous work.

Animal Observations

For another purpose, in conjunction with Mr E. T. Halnan of the Department of Agriculture, I have recently been studying the intestinal tract of the hen. Among the radiographs that were taken I happened to obtain pictures of the various phases of swallowing, and these seem to throw some light on the process in man. The larynx rises in a most extraordinary manner until it seems to disappear into the base of the tongue; the pharynx is completely obliterated and, just as it opens out again, the bolus of food is apparently sucked into the pharynx. This bird (see Figs. 125–128) appears to obtain the negative pressure by relaxing and then contracting the anterior wall of the pharynx until it becomes like the string of a bow across the arch of the neck. After the bolus has passed down, the larynx descends to its normal position (Fig. 128). The relatively large size of the pharyngeal space probably accounts for the fact that the hen swallows a great deal of air and distends its crop with it. So far as I have yet noted, however, the swallowed air never goes beyond the crop.

I have also watched the dog swallow and have some records, but have as yet obtained little, if any, information from this source. The rate at which a dog gulps food down makes direct observation almost valueless.

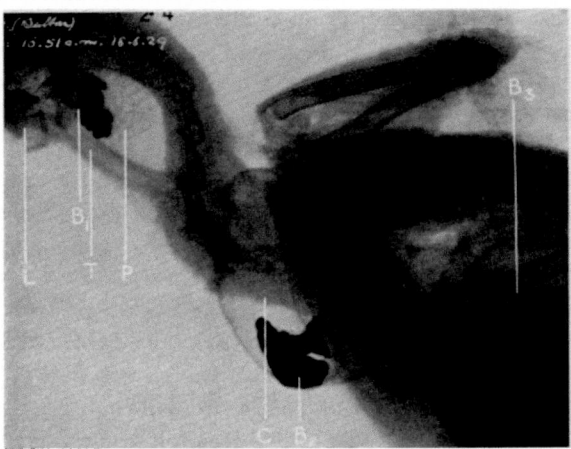

Fig. 127. The hen is just swallowing. Note the large cavity of the pharynx, P, into which the food is, apparently, being sucked. In the hen, the cavity seems to be formed by the straightening out of the trachea, T, like the string of a bow. The larynx, L, remains high up under the back of the tongue. Some food can be seen on the tongue, and the bolus, B_1, gives the impression of being sucked into the cavity of the pharynx. The crop, C, is full of air with some opaque food, B_2, in the lower part. A bolus, B_3, is passing on to the gizzard under the pressure of peristalsis.

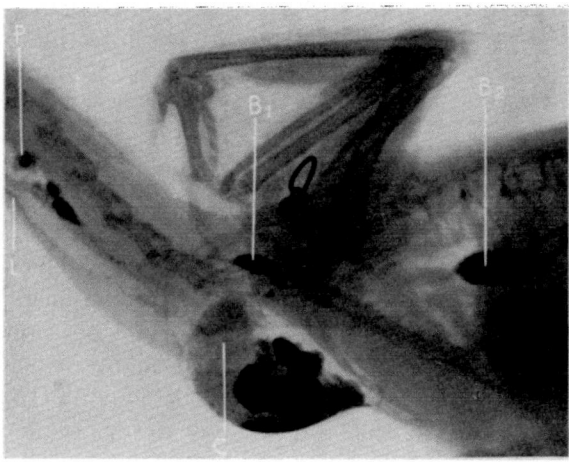

Fig. 128. The act of swallowing is over; the pharynx, P, again contains air with bits of sticky food adhering to the walls. The larynx, L, has come down to the normal position. The crop, C, contains a good deal of air and opaque food; under observation the bolus divided at the crop, part, B_1, remaining there, and the rest, B_2, passing on to the gizzard.

THE CONCEPT OF NEGATIVE PRESSURE

When I come to interpret the observations in terms of the dissected larynx, this new conception seems impossible. For instance, how can I explain such appearances as that the tongue is apparently swallowed by the hyoid, and that the epiglottis manages to move so far from the thyroid and hyoid, to which it is attached anatomically by elastic ligaments? I can see how by closing the apertures a negative pressure is produced in the pharynx, but how is it produced in the oesophagus and how far down does it extend? I can see that the so-called constrictors of the pharynx with their oblique, criss-cross fibres, and some of the other muscles which are directly and indirectly attached to the laryngeal pharynx and oesophagus, would tend to open the pharynx out as they pull upward; that is, act as levators rather than constrictors. These suggestions, however, only go a very short way towards explaining the mechanism. As a radiologist, I can but record observed facts and leave it to others to follow up and complete the story.

Anderson, Lockhart and Souter [19] recently described a case of thrombosis of the posterior inferior cerebellar artery with paralysis of the right superior constrictor of the pharynx and spasm of the oesophageal entrance. The man was quite unable to swallow either solids or fluids, and when he tried to swallow, the hyoid bone and thyroid cartilage moved strongly. The paralysis gradually subsided after about three weeks and the inability during that time to swallow even water makes the case unique. The authors find it a complete puzzle when they attempt to explain it on the basis of the conventional theory of swallowing. "The hemiparetic pharynx may be unable to negotiate a rough bolus", they say, "but why should the healthy side not function enough to transmit at least a trickle of water?" If the mechanism of swallowing demands first of all the production of a negative pressure in the pharynx, the explanation seems simple. If any portion of a tube is paralysed it will be impossible to obliterate the lumen completely, and therefore no vacuum can be produced in it.

I do not for one moment believe that the negative pressure mechanism is the one and only method of swallowing; it is, however, the one that most people usually employ. Nature provides alternatives in this as in other functions. She has no hard and fast rules. Taylor [308] has said of the chemical aspect of digestion that we are provided with "duplicate plants", and Alvarez [12] writes: "If pepsin fails, the pancreatic ferment can come to the rescue, and when that is shut off, the gastric and intestinal ferments can, between them, do remarkably well. On the chemical side, the factors of safety are large; on the mechanical side, there is only the one muscular tube which cannot be replaced." But Nature provides a margin of safety by endowing her muscular system with a twofold action: contractile and tonic. These interplay and balance one with another to achieve the same purpose in different ways. So also in swallowing: although I hold that negative pressure is the main force, yet propulsive action is latent, ready to come into play if the negative pressure is not sufficient to accomplish the swallowing of the bolus. Hence, whenever obstruction is present propulsion is likely to be invoked.

It was purely on X-ray observation of the natural swallowing of ordinary opaque foods by healthy students that I came to the conclusion that the mechanism I saw was produced by negative pressure. In some cases the mechanism was obvious, in others it was very difficult to see, and in a few I was doubtful of its existence. In some students one can actually demonstrate the whole of the mechanism as I have described it; in others it looks as if there are wide variations from what I have described and that they only use suction to a relatively small extent. Some subjects obviously use suction far more than others. But in all the cases in which I obtained manometer readings, negative pressures of considerable magnitude were recorded. The conclusions I arrived at were entirely the product of radiographic methods applied to normal persons. Only when this work had been done did Prof. Anrep very kindly undertake the work of recording on graphs the actual negative pressure, and in spite of the graphs my real conviction rests on the actual observations made when no abnormal recording instruments were introduced.

CHAPTER XI

THE OESOPHAGUS AND STOMACH

The gullet has been described in text-books as a tubular organ of definite diameter, but in fact its diameter varies from a potential space to the size needed to accommodate a given bolus. It is possible for a complete upper set of false teeth to pass down without causing more than discomfort! Normally, however, as Prof. Wingate Todd pointed out to me many years ago, the lower part of the oesophagus is wider than the upper, and the increased width at the lower end practically amounts to an ampulla where food, if swallowed too hastily, tends to lie for a few moments until the narrow cardiac orifice has allowed that in front to pass into the stomach. This "back-pressure" dilatation of the ampulla is best seen when the patient swallows rapidly. If the normal diameter of the upper part of the oesophagus be taken as half an inch, then the ampulla has a diameter of three-quarters of an inch, but can be distended to about an inch without discomfort.

The first large drop of a thick opaque food enters the lower two-thirds of the oesophagus with a rounded end which flattens out a little further down and tends to show the vertical folds of the mucosa. It seems to traverse the whole length down to the cardiac orifice, usually at about the same speed, with more or less undiminished and often almost uniform calibre, with no indication of being cut off into sections and urged along by peristaltic waves. Yet the food passes on. Many years ago Jordan (187) maintained that the food passed down by its own weight, his contention being that peristalsis plays a very small part in the propulsion of the food. As, however, the same appearance and approximately the same rate of progress are noted when the patient lies down, gravity can play very little, if any, part in the normal mechanism of oesophageal progression. Lexer (219) replaced the oesophagus with a skin tube in cases of obstruction and noted that swallowing took place quite satisfactorily. This disproves the belief that solid food cannot pass down a tube devoid of peristalsis. Moreover, Sampson (288) has published a radiograph of a patient with an artificial oesophagus in which the food is seen passing "uphill", the patient having been inverted!

If fairly hard lumps are swallowed quickly, the picture may be different and may correspond to that seen if the patient is tilted head-downwards. The food often comes to a certain point and pauses: the first halt is usually at the level of the clavicle, and the next is about midway between this level and the cardiac orifice. At these points the food sticks, and a narrowing—a peristaltic wave—

takes place above it and progresses downwards, following the food. Generally speaking, this narrowing is not very marked and does not segment the shadow unless it fails to propel the food on.

Where there is marked obstruction this picture is exaggerated. The opaque food comes down to the obstruction and, if the channel is blocked either by a bolus or by spasmodic or organic narrowing, the oesophagus becomes dilated above and the screen shows evidence of a powerful wave of peristalsis descending on the food and attempting to push it through. A large proportion of the food escapes backwards through the peristaltic ring as this descends. The movement was, in the early days, mistaken for reverse peristalsis, a condition which I have never seen in the oesophagus.

The Cardiac Orifice

Even thin opaque food almost invariably pauses as it reaches the ampulla, which bends backwards and to the left to enter the stomach. This bend varies considerably in different individuals, from an almost straight line to a very marked angle, especially when there is obstruction at the cardiac orifice and dilatation of the lower end; the oesophagus appears to be lengthened as well as dilated.

The mechanism that controls the opening of the cardiac orifice is not clear, though presumably some question of pressure is involved. Although there does not appear to be any anatomical sphincter at the cardia, yet, radiographically, sphincteric action is obvious. Moreover, Knight and Adamson [207] have shown that this sphincteric action is subject to the vagus and sympathetic nerves (p. 210). Normally it seems to open irrespective of the fullness or emptiness of the stomach, and its opening does not seem to be associated with the intragastric pressure; there is just a little pause, a little accumulation of food behind the cardiac orifice, and then the food slides into the stomach.

Its passage, apart from the pressure of more food coming down the oesophagus, does not seem to be markedly influenced by the act of swallowing. The mechanism is, to a certain extent, associated with the respiratory movements and the position of the diaphragm, but what the relationship is I have not made out. The diaphragm has been said to move in relation to swallowing (diaphragmatic swallowing), but does not appear to me to do so. During the act of swallowing, when the food is passing through the pharynx, the larynx is automatically and completely closed, and naturally the diaphragm must remain stationary. There is no indication, so far as I can see, that the diaphragm tends to compress the air in the lungs against the laryngeal closure in order to prevent food from entering the larynx, as has been suggested. I think the diaphragm remains stationary simply because the laryngeal opening is closed.

When relative obstruction occurs, the resistance of the cardiac orifice appears to be overcome by the piston pressure of the food forced against it by the waves of peristalsis as they descend. Powerful waves then produce a marked increase of tension, and it is this that causes the pain after swallowing that occurs in the middle stage of oesophageal obstruction. In the later stages, when the oesophagus has become dilated and the peristalsis can no longer produce effectual pressure on the contents, the pain diminishes. It is probable that oesophageal, like abdominal, pain is only experienced in response to tension.

Normally the food slides into the stomach as if through a patulous tube, but if there is a hold-up it is usually an inch above the cardiac orifice, i.e. about the level of the dome of the diaphragm. In normal subjects a delay of seconds or even minutes is quite often seen at this place, suggesting the presence of a sphincter at the level of the diaphragm, or at any rate a sphincteric action involving the last two inches of the oesophagus, rather than any sharply-defined sphincter at the cardia itself. It often looks as if the sphincter opened in response to peristaltic pressure.

There also appears to be a third mechanism: one that is the last reserve in cases of obstruction at the cardiac orifice. Payne and Poulton (265) have made some most interesting observations on rabbits and on themselves, but their work does not seem to have been widely noticed. In newly-killed rabbits they found that the lower end of the oesophagus invaginated through the cardia whenever the cardia was touched or the vagus was stimulated. They say: "The appearance is reminiscent of the firm closure of the anus that occurs after defaecation; the whole action is in fact very similar to what can be seen immediately after defaecation in the horse". They also obtained some evidence of a similar mechanism in man. One of them swallowed a balloon in which a piece of metal was contained; this was seen by X rays to be in the oesophagus, well above the cardiac orifice, to be apparently carried into the stomach when the subject swallowed, and then (presumably after a definite interval) to be returned to its original position. At the same time the catheter to which the balloon was attached was felt to be pulled down and returned. "Although these observations are compatible with the theory of the cardiac sphincter described above, they do not prove that the oesophagus is invaginated into the stomach."

Since reading this, I have watched a number of students and, in most cases, the opaque food just flows through, giving no suggestion of a sphincter, but in a few, and in one man in particular—a healthy student who was quite unaware that the whole of the food had not passed into the stomach—I noted the appearances recorded in the accompanying diagram (Fig. 129). The striking point was the complete absence of any suggestion of a sphincter, an appearance utterly unlike the way in which the food passes through the pylorus. This observation does not prove that the suggestion of Payne and Poulton is correct but, to my mind, it goes far in the direction of indicating that in man an alternative mechanism of this kind is in reserve, and is used when there is some difficulty. I gather that their impression of the action of the cardia is that the lower end of the oesophagus is itself the sphincter, in much the same way that the anal canal is the sphincter of the rectum. Their theory is particularly interesting to me because it explains what I saw in a case of cardiospasm with extreme dilatation (cf. p. 212) the mechanism of which entirely baffled all those who saw it: the whole column of food was pushed straight through into the stomach *en masse* when once the obstruction was overcome. There was no suggestion of narrowing at the cardiac orifice. I always narrated this case to my classes, and the description that I gave to the appearance was that the progress of the shadow resembled the process of defaecation in the horse.

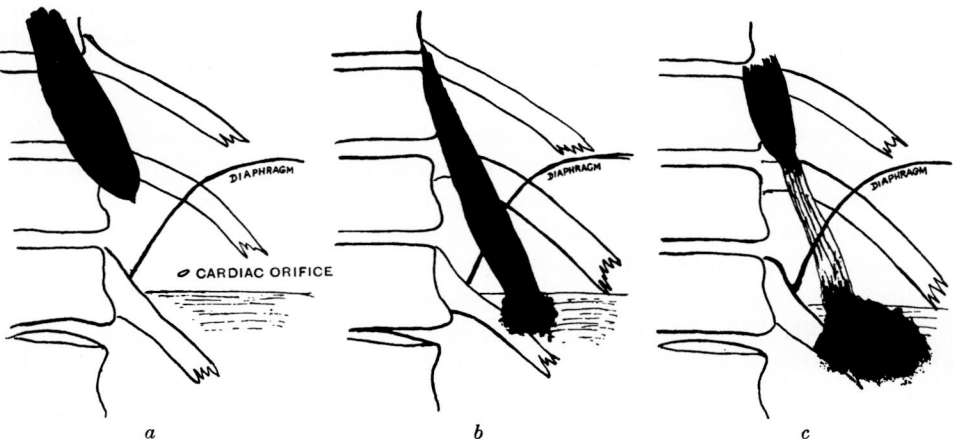

a　　　　　　　　*b*　　　　　　　　*c*

Fig. 129. Unusual action of cardiac orifice seen in a healthy student. *a*. Food was seen retained in the lower end of the oesophagus about 2 in. above the cardiac orifice. *b*. The subject swallowed again and the whole mass moved into the stomach with undiminished calibre, leaving an appearance, *c*, in which the rugae were seen but there was no indication of the narrowing of a sphincter.

In one medical student whom I watched a small part of the bolus seemed to pass into the stomach and then to retreat again, and to go on advancing and retreating through the cardiac orifice for about five minutes. The appearances suggested that the cardiac orifice with the food contained in it moved up and down—possibly independently of the movements of the diaphragm.

It is probable that the crura of the diaphragm exert influence, as food is seldom seen passing during expiration. It looks as if the crura, extended in expiration, exert pressure and as if the lower end of the oesophagus, which has no anatomical structure comparable with a sphincter, is freed during inspiration or the mid-phase of respiration.

Probably the lower end of the oesophagus can act in various ways, and this particular mechanism is merely one of them—one that can be brought into play when the cardiac end of the oesophagus is not sufficiently relaxed to allow the food to pass through or when the bolus to be dealt with calls for something more than the usual mechanism. The balloon used by Payne and Poulton would have the effect of an abnormal bolus and automatically call up a reserve mechanism for overcoming difficulties.

To sum up: the cardiac orifice may function in three ways:

(a) as a patulous canal,

(b) as a sphincter that responds to peristalsis,

(c) by invaginating its contents into the stomach.

THE STOMACH

Before the advent of the opaque meal and the examination of the stomach as it performed its functions, teachers described it as an organ consisting of two parts: the upper acting as a hopper, in which the food was stored, and the lower as a mill, in which it was thoroughly mixed and churned until a given degree of acidity was produced; this influenced the pylorus, which opened to allow the food to pass. This idea is now completely discredited. It is essential to conceive the normal stomach as a living tubular muscle, as a sensitive organ, and as perhaps the most sensitive muscular organ in the whole body. Its shape depends on its tone, and tone may alter from moment to moment in response to a great variety of physical and psychical stimuli.

The stomach is a "fluid" organ, if one may use the term in this sense. It may be displaced across the abdomen by a collection of gas in the colon; it is easily pushed upwards by pressure on the abdomen, pelvic tumours and such agents, and in spite of gross displacements—even that of full-term pregnancy—it may not give the smallest sign that the distortion is causing any embarrassment of its functions. How some of the ladies existed who "tight-laced", and thus nipped atonic stomachs in the middle, is a problem which, when that fashion recurs, will be worth studying. The fact that this was done and that there are survivors to tell the tale is sufficient to show how wonderful is its adaptability.

The cardiac end of the stomach naturally varies in size according to the quantity of air it contains. When there is no fluid in it the air appears as an oval clear area, but if the usual small quantity of secretion is present, the air space is the arc of a circle bounded below by a short, straight fluid line (Fig. 130).

Jefferson [185] studied the canalisation of the empty stomach and found that the liquid food passed down the lesser curvature. He attributed this course to the very marked band of oblique fibres that, curving over the cardiac orifice, runs down on either side of the lesser curvature, forming more or less the "canalis gastricus" described by Lewis. It is said that such a channel is present in certain animals and that its function is associated with rumination. These observations I have confirmed, but I do not think that Jefferson's explanation is correct. My own impression is rather that food usually takes this route because it is the nearest to the straight line of gravity. That there is no definite channel down the lesser curvature in the empty stomach can readily be shown by giving a spoonful of ordinary food as solid as the patient can swallow and following it up with a watery suspension of barium; the watery fluid will flow over the solid

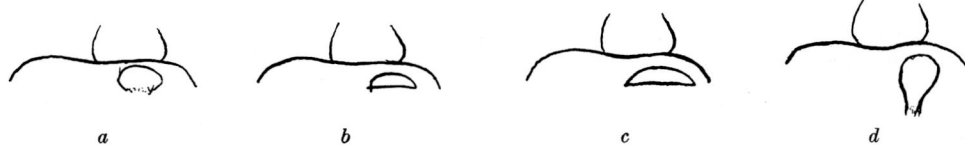

Fig. 130. The air space in the stomach. *a*. The stomach empty. Perhaps a small line of secretion bounding the air below. *b*. A certain amount of food in the stomach. Probably a J-shaped stomach. *c*. A large quantity of food in the stomach. Probably a J-shaped stomach. *d*. An atonic stomach. Lower limit of air space drawn out. Perhaps a little fluid is seen where the walls come in contact.

bodies and may take any one or all of the alternative courses down between the rugae, which can usually be seen as separate shadowy lines, some seven or eight in number, running straight down to the lowest part of the stomach (Fig. 131). The orderly arrangement of the rugae in a series of channels down the stomach and around the food is in striking contrast to the conception of the mucous membrane we obtain from the dead body, or even from the stomach in the operating theatre.

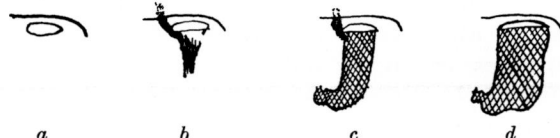

Fig. 131. Canalisation of normal empty stomach. *a*. Air space. *b*. The first mouthful enters, showing the rugae. *c*. The J-shaped stomach is full. *d*. The increased capacity for more food is obtained chiefly by lateral expansion.

As filling takes place, the capacity for moderate quantities is obtained almost wholly by lateral expansion. The organ maintains its tubular form and this tube widens out as more food is taken. The maintenance of the tubular form is the function of the tonic action of the walls and is automatic. It is compensatory to the influence of gravity on the contents. In the recumbent position the action is not required to counteract gravity, and to a large extent disappears. When the patient lies down, the gastric contents all tend to fall into the cardiac end of the stomach, which is naturally very much lower, leaving the pyloric portion quite empty or filled with air.

Foods pass down to the pyloric antrum in the order in which they are taken *unless* a heavier food should succeed a lighter, in which case the heavier sinks in the mass till it finds its level, and the whole is bathed by the gastric juices. These can flow freely around the food mass, but do not mix to any great extent except near the pylorus where the channel narrows (Fig. 132). Possibly this explains the indigestibility of plum pudding: the heavy carbohydrate food falls to the pyloric end and demands passage before it has had time to be acted on by the secretion.

Although no definite difference can be seen with the naked eye, it has been stated that the upper two-thirds of the human stomach corresponds to the crop and the pyloric portion to the gizzard of the bird. The muscle of the pyloric portion is certainly thicker and tougher than that of the rest of the stomach, its blood supply is differently arranged, and the nerve supply of the lesser curvature comes from a separate branch (Fig. 53, p. 64).

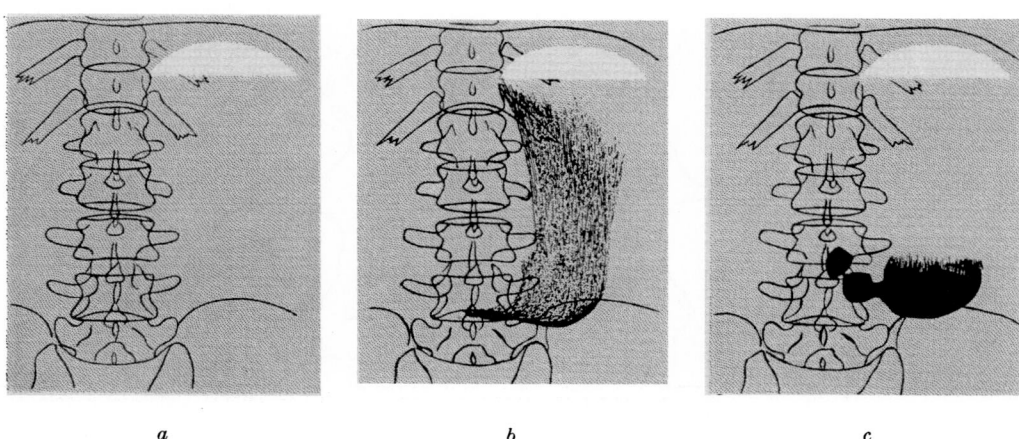

a   b   c

Fig. 132. Passage of a fluid opaque meal into a full stomach. *a*. A normal stomach that contains ordinary food. The air space only is seen. *b*. A watery suspension of barium is given. This flows around and through the non-opaque food, giving a veil-like appearance. *c*. The opaque fluid settles out and lies at the bottom of the stomach.

GASTRIC PERISTALSIS

The earliest and most satisfactory study of the peristalsis of the stomach, one that is still a standard, was published by Kaestle, Rieder and Rosenthal[190] (Figs. 133 and 134), who succeeded in obtaining twelve to thirteen plates in the period of a single gastric peristaltic wave, i.e. twenty-two seconds. Tracings were made of each outline and, in addition, composite pictures were obtained by superimposing these outlines. This article is still worth study and the description has not, to my knowledge, been surpassed, although two years later L. G. Cole [101] made an intensive study by means of rapid serial radiography. He, like Kaestle, Rieder and Rosenthal, avoids the fallacy of describing peristalsis as "normal"

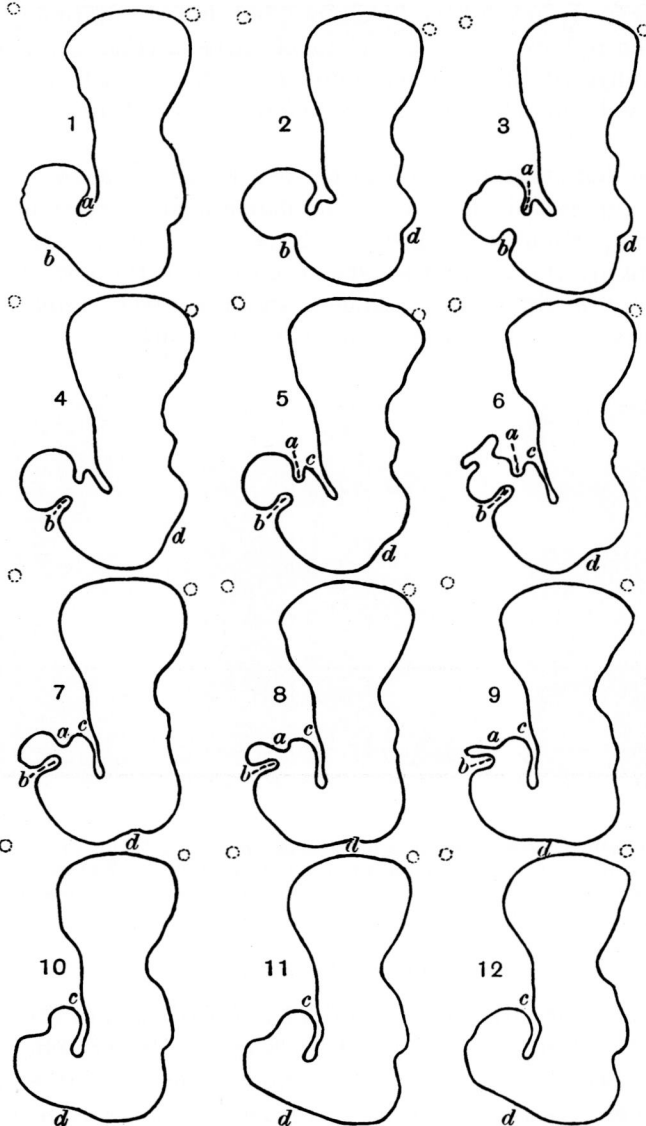

Fig. 133. A series of tracings from cinematograph X-ray pictures of the human stomach in one phase of its motion. Each of the letters *a*, *b*, *c* and *d* indicates a peristaltic wave. (From Kaestle, Rieder and Rosenthal.)

and speaks of obstructed and unobstructed peristalsis. He speaks of a gastric cycle in which there is a systole and a diastole of the stomach in addition to the peristaltic contraction passing pylorus-ward. He classifies gastric peristalsis under five types, according to the number of waves present at any given moment:

(1) One-cycle type: described by Holzknecht as normal. (Cole regards this as exceedingly rare.)

(2) One-and-a-half-cycle type: claimed by Holzknecht as belonging to the preceding type, and by Kaestle, Rieder and Rosenthal as belonging to the following type.

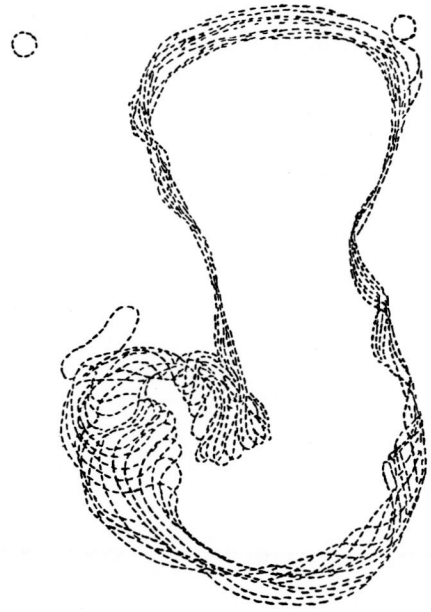

Fig. 134. Composite figure made from tracings in Fig. 133, showing the progression of the waves on the walls of the stomach during a whole cycle. Comparison with Fig. 133 shows that during the gastric cycle the whole stomach was displaced vertically, probably by an accidental respiratory movement. The waves of contraction appear to continue to the pylorus, but this does not always happen. (From Kaestle, Rieder and Rosenthal.)

(3) Two-cycle type: described by Kaestle, Rieder and Rosenthal as normal.

(4) Three- and four-cycle types: considered by Cole to be more common than all the other types combined. Of these two types, the four-cycle type is the more common.

(5) A group representing an active peristalsis in which more than four cycles are required for the progression of a contraction. A similar condition has recently been described by a French author as the "choreic type".

Groedel (144), with an apparatus for rapid serial radiography, also compiled an exhaustive study of gastric movement and peristalsis (Figs. 135 and 136). The Cole Collaborators now have available a direct cinematograph apparatus that takes a length of film ten inches wide. Some of their records will well repay study. Apparatus on a smaller scale has also been built by Jarre, Alvarez, van der Maele and myself.

The cost of film records of such a large size is, of course, very great, but we are within measurable distance of satisfactory indirect films that will make the study of peristalsis really possible. Several workers, notably Russell Reynolds (280a), are rapidly perfecting the technique. Kymography may also be used, not only to analyse the peristaltic waves of the stomach but also to record changes of the mucous membrane pattern. The method consists of exposing an ordinary radiographic film for a few seconds, during which period a grid containing a number of horizontal slits is moved vertically across the film a distance corresponding to the interval between two slits. The resulting picture is a number of bands each showing a representation of the portion of the stomach opposite the slit through which it was taken, with the lateral motion translated into a wave form. The apparatus is now more or less standardised but the interpretation of the results is difficult and requires considerable practice. One of the chief pioneers and exponents of the method is Dr Pleikart Stumpf(306a) of Munich.

My own views on gastric peristalsis are that it varies so enormously, not only with the individual and the contents of the stomach but from time to time in the same individual, that to attempt by a description or even a number of descriptions to represent the normal would not be satisfactory and the radiologist can only report that the stomach appears to be active, or that its movements are poor or absent. Groedel (144) said many years ago: "In healthy people with normal stomachs there is very little peristaltic movement". In other words, the forceful churning waves that were described in the physiological literature, chiefly that of Cannon, are not the usual type of movement seen in man under normal conditions. Peristalsis in the normal subject does not appear to be a forcible movement. It suggests the waves that running shorewards help the sea-drift on its way, rather than the breakers beating upon the rocks.

"*Churning*"

The idea that there is general churning of the food in the stomach with the gastric juice is extinct now that X rays have revealed something of the true state of things. Cannon stated that the food was pressed into the pyloric antrum, that here it was thoroughly churned by its rush to and fro through the rings of peristaltic contraction, and that finally when it had been thoroughly triturated by this method the pylorus opened. I fear, however, that Cannon's conceptions and deductions were made from animal and not from human observation. They certainly do not hold good for what the radiologist sees. Hurst describes each bolus as coming from the oesophagus and entering into the midst of the rest of the food, thus being protected from the gastric juice, which would otherwise check the action of the ptyalin on the carbohydrates (172).

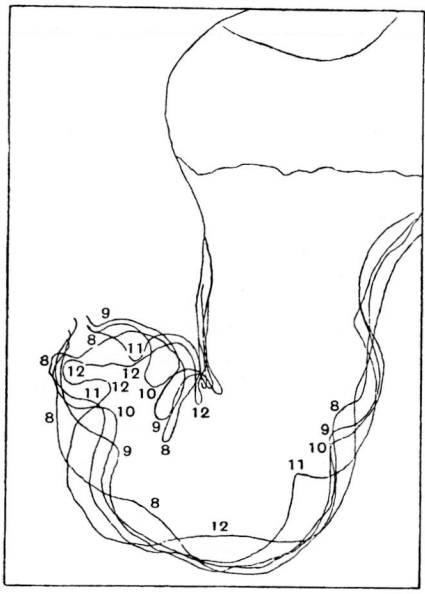
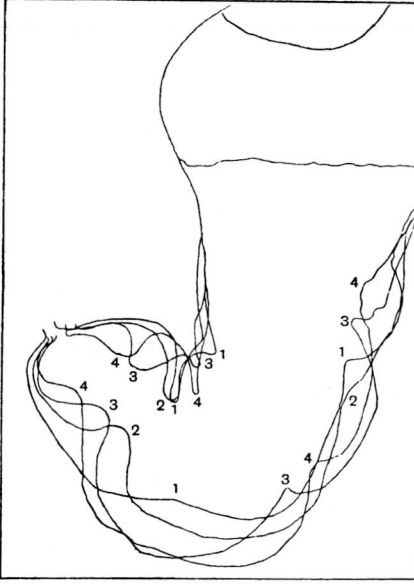

Fig. 135.   Fig. 136.

Fig. 135. Very active peristalsis of the stomach and propulsive movements of the antrum associated with hypersecretion. The deep "shovel-shaped" wave which appears to be travelling along the lesser curvature (No. 8) is really an indentation produced by the incisura angularis. The contraction passing over the incisura angularis displaces the direction of this fold. (Contributed by F. M. Groedel.)

Fig. 136. The same case showing another phase of the peristaltic cycle. (Contributed by F. M. Groedel.)

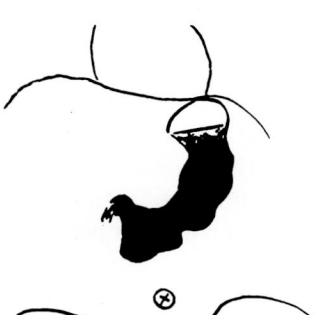
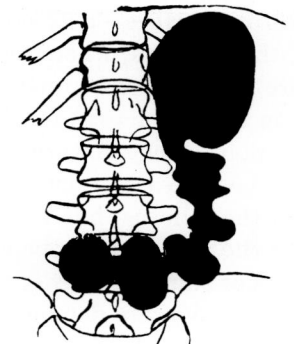

Fig. 137. A small stomach exhibiting rather active peristalsis. The duodenum is not seen, as it passes backwards.

Fig. 138. Tracing of a radiograph (Plate fig. 192). Recumbent position. It shows extremely active peristalsis. The patient had a small ulcer in the pyloric canal.

One of the earliest experiments I made was on this point. I gave a mouthful of opaque food and followed it by a meal of ordinary food: the opaque food outlined the lower border and did not mix. I then gave a watery suspension of bismuth. This outlined the non-opaque contents, flowing mostly around them, and in a short time all the opaque food, i.e. the heaviest gastric contents, had sunk to the lowest part (cf. Fig. 132). I think from this and other experiments that fluids can pass at all times round the food mass to the pylorus. Vice versa, the secretions, being lighter than the food, can flow up at all times and may usually be seen gathering as a non-opaque area between the air and the opaque food. I have never observed anything in the normal stomach suggestive of churning, though of course it occurs under abnormal conditions such as excessive peristalsis and retching. Some mixing in the pyloric antrum is brought about by the more powerful peristalsis caused by the relative obstruction of unmasticated lumps, but with the type of food now used this is not likely to be observed on the screen. Normally the foodstuffs in the stomach, having taken up positions according to their specific gravity, are gently stroked by the secretion-bearing mucous membrane as each successive wave of contraction passes along. The usual indentations of peristalsis do not appear to disturb the body of the food; they merely mould the surface. The mucous membrane also has independent movement (cf. p. 71 and Fig. 61).

The peristaltic movement is a ring contraction which travels at a regular pace down the length of the stomach. The rate is about three waves a minute, and each takes about twenty seconds to pass from end to end. The depth of the waves varies within wide limits (Figs. 135 to 138). A wave is first seen as an indentation on the greater curvature only, starting high up—perhaps as high as the cardiac orifice—and slowly progressing downwards as far as the lower third of the stomach, where an indentation also becomes definite on the lesser curvature. This is comparatively shallow because the muscle wall is so much thicker on the lesser than on the greater curvature; as the circular fibres have no fixed point, they naturally contract towards the most fixed part of the stomach, i.e. the lesser curvature. The indentations become deeper as they approach the pylorus, but I have made out no difference in their depth before and after the pylorus has opened to let some of the contents pass.

All sorts of combinations of peristaltic waves, systoles, tonus waves, wavelets and reverse waves are demonstrated by mechanical recorders, and recent work has shown more and more that the muscular movements of the stomach are by no means simple. Reverse peristalsis is sometimes seen on the screen, but only in cases of marked obstruction and, in my experience, in association with fairly extensive lesions involving the last inch of the lesser curvature (see p. 267). When there is definite obstruction, the usual appearance is a succession of powerful waves that gradually diminish in force as if the stomach wall were becoming exhausted. Then follows a period of rest during which no peristalsis or movement of any kind is noted other than occasional faint indications of waves that begin like ordinary waves but just die out and give the impression of futile attempts to continue the habitual routine of a lifetime.

Factors affecting Peristalsis

Generally speaking, the small type of stomach exhibits much less prominent peristalsis than does the average J-shape, and may in fact hardly show any at all. In an atonic stomach the waves are often no more than faint notches on the outline of the opaque food. In the recumbent position there is often no evidence of peristalsis affecting the stomach contents, but if the pyloric portion is filled by posturing the patient, by making him sit up and then holding the contents in position by pressure while he lies down again, the peristalsis can often be seen very plainly. There does not seem to be any appreciable difference between its actions in the upright position and in the horizontal position respectively, except that the waves tend to segment the food more in the horizontal position.

The normal stomach under normal conditions always exhibits peristalsis when it contains any food. A single mouthful of barium water given on an empty stomach will nearly always reveal a peristaltic wave. During the digestion of a fairly big meal, however, there are periods of rest or, at any rate, intervals in the activity. Whether the cause of this interruption is psychical, associated with the visit to an X-ray department or with the opaque meal, or whether it is part of the process of normal digestion, I do not know. It is, however, a constant feature when, owing to rapid emptying—perhaps associated with the continued action of a purgative—the small intestine becomes overloaded. The slowing-down or absence of peristalsis associated with the ileal stasis of a chronic inflammation in the appendicular region is described on p. 168. When gastric peristalsis is watched, its force is often seen to vary although its normal rhythm, one wave about every twenty seconds, is unaltered. Wingate Todd and his colleagues (213) have made many studies of the effect of the stomach contents on peristalsis in the normal subject. They say that a drink of water tends to increase the depth of the contractions but that the rhythm is undisturbed. Milk, on the other hand (301), tended to diminish the force of the waves, and to slow the rate of their travel in the body of the stomach. Buttermilk had a more definite slowing action. Waves induced by a soda meal were deep and forceful, and the effect on the rhythm was similar to that of buttermilk. Peppermint had little effect on the rhythm in the pyloric part but slowed the waves in the body; they were larger and more vigorous than usual. Soda and peppermint (314) tended to relieve undue closure, i.e. spasm, and thus assisted the passage of the food from the stomach to the duodenum. Heat and cold produced a marked increase not only in the depth of the contractions but also in the rhythm.

The study of the effect of the gastric contents is only one side of the picture, for other influences are at work. In severe headache, peristalsis often stops altogether. When the terminal ileum is overloaded, gastric peristalsis is diminished and there is delay in emptying. Again, when a patient has diarrhoea, although the intestine may be empty, yet gastric peristalsis is often weak or absent. Whether this is due to a reflex from the intestine or to psychic influences, I do not know. I mention these few instances to show how extremely complex the whole problem is, and to suggest that, valuable as individual studies may be, radiologists must not imagine that because they can trace a definite influence in one set of circumstances, they are even on the fringe of explaining the problem as a whole. There are many influences at work, and these are variables that can be balanced one against the other in order to achieve the desired result—i.e. efficient function in the conditions with which Nature is called upon to deal at the moment.

Hunger Movements

Peristalsis probably persists in a mild degree even when the stomach is empty. According to Alvarez [11], there are three types of hunger activity in the stomach of the dog. If the tone is poor the contractions last about 30 seconds and occur at about half-minute to 4-minute intervals. If the tone is good the contractions follow in close succession and are frequently interrupted by periods of incomplete tetany, which in man cause a continuous sensation of hunger. The third type shows periods of tetany with a series of rapid contractions superimposed, lasting from 1 to 10 minutes. Carlson [79] says that the hunger contractions in man are actual peristaltic waves coursing from one end of the stomach to the other. There has been much dispute whether or not the pain felt by patients suffering from ulcer is produced by these hunger movements. It seems clear that the essential feature in the production of pain is not an increase in the depth of the hunger contractions but an increase in the sensitiveness of the nerve endings. It is certain that the stomach cannot be put at rest by withholding food.

The Control of Peristalsis

Alvarez [13] believes that "the forces which bring about, modify and control peristalsis must be looked for mainly within the walls of the gut itself". He is sceptical of Bayliss and Starling's law that "a wave of contraction is preceded by a wave of relaxation when peristalsis passes down a muscular tube". By means of motion pictures he has shown that in the dog the peristaltic wave in the longitudinal muscle runs to the pyloric line, but the wave in the circular muscle changes at the pylorus into a systole. Further, the muscle next to the pylorus contracts so much more slowly than the segment just above it that the impression given by a study of the record may be that of a simple peristaltic wave, whereas in fact it is a systolic contraction of the circular fibres in the last centimetre or so. Alvarez attributes the hesitation of peristaltic waves between the body of the stomach and the pyloric portion to the difference in the rate of wave conduction in the two parts. At present little is known about the exact method of conduction of the wave of gastric contraction.

"The Gradient"

Alvarez[11], who has devoted an enormous amount of patient study to these movements, has formulated the theory—from animal experiments—that the response of the alimentary tract to stimulus is progressively slower from top to bottom; that the canal manifests, in fact, a "gradient" of activity. When a stimulus is applied to an excised segment of muscle taken from the upper end of the stomach, it responds much more rapidly than a similar segment taken from the lower end; the lower the place in the tract from which a segment is taken, the slower is its response. Whenever, therefore, the tract or any part of

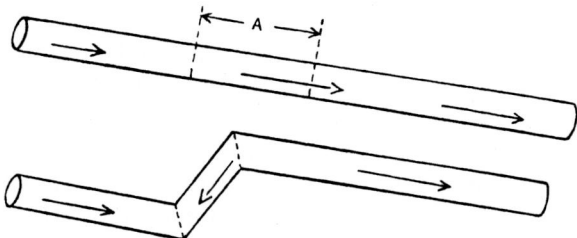

Fig. 139. Diagram to illustrate Alvarez's theory. The slope of the upper figure suggests the normal gradient down the alimentary tract. If a section, A, is excised and reinserted in the opposite direction, as in the lower figure, the grade is reversed in this section and it acts as a drain-trap. Fluids, it is found, are able to pass along, but solids cannot pass and obstruction occurs at the proximal end of the insertion.

it is stimulated, it responds not by a simultaneous contraction but by a descending wave of contraction. His theory is supported by the results of experiments on intestinal muscle excised from animals. If a short section of an animal's intestine is excised and reinserted the wrong way round, solids are invariably blocked at the upper union, though fluids may pass through. The reversed section, he infers, acts like the trap of a drain, interposing a short up-grade into the otherwise uniform down-grade of the tract. The pressure behind the food will lift fluids over the adverse grade but is not powerful enough to transmit solids (Fig. 139). He invokes this theory to explain coincident vomiting and diarrhoea. Some irritation or other stimulus, he suggests, disturbs the alimentary gradient in its course. When it reverses the gradient the patient vomits, and when it accentuates the ordinary declivity the faeces run through at an abnormal speed. Hence the diarrhoea and vomiting so frequently associated with abdominal conditions.

In my view this theory represents a distinct advance, and comes nearer than any other I know to explaining some of the puzzling things the radiologist sees. For instance, it suggests the reason why food is nearly always driven away from the site of an acute or semi-acute lesion. In conditions such as acute appendicitis and tuberculous caecum it is common to find the terminal ileum and ascending colon practically empty. In lesions of the colon the neighbouring lumen is nearly always found empty, and it is only in the later stages of obstruction that a coil of gut distended with food is found behind the block. Obviously, an inflamed section will respond more actively to stimulus and will therefore have a shorter reaction time than the healthy section above it—instead of a slightly longer one, as Alvarez has shown to be normal. Therefore it will interrupt the smooth gradient down the intestine.

THE CONTROL OF THE PYLORIC SPHINCTER

Why does the food go through the pylorus? It has been generally accepted that peristalsis is the chief motive power in the propulsion of food through the stomach and intestinal tract, but X-ray observation suggests very strongly that, although in obstruction it plays an important part, under ordinary conditions it is not so important as was formerly supposed. For instance, the food is often seen passing out of the stomach when practically no peristalsis is visible, and it is quite clear that other factors must be of equal, if not of greater, importance. One of these may be the increased gastric pressure due to tone; possibly the action of the muscularis mucosae also exerts a definite influence. In the normal subject in the upright position under normal conditions and with thoroughly masticated food there is very little suggestion of propulsion, and yet the food goes through intermittently. The relationship of its passage to the dictates of peristalsis is not causal. The first part of the opaque food to reach the pylorus may go straight through into the duodenum, but more frequently there is a delay of some minutes. The delay depends of course to a considerable extent on the type of food, the modern emulsion going through much more freely than the bread and milk opaque meal of other days.

Under ordinary conditions the opening of the pylorus does not seem to be controlled by the intragastric pressure, although under obstructive conditions the peristaltic action takes on such a forceful character that it is obviously trying to overcome resistance. In the body of the stomach the peristalsis is certainly not definitely propulsive; towards the pylorus the waves tend to segment the food shadow and give some appearance of propelling the food gently against the pylorus, but in most cases the food seems to slide back through the peristaltic wave and remain in the stomach, for the pylorus does not open at the call of each peristaltic wave, nor necessarily at the bidding of one wave that is more powerful than another.

Gravity and tonic action appear to play a part, but what determines whether the pylorus will open or not I do not know, for the waves appear identical in force, whether it relaxes or not. The artificial stoma of a gastro-jejunostomy sometimes acts in the same way as the pylorus after a few months, though at first the food passes through it more rapidly.

To obtain a satisfactory view of the duodenal cap the radiologist often attempts to push food through the pylorus. Experience shows that the period in the peristaltic cycle at which this manœuvre will most probably be successful is when a wave is about two inches from the pylorus. If at this moment the contents of the stomach are suddenly pushed against the pylorus and held there, the food will often pass through and fill the duodenum. Sometimes the manœuvre persistently fails in the upright position but is successful when the patient lies down. When the pylorus relaxes in these circumstances it does so in a most whole-hearted way and allows a gush of food to pass through that may fill not only the cap but the whole loop of the duodenum.

The peristaltic waves passing down the stomach stop at the pylorus and do not extend to the duodenum; Alvarez suggests that the separation of the two peristaltic activities is due to the strong admixture of fibrous tissue with the muscle in the pyloric ring. In most places the thick layer of sub-mucous fibrous tissue in this part divides the muscular sheets of the stomach and duodenum quite sharply from one another (Horton (162)). Auerbach's plexus, on the other hand, crosses from stomach to bowel without much break and thus effects co-ordination. There is a dynamic balance between the two viscera. That the contraction of the sphincter is not all-important in the mechanism of emptying is shown by the fact that after a time the stomach empties fairly normally even though the sphincter has been excised. The fact that the circular fibres of the stomach end abruptly at the pylorus and do not reappear as a definite layer till near the head of the duodenal cap (see p. 71) seems, however, to be a satisfactory explanation of the differences that are seen on the two sides of the pylorus.

One of the important factors determining whether or not a gastric wave forces food through the sphincter may be the way in which the wave approaches the pylorus. Deep peristaltic waves that pass right to the end of the stomach would seem more able to push food through than shallow waves that fade away or waves that end in systoles. Gianturco (132) has shown that the pylorus responds to approaching waves of peristalsis much as does the adjacent part of the pars pylorica; that food leaves the stomach when the pylorus and the duodenum are relaxed at the same time; and that relaxation of the pylorus alone is not followed by passage of food.

It is fairly definite that hunger is a factor in the opening of the pylorus. If the patient is more or less starved, as he usually is by the time the opaque examinations are made, the food will tend to pass out much more rapidly than when the intestines are filled. It is not uncommon to see the food passing out of the stomach rapidly—perhaps unduly rapidly—at the beginning of an examination, even in such quantities that the intestines become overloaded, and yet to find a considerable residue in the stomach after five hours. This phenomenon is often associated with delay behind the ileo-caecal valve (see p. 167), although it may be due to other causes. It has been attributed to an "ileo-pyloric reflex"(44), analogous to the reflex described by Hurst which determines the passage of food from the terminal ileum into the caecum when fresh food is taken. These observations seem to me to indicate that one very potent factor in the control of the pylorus is reflex from stimuli perhaps far remote from the pylorus itself. My impression is that the terminal ileum is very specially and intimately concerned but probably there is interconnection with the whole tract. I have even attributed delay in emptying of the stomach to a loaded rectum, but whether this was actually a reflex from the rectum or from the delay in the colon is merely conjectural. The various factors that have been associated with delayed emptying are considered with pyloric obstruction (p. 263).

Certainly the opening of the pylorus does not depend on the acidity or alkalinity of the food. Neither tartaric acid nor sodium bicarbonate seems to have any definite effect. Hurst(171) thought that the bismuth carbonate at one time used as an opaque medium neutralised the hydrochloric acid of the stomach, and he substituted the oxychloride. But, as far as I could tell, neither of these salts made any difference in the wayward response of the pylorus to the advances of peristalsis. Carman(80) added a routine quantity of sodium bicarbonate to the opaque food in the belief that it would ensure satisfactory filling of the duodenum. I followed this practice for some years, but eventually abandoned it because I did not think that it made any appreciable difference. Moreover, it had the disadvantage of neutralising the free acid so that the acidity of the contents could not subsequently be tested by estimating the evolution of gas after the administration of sodium bicarbonate—a test which has a certain very limited value in the diagnosis of malignancy. The secretion of acid is largely the function of the upper part of the stomach and only to a very limited extent of the pyloric portion. Meulengracht(235) has recently shown that the pyloric portion of the gastric glandular system is concerned with the production of the anti-anaemic factor and not with the digestive juices at all. Yet after pylorectomy, for some unknown reason, gastric acidity seems to be lowered. Watson(330a) makes the astonishing statement that two-thirds of the mucous membrane (four-fifths of the acid-secreting cells) can be removed without greatly influencing the gastric acidity.

That variations in gastric acidity occur in normal persons from day to day and hour to hour is brought out by Vanzant and Alvarez(18), who quote Lyon, Bartle and Ellison(223): "If the stomach contents of the same individual are examined daily...great variations will often be found in the gastric acidity";

pointing out, however, that these authors did not publish their data. They also quote Bell and MacAdam (57), who, "with a normal person as a subject, studied the gastric secretion for twenty consecutive days and treated the data statistically, but unfortunately, not in such a way as to answer our question". They gave figures for daily observations on two healthy young women and found such a large range of "individual variation that a single estimation of gastric acidity might well be very misleading". Moreover, "the total acidity varied as much as did the free acidity". They sum up as follows: "In the individual the daily range of variation in gastric acidity is so great that a single estimation may be very misleading. Apprehension over swallowing the tube the first few times did not seem to be a factor in modifying gastric acidity. In one of the subjects studied, painful emotion caused first a marked upward swing in the acidity and then a downward one. It may be that such upward swings, produced emotionally, can account for some of the flare-ups so often seen in the symptoms of peptic ulcer. There is some evidence that in women the degree of gastric acidity follows monthly cycles".

Shay and Gershon-Cohen (298), in attempting to solve the riddle of the control of the pylorus, have made many radiographically controlled experiments and, as would be expected, cannot come to any very definite conclusions. They maintain that gastric tonus is probably a more potent factor than peristalsis under normal conditions but that both are entirely dependent on the state of the pylorus. They have especially studied the effects of acids and alkalies in the stomach and believe that hydrochloric acid is the natural intrinsic agent responsible for pyloric action, although they disclaim any suggestion that it is the sole factor. Their work suggests that the gastric and duodenal contents do play a definite part in pyloric control, the stomach being, up to a point, a preparer of the food, which is not presented to the duodenum until it is suitable, the duodenum being a sensitive connoisseur.

No doubt chemical stimulation and food being prepared to the taste of the fastidious duodenum is one factor, but there are many others which are probably of far greater importance: food is often seen to pass into and through the duodenum with practically no pause in the stomach and certainly no opportunity for being prepared to the taste of the duodenum. Preparation may be a part of the story, but it seems to me a part of relatively little importance as compared with the more remote reflex influences controlling the pylorus.

I have already mentioned the effect of hunger and of accumulations of food behind the ileo-caecal valve, but also relevant in this connection are dental sepsis, sinus infection, reflex delay from gall-bladder trouble, constipation, diarrhoea (which may be associated either with very rapid emptying of the stomach or with delay), headache, fear and other psychical influences.

There is more than a tendency nowadays to belittle the digestive functions of the stomach. They appear to be of minor importance. In fact operation has shown that we can digest perfectly without the stomach and its secretions. It is just one more instance of the way in which Nature balances the various forces she has in reserve in order to arrive at the same result. The more one thinks of the control of the pylorus the more complex and incomprehensible it seems to be. Descriptive terms seem useless and even dangerous in a problem that is full of cross-references which all give the same answer but which all have floating values in the general scheme. A description of any one, or of any group, becomes, in the circumstances, little more than a half truth.

Boyd Orr[262], in summing up a lecture on secretion in the stomach, said: "It is obvious that the disorders of secretion, whether in excess or deficiency, are of much less importance in the aetiology of disease than was formerly supposed, but that movement is the function which plays the most significant part in the maintenance of health and in the causation of disease".

CHAPTER XII

THE INTESTINES

THE DUODENUM AND SMALL INTESTINE

In the first part of the duodenum the food forms a definite shadow, filling it out into a triangular cocked-hat shape—known to radiologists as the duodenal cap or bulb. The shadow tends to remain in this portion more or less as long as there is food in the stomach, but passes on from time to time. No peristalsis is noted in this segment, and its shape is often unchanged over quite long periods. We do not know why it empties, but the manner of the emptying appears to be less by a peristaltic wave than by a general contraction which, with the pylorus closed, pushes the food into the second part of the duodenum. Sometimes the oncoming of food from the stomach seems to project the duodenal contents onwards.

Beyond the duodenal cap there is a complete change: the comparative inaction of the stomach and the first part of the duodenum is succeeded by a restless and extremely efficient activity. It is difficult to see what happens, but the sharp, well-defined shadow of the first part of the duodenum is followed by an ill-defined and very much diffused outline, in which it is apparent that the mass of the food has been rapidly broken up and hurried off round the loop of the duodenum into the jejunum (Fig. 140). Some fragmenting action must be in progress to account for the extraordinarily fine sub-division. Whether this fragmentation is entirely due to a very active movement of the mucous membrane in co-ordinated association with the contractions of the duodenum itself, or whether to some other mechanism, is as yet impossible to say. It is certainly not due to peristalsis.

Fragmentation is observed in most cases but not by any means in all, for in a considerable proportion the food passes on from the first part of the duodenum in such large quantities that it cannot be dealt with by the fragmentation process, and therefore gives a fairly good shadow in the outline of the second and third parts of the duodenum. It may even pass on round the duodeno-jejunal flexure and some distance into the jejunum before it is fragmented and loses its solid outline. This behaviour is probably a variation of the normal rather than a pathological condition, although it is always marked when there is some obstruction at the duodeno-jejunal flexure. In that case the observer sees the food tossed backwards and forwards in the duodenum; there is something in the nature of peristalsis but the waves do not appear to be so much rhythmically and slowly progressive as intermittent and spasmodic types of contraction. Moreover, even when there is no definite obstruction, the food may be seen to collect in one part and pass backwards, sometimes into the duodenal cap and occasionally into the stomach itself. Bolton and Salmond (66), taking this appearance as normal, recognise four movements in the duodenum:

(1) Contraction of the cap (first part of the duodenum).

(2) Peristaltic contraction of the duodenum (other than the cap), propelling the contents forwards.

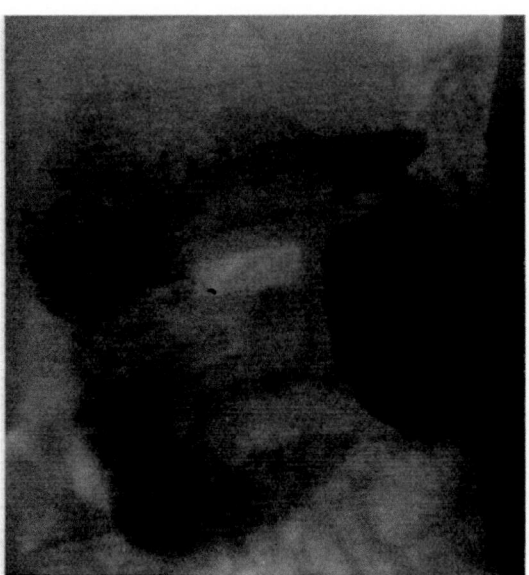

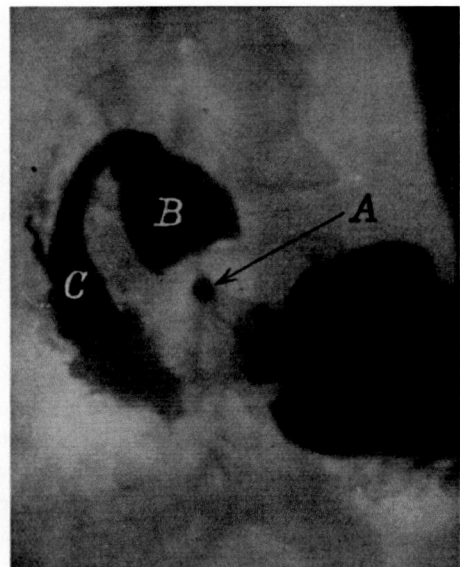

Fig. 140.   Fig. 141.

Fig. 140. Normal duodenal cap partially emptied, with the food fragmented in the second and third parts. Note the entire absence of any suggestion of peristalsis in the duodenum to account for this fragmentation. (Contributed by G. Harrison Orton).

Fig. 141. Normal duodenal cap (*B*). A peristaltic wave has just emptied the pyloric antrum, in which a small fragment, *A*, remains; in another moment it would have passed back into the stomach. It simulates a pyloric ulcer. The duodenal cap, *B*, has just been completely filled to replace the contents that have been projected en masse into the second part, *C*, in such quantity that they have not been fragmented.

(3) Contraction of the duodenum (other than the cap), forcing the contents backwards, presumably anti-peristalsis.

They maintain that anti-peristaltic movements are normal in the duodenum and tend to delay the passage of the food and to promote its disintegration.

(4) Segmentation, or mixing movements.

The division of the opaque food is so fine and its movements so rapid that I do not believe satisfactory information on the movements of this part of the tract will ever be obtained until effective cinematograph records of normal digestion in man are made. Such scanty radiographic information as there is about the function of the human intestine under normal conditions seems to

PLATE IV

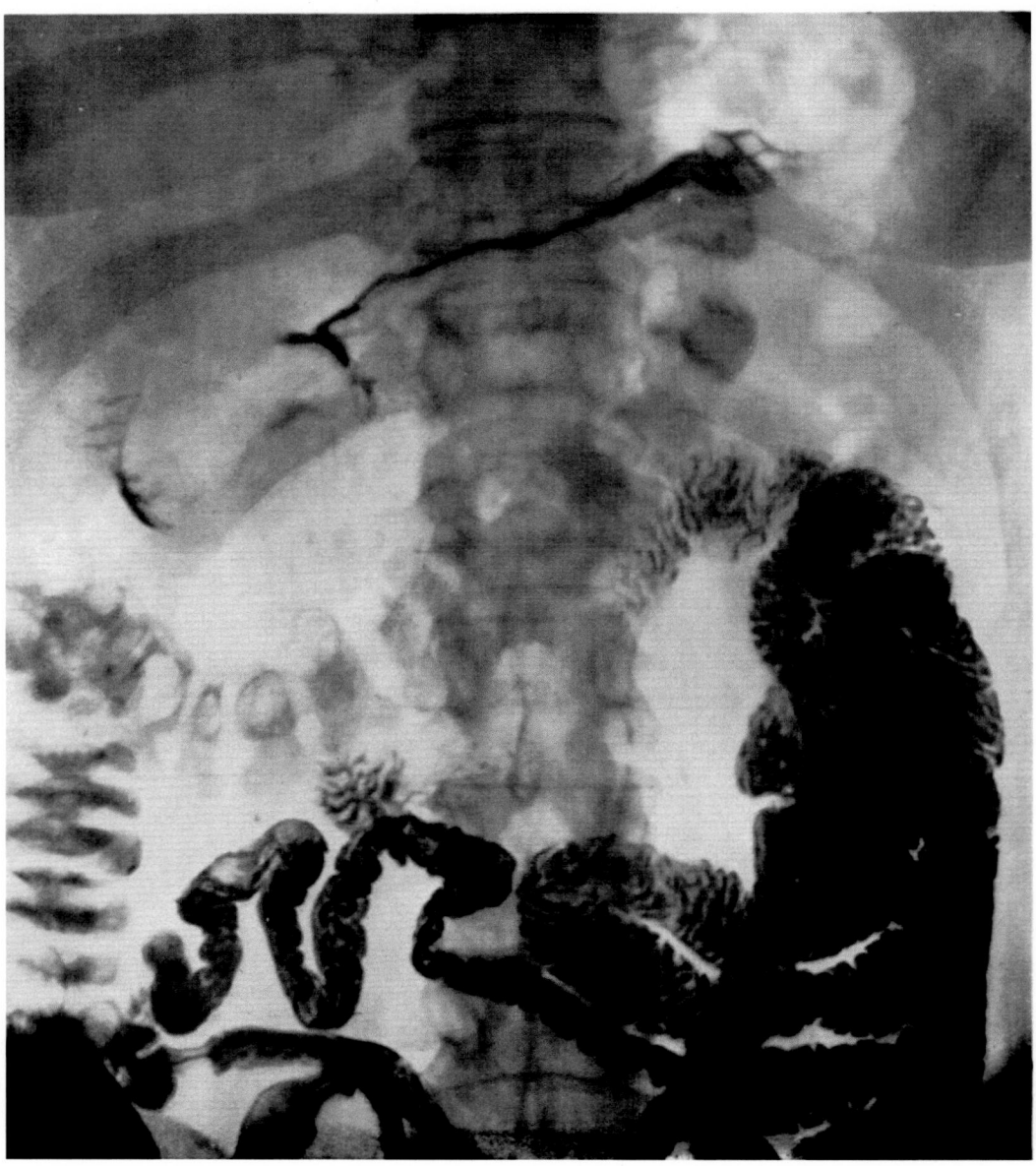

Fig. 142. Small intestine. Shows food passing through the small intestine and fairly evenly distributed. Note that the rugae are disposed on the whole transversely, but that towards the ileo-caecal valve they are in the line of the lumen of the gut. (The case is one of a fibroma of the stomach. See Fig. 223. Traces of the food are seen near the pyloric end surrounding the fibroma.) (Contributed by H. Graham Hodgson.)

confirm singularly little of the current teaching on its movements. The mechanism that fragments the food at the top of the duodenal cap seems comparable with a mincing machine. It tears and shreds the bolus most rapidly and effectively. There is no suggestion in the radiographs that this fragmentation is due to powerful contractions of the muscularis propria for, unless the duodenum is overloaded, there is certainly no peristalsis. The general outline is indicated by the scattered flocculent shadows of the divided opaque food (Figs. 140 and 198) and there is no indication of narrowings, progressive or otherwise. We are therefore driven to the conclusion that other forces are responsible, and the most likely would seem to be active movements of the muscularis mucosae. I made one short cinematographic record that seems to suggest two types of movement in the mucous membrane, i.e. a slow change in form of the rugae, and one that is extremely rapid but perhaps infrequent. In the series of pictures the mucous membrane pattern changes slowly; then there come one or two pictures that are blurred in detail, while the next ones, showing a changed pattern, are quite sharply defined again. When opportunity occurs I hope to confirm and repeat observations such as this on other subjects.

From the duodeno-jejunal flexure onwards it is impossible to observe what happens under normal conditions, for the fragmentation of the food is so fine that it is not seen as a definite shadow upon the screen, but as a cloudy opacity. If the observer analyses a section of it, he will find what appear to be small collections of the barium lodged between the folds of the mucous membrane. In contradistinction to the gastric folds, those in the duodenum and small intestine seem for the most part to be disposed irregularly across the lumen of the gut. The shadows suggest myriads of snowflakes arranged transversely rather than longitudinally, but in Plate fig. 142 the food has passed through so rapidly that the intestine has been overloaded and the normal appearance of a multitude of finely-divided shadows is lost. Although the gut itself seems to move about, it does not necessarily dislodge these collections. Sometimes, when food has collected in a coil, there is evidence of peristaltic waves sweeping along sections of the gut; they may or may not disturb these small collections, although they seem to drive on the larger collections.

The movements of the muscularis mucosae are probably of far greater importance than would have been expected. It is likely that they are capable of dealing with the propulsion, fragmentation and turning over of the intestinal contents quite effectively under easy conditions. The function of the muscularis propria seems to be that of a "stand-by", a reserve mechanism that comes to the rescue if called upon. The two mechanisms might be likened to the weir and flood-gates of a river. One or more of the flood-gates are used to relieve the weir. If a block of wood will not pass over the weir it is let down through a flood-gate, or, if it is necessary to flush out the bed of the stream, all the flood-gates are opened. Only in emergency are all the possible channels used to full capacity. The analogy should not be taken too far, but it gives my meaning, i.e. that throughout the intestinal tract peristalsis can be regarded not as the main factor but as one of the main reserve mechanisms. It is the heavy duty machine that stands behind the light duty mechanism of the action of the muscularis mucosae, aided perhaps by other factors.

When the small intestine becomes overloaded, owing to over-rapid emptying of the stomach, there is evidence of peristaltic waves which push the food on-ward but seem to involve only a small section of gut before they die away, to be followed by other waves in the same section driving the contents in the reverse direction. Whether this phenomenon is normal or not it is difficult to say, for the mere presence of masses of any size may be abnormal, but the effect upon the food is apparently to drive a bolus some distance in one direction and then to return it over part of its course.

In the intestine the opaque shadows are exceedingly difficult to interpret, but they convey the impression that peristalsis is much less important than the constant motion of the muscularis mucosae. Moreover, an observer with the mechanism of swallowing in mind will suspect that negative pressure may also play a part. Alvarez very kindly placed at my disposal his cinematograph film of exposed rabbit and cat intestines, and I studied the motions to see if I could find any signs of it; certain sections of the film show flattened, collapsed coils into which the food rushes in a manner quite compatible with a mechanism that might be imagined to produce negative pressure. The coils behave, in fact, just like an india-rubber tube which flattens when the air is sucked out of it and expands when fluid is allowed to enter it from above. At present, however, there is no means of confirming this suggestion, for the conditions in the open abdomen are necessarily abnormal, and instruments inserted into a hollow viscus may bring into action mechanisms which play no part in its ordinary life. When efficient cinematographic X-ray studies are possible, they will give a better idea of the movement of food along the tract.

The Terminal Ileum

The activity of the movements, both of peristalsis and probably also of seg-mentation, which give rise to the fragmentation of the food in the whole of the jejunum is very marked. Only when the ileum is reached do definite shadows of the opaque food begin to collect and remain more or less inert. This quiescence of the terminal ileum calls for comment; waves of peristalsis are comparatively seldom seen, and the picture there is a very different one from the restlessness of the duodenum and jejunum. I do not recollect ever having seen powerful waves in the terminal ileum, although I have seen twisting movements.

The last coils before the ileo-caecal valve are almost as inert as the caecum and large intestine, and it seems as if the last few inches were different in function from the rest. This portion is not tortuous, but runs more or less straight upwards and outwards to the caecum. Its calibre is smaller, and the chyme in it forms a continuous shadow which looks different from that in other parts of the small intestine. The appearances suggest that the circular muscle fibres are more evenly developed and that tonic action is a more persistent feature of the muscular function. In this region the mucosal rugae run more or less regularly along the axis of the gut, forming half a dozen lines. The whole of this terminal portion appears to be closely associated with the sphincteric and valvular action that is ascribed to the ileo-caecal valve itself. Possibly its mechanism is similar to that of the cardia, and ileal stasis should be called "achalasia of the ileo-caecal valve", but there is not yet sufficient knowledge to justify this description.

Normally delay occurs at the ileo-caecal valve, which the opaque food may reach in anything from a quarter of an hour onwards. Hunger, irritability, drugs and various other factors may speed up the passage of the food and give the impression of a much earlier arrival at this point than is actually normal in ordinary life. In the routine that I employ, I do not as a rule see the patient at the time when the first food passes through the ileo-caecal valve, but whenever I have made observations on this point, under the most normal conditions that I can obtain, I have seen the first of the food in the caecum at about $1\frac{1}{2}$ to 2 hours.

The mechanism of the filling of the caecum from the terminal ileum is not understood, but it is certain that the food gradually fills up the caecum, although no marked movement to produce filling is visible.

I have only once seen definite movement in this section of intestine; the observation was made in a normal male student during a demonstration. The caecum was well filled and the terminal ileum formed a uniform tubular shadow running into it. As I watched, I saw a segmenting constriction in this shadow about half an inch from the caecum, and almost immediately a similar constriction appeared about two inches further back. The shadow between the two constrictions was fusiform, tailing off at both ends; it remained stationary for a few seconds and was then projected into the caecum. The movement was over in perhaps 15 seconds, and after it the terminal ileum was empty. I did not observe its refilling, which took place within the next 10 minutes.

The Gastro-ileac and Ileo-gastric Reflexes

Moynihan, I believe, made an epigram to the effect that the most frequent seat of a gastric ulcer is in the right iliac fossa. All surgeons must now appreciate the underlying truth of this. Observations have gradually accumulated to indicate a very close connection between the ileo-caecal region and the duodenum. Radiography shows that the entrance of food into the stomach tends to make the ileum empty into the caecum (the gastro-ileac reflex of Hurst).

I have described (48) a series of cases which indicate another type of connection, i.e. a definite ileo-gastric reflex, back from the terminal ileum to the stomach:

In certain cases of the duodenal irritation or ulcer type the stomach began to empty very rapidly, overloading the small intestine. In a short time (say three-quarters of an hour), if the quantity of the food was small, the stomach was empty. Yet, when a reasonably large meal was given, it was found that, instead of the stomach being empty in the usual four hours, there was actual delayed emptying, and that in some cases quite half the food was still present after seven or eight hours. On again watching the progress of the food, I noticed that, so far as could be determined, this rapid emptying and general activity of the stomach ceased when the shadows reached the terminal ileum, and that in each case there was quite well-defined ileal stasis and very little, if any, food seemed to be passing on into the caecum.

These observations give the impression that any abnormality of the terminal ileum may cause a reflex closure of the pylorus and a quieting down of the gastric activity; in other words, a message is sent from a nervous centre in the ileo-caecal region to the centre in the duodeno-pyloric region stating that as much food has come down as can be dealt with, and requesting that supplies be shut off. In nearly all these cases I found at a seven hours' examination that there was a complete gap between the food in the stomach and that which was collected in a mass behind the ileo-caecal valve. All the cases submitted to operation showed definite evidence of old inflammatory changes in the ileo-caecal region. The importance of this observation is plain; it throws light on that curious manifestation, appendix dyspepsia, and also on the comparative frequency with which these patients complain of pain in the duodenal region when pressure or manipulation is applied over the site of the appendix.

Lane's kink I have not recognised radiographically, and I am far from convinced that it is a cause of either ileal stasis or of this ileo-pyloric reflex.

The ileo-caecal valve

The ileo-caecal valve has been very carefully studied by Hurst, Case, Cole and others, both by feeding methods and by means of opaque enemata. Hunter (164) maintains that the lower fold of the frenulum coli acts as a valve and that the caeco-colic sphincter is incorporated with it. The valve action therefore depends on the position of the terminal portion of the ileum; when it is raised there is no valve action and the sphincter opens and permits food to pass from ileum to caecum. Freedom of movement from the terminal ileum is therefore essential for the free passage of food to the large intestine. Earlier writers suggested that the ileo-caecal valve, if normal, should be quite resistant to the injected enema and that no leakage should take place into the ileum. In at least 16 per cent. of cases, however, some of the injection does pass through, i.e. the valvular action is incompetent. In one of my own cases I saw an injection flow quite freely, not only into the ileum but also into the jejunum; some of it I actually located in the duodenum! Case (89) states that when this phenomenon is noted radio-scopically, the incompetence can be confirmed at the operation by "milking" the food or air in either direction, and Kellogg (195) has devised an operation for the repair of the valve or the formation of a new one.

As a cause of ileal stasis this defect is well worthy of consideration, and Cole (101) asks if it is likely that the small intestine will tolerate regurgitated faecal matter without giving rise to symptoms of some kind, probably referred to the stomach. This incompetency of the ileo-caecal valve probably explains why patients sometimes state that they can taste a soap enema. A patient is stated to have actually vomited a part of an oil enema within half an hour (77).

Alvarez (12) says: "I have talked with a number of intelligent persons who objected to their nutrient enemas because of the bitter taste of the peptones given. Dr Emge...tells me it has been his custom to give coffee enemas, which soon tinge the vomitus;...chemical analysis showed that it was coffee and not blood. This article could be filled with such observations culled from medical literature". An interesting paper on the subject was published in 1924 by Parkes Weber (333).

My considered opinion is that the competence or incompetence of the ileo-caecal valve is of no significance in diagnosis.

THE LARGE INTESTINE

THE APPENDIX

The appendix is readily recognised when it is filled with opaque food, and, in a systematic examination, is always sought with the patient lying down. By posturing the patient and using a wooden spoon, as suggested by Holzknecht (161), the shadows can be manipulated, and the caecum can be brought up out of the pelvis, as described by Case (89), so that the lower end of the organ is quite clear of the shadows of the ileum. In one patient I had the opportunity of watching various movements in an appendix nearly six inches long and completely filled. I saw the shadow cut up into five oval beads, and then the organ emptied itself; a few minutes later the shadow again appeared and remained stationary, with the exception of worm-like writhing movements while the food canalised it; these persisted for a few minutes after it was completely filled.

In my early hospital cases I used to find the appendix in about 30 per cent. only. Case found it in about 50 per cent. of all patients; while George (128) gave a figure as high as 80 per cent. A third day examination often reveals an appendix that has not previously been visualised. Those who have employed magnesium sulphate after the opaque meal (p. 15) state that by this technique they can visualise the appendix in most cases. Case states that he can sometimes "milk" the food into the empty appendix, a manœuvre in which I have only once been successful.

CÆCUM AND COLON

In the caecum the food collects and forms a very heavy indented shadow, but there are no peristaltic waves and no movement that is easily detected on the fluorescent screen (Fig. 143). Serial radiographs show alterations in the contour but they do not show what the radiologist usually pictures as peristaltic waves. How the food passes upwards from the caecum and into the ascending colon is obscure. Sometimes the colon almost appears to fill by pressure from behind. No sudden change of picture is observed in the terminal ileum, caecum and ascending colon. Whatever change there is in the distribution of the food seems to take place slowly, and it is possible that filling depends to some extent upon respiratory movement, for this portion of the intestine, like all others, is affected by respiration; the alternate lifting and lowering of the ascending colon may have some pumping or suction effect.

"MASS" MOVEMENT

It is evident that the slow peristalsis which used to be described in the large bowel does not take place—at any rate it is never seen—and the only change in the shadow is that occasionally a small bolus rolls from one saccule into another in a manner which does not suggest any action that could accomplish the normal passage of faeces. Certainly such a movement could not account for the fact that from time to time the shadow is found to have extended many inches or even feet farther along the colon during a short interval—possibly one of a few minutes only—between two examinations of the abdomen.

More than twenty years ago Holzknecht (161), who had already performed a vast number of examinations, published his observations on two cases in which he had seen certain movements that would account for these changes (Fig. 144). He twice saw the faecal shadow traverse suddenly a length of the colon, and this change in the position of the faeces was unaccompanied by any subjective sensation. From these two observations he propounded the theory that this phenomenon was normal, and that the progress from the caecum to the anus was accomplished by these movements. He said:

"Suddenly, during the examination, the segmentation in the transverse colon disappeared so rapidly that the eye could hardly follow the movement. We had the impression that the haustral segmentation disappeared at the same instant along the whole of this part of the intestine. On the other hand, the ascending colon in no wise altered its appearance. The outline of the transverse colon became smooth, like that of a ribbon with parallel borders, with no trace of segmentation edging. Almost immediately this ribbon broke at the hepatic flexure, and was forced forwards, without altering its length, into the descending colon, which up to that time had been empty. The passage from one portion of the colon to the next was extraordinarily rapid when compared with our former conception of the peristaltic contraction of the colon. According to our estimation, the movement occupied at most three seconds. At first the newly-filled descending colon also presented the appearance of a ribbon with parallel edges without fringes. Immediately the transference was accomplished, however, the haustral segmentation reappeared and, as far as we could make out, over the whole length of the descending colon at the same moment. Although the observation was continued for some time, no further movement was visible; the transverse colon remained empty, and the contents of the ascending and descending portions

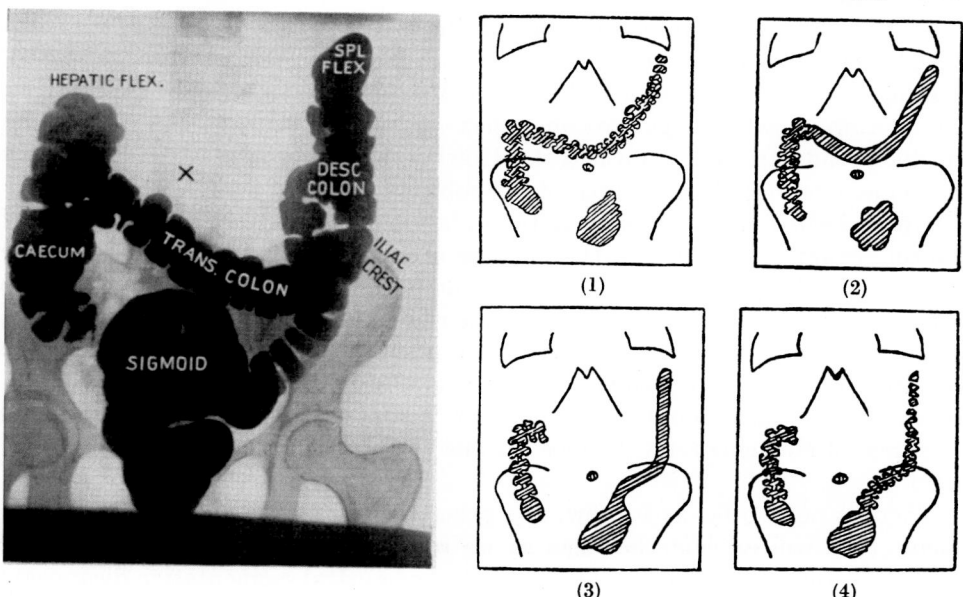

Fig. 143. Normal large intestine, particularly well filled from end to end.

Fig. 144. Mass movement. (From Holzknecht's original paper.)

remained undisturbed. During the whole time the patient was not aware of any subjective sensation of any description."

Two years later I reported (30) two cases which confirmed these observations. The following is the description given at the time:

"As is my custom, I examined the patient again after twenty-four hours to confirm the diagnosis. The bismuth food had all passed into the large intestine, and filled the caecum and the ascending and transverse colon to a point about six inches from the splenic flexure. The patient swallowed a mouthful of bismuth food.... It was as the first food entered the stomach that the faecal shadows suddenly moved on, so quickly that the eye could hardly follow the movement, although the X-ray tube was working perfectly. In less than three seconds, I judged, the shadows in the colon again showed the usual picture of still-life to which we are accustomed. Nevertheless in this short time the faeces had passed on through some 12 inches of the large intestine, including the splenic flexure. It appeared to be a movement of the whole of the contents from the caecum onwards, and on examination I found no break in the shadow from the caecum to nearly six inches beyond the splenic flexure. So far as I could make out, the haustral segmentation disappeared during this movement, but on this point I am not certain. Beyond this there is nothing to record; the bowels were opened naturally next day and, although I made persistent attempts to see the phenomenon again, I failed."

In the second case I happened to take plates before, during and after a mass movement.

It was not until Hurst (168) studied the phenomenon systematically that Holzknecht's somewhat revolutionary theory became more or less established. Taking advantage of the fact that the call to stool usually follows close after the morning meal—the gastro-colic reflex—he made a series of observations on medical students, and confirmed the Holzknecht theory. He actually saw the movement taking place in three of the subjects.

Up to 1915 I had only seen it take place some ten times in the course of routine examination but, in the absence of any other explanation, I became entirely convinced that it is the natural and normal movement. In one of three students whom I examined as they ate their breakfast and for a time afterwards, I saw the movement most perfectly; and in another I happened to look at the intestine just as the movement was ending. Jordan (188) has also recorded observations on these movements, but Case's report to the 17th International Congress of Medicine (89) is the most extensive and scientific treatise that I have seen.

There is not, so far as I know, any other theory, except this of mass movement, that will explain the facts as we see them. All observers agree that, without subjective sensations of any kind, the haustral segmentation disappears and the whole mass rushes suddenly—in three seconds, Holzknecht suggested—through a length of colon. In all my cases it happened that the head of the column was in the transverse colon and, when the movement had finished, the head of the shadow had passed round to the splenic flexure and some distance down the descending colon.

On one occasion I saw a portion of the shadow in the ascending colon detach itself and traverse the whole length of the colon into the sigmoid. When the movement was over, a slight anti-peristaltic mass movement took place, in the nature of a rebound, and part of the shadow returned through the iliac colon to just above the iliac crest. The whole movement occupied about ten seconds.

The complete process is over in a very short time, and the haustral segmentation returns in a few moments, the general picture of still-life being almost immediately restored. My impression is that the perfectly natural movement is somewhat slower; at any rate it has appeared to be so since I had my patients prepared sixty hours before I proposed to observe the large bowel. In one instance I timed the passage from the middle of the transverse colon to the pelvic brim as 15 seconds; but in all the other cases the passage was so unexpected that it was almost completed before I had time to realise what was happening.

The mechanism appears to be: (1) a relaxation of the tonic action of the muscular coats so that the haustral segmentations disappear; followed by (2) a big peristaltic wave that sweeps the whole contents along. How often this movement takes place we do not know. Like defaecation, it is probably an individual habit. Incidentally, it is interesting to note that the firm and solid appearance of the colon shadows, both on the film and also on palpation, is due to the tonic action holding the more or less fluid faeces in definite form.

The Mechanism of Mass Movement

I have often noted the formation of a definite constriction, a *point d'appui*, such as I suspect is necessary for the efficiency of the mass movement. In the majority of cases it was near the hepatic flexure, and was not evident until this was palpated out with the spoon. I am not absolutely certain on the point, but I believe that the sphincter tended to appear after palpation of the caecum in the exploration of the appendicular region. The colon distal to the constriction lost its haustral segmentation, and the contents seemed to back up to the *point d'appui*, as if forming a mass ready to be propelled onwards when the mass movement took place. In some of these cases a strong mass movement occurred within half an hour, but I did not actually see it. The whole column on the distal side of the *point d'appui* was swept along. In one or two instances about half of it was left behind, but these colons did not look healthy and, in fact, there was said to be mucous colitis.

On other occasions, I have seen the *point d'appui* in the splenic end of the transverse colon. The haustral segmentations first disappeared, leaving a fat sausage-shaped mass in which a constriction developed after a few minutes. Shortly after the formation of this sphincter, the mass distal to it started and moved comparatively slowly, in about 45 seconds I should say, round the splenic flexure and down to the rectum.

I am convinced that the keystone to the efficiency of this mass movement of the large intestine lies in the competence of the *point d'appui*.

The problem of the passage of food through the large intestine is full of difficulty, not only because the observations are few and far between, in spite of the vast number of patients examined, but also because the whole conception of mass movement is revolutionary and alien to the traditional line of thought.

It would be easier if we had not been brought up on armchair conceptions of what takes place, for unconsciously we attempt to make our observations fit in with our preconceived notions.

OTHER MOVEMENTS

Case (89) gives incontrovertible proof of anti-peristalsis in the large intestine, and it can probably occur in the normal healthy subject; in fact I have actually seen it after a mass movement (see above). Probably anti-peristalsis is exactly analogous with the usual forward mass movement, but in the opposite direction.

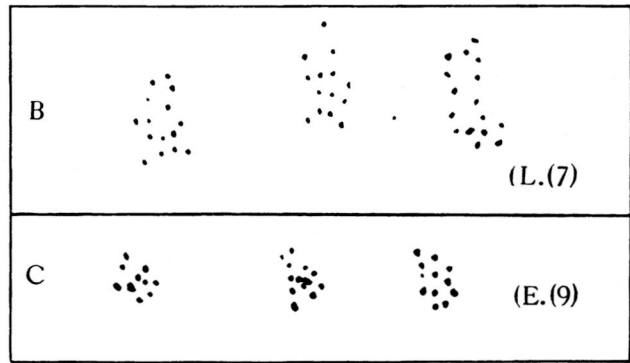

Fig. 145. *B*, movements of opaque seeds in the ascending colon. (Films taken at the rate of 1 in ten seconds.) Probably about half of the movement recorded in the vertical direction is due to respiration. *C*, movements of opaque seeds in the descending colon. (Films taken at the rate of 1 in seven and a half seconds.) Little, if any, respiratory movement appears to be included in the excursion of the shadows of the pellets, which seem, on the whole, to be moved more or less in circles. No indication is, of course, obtained of the movements in the third dimension.

It is not actually seen on injecting an enema, but in most cases as much as a pint will be carried back to the caecum, especially if the patient is suitably postured, which seems to suggest an anti-peristaltic action.

Besides the mass movement, changes are from time to time seen in the shape of the haustral segments of the large intestine, especially of the transverse and descending colon. This movement is not at all conspicuous, and probably has no connection with the progress of food along the intestine. The Cole Collaborators(102a) maintain that the haustra do in fact pass slowly along. Their movements cannot be seen on the screen, and can only be recorded by making a series of exposures at relatively long intervals. The technique is difficult, owing to the effects of respiration, and there is a possibility of misinterpretation.

I attempted to record the movements of the haustra using a direct cinematograph apparatus* taking pictures 5 in. square capable of making eight pictures a

* I am indebted to the Medical Research Council for a substantial grant towards the building of this apparatus.

second, but, for this study, operating at only about four a minute. These movements are slow and intermittent, and may be localised to individual haustra. They are not in the nature of propulsive peristaltic waves and do not appear either to produce definite progression in the intestinal contents or to have directional intention. The waves may progress over a certain distance and then come back over the same course. Often they are entirely absent. They seem to be concerned solely with the turning-over of the intestinal contents and, one would imagine, with the mixing and dehydrating process that tends to give a uniform consistency to the stools. These observations are very incomplete and tentative, and I hope to continue them as soon as opportunity offers. Some experiments, however, have been made with bismuth pills coated with celluloid. When the records so far obtained were transferred to a chart (Fig. 145) they showed that the pillules that moved (apart from the transmitted movements of respiration) followed a more or less circular course.

Rieder described "large pendulum" movements, which appear to be much the same as the smaller haustral churning of which evidence is often obtained. Case[89] states that every time he has seen the larger type of movement it has been the precursor of a mass movement.

Recent Work with Cinematograph Films

I have not been able to do more direct cinematography but I have transferred strips of serial film to 16 mm. cinematographic film making several frames from each serial picture. The resulting ciné-picture is rather jerky but confirms the movements that I had deduced from charting on transparent films and has also revealed a new movement in the caecum. In my original film I had not detected any definite movement as I was looking for changes in the haustra, but in the new films a definite systole and diastole can clearly be seen: a general contraction and expansion of the caecum without change in the haustra. This might possibly be due to transmission of respiratory movement, but it looks more like a slow, intrinsic pumping action.

Defaecation

A mass movement does not necessarily induce a call to stool; it has never done so when I have seen it, even though the faecal column has passed well down the sigmoid. Distention of the rectum is generally held to be the exciting cause of a call to stool.

When the colon is examined after a motion, it is usually found to have been voided from the splenic flexure onwards. Hurst[168] described the mechanism and his X-ray observations of the process, but before the absence of colonic peristalsis and the nature of the mass movement had been discovered.

The raised intra-abdominal pressure due to the action of the diaphragm and abdominal muscles plays a very large part. Whether the colon functions in the same way as in the mass movement has not yet been observed, so far as I am aware, but this seems likely.

In the hen the mechanism has been observed by me fairly frequently. The colon loses the haustral segmentation and its curves straighten out, giving the impression that its length is diminished while its calibre remains constant; i.e. it looks as if the circular fibres are fixed in tonic contraction while the longitudinal fibres contract, shortening the tube and extruding the contents through the rectum. Possibly the same occurs in man, but one would expect that, after a preparatory mechanism of this kind, there would also be some form of peristaltic wave to expel the column.

CONSTIPATION

There is a vast literature on the colon and its diseases, but extraordinarily little has been written in recent years on its physiology. Glancing through the titles, one is struck by the fact that the papers are mainly written by radiologists and clinicians. The whole subject of the physiology of the colon seems to be in chaos, and there is no satisfactory basic knowledge. Because we do not know the normal, we derive little profit from either the clinical or the radiological study of the large intestine, except in a few very definite and specified conditions, such as neoplasm, diverticulitis and polyposis. Even the subject of constipation, which is of such universal interest and importance, is still extremely confused. The ubiquitous advertising of proprietary drugs for the treatment of constipation, real or imagined, has made the public "bowel conscious", and the wide variations that are possible within the limits of normality and the indefinable borderlands are misinterpreted as definitely pathological. It is more than likely that the persistent use of purgatives so disturbs the natural variations that Nature has difficulty in coping with these interferences and a definite pathological condition results.

Whether constipation should be regarded as a pathological condition or as a disorder of physiology is a debatable question. I have treated it here, rather than in Part III, because it is so closely bound up with physiology as to be inseparable from it.

X-ray observations constantly reveal the unreliability of a patient's statements as to constipation. Some who deny constipation show conditions that appear quite incompatible with free bowel movement, while others who complain of constipation show the opaque food passing through without apparent delay. The variations observed in healthy subjects are so wide that it is little wonder that no satisfactory definition of constipation has ever been framed. The individual habit and the effect, both physical and mental, of the presence of food in the large bowel are so diverse that there can be no standard, and each subject must be a law unto himself. Constipation, or rather the complaint of constipation, depends very largely on the patient's outlook and upbringing. The infant strictly schooled in a certain habit will attempt to conform to this habit throughout life, no matter what routine Nature may have designed as the correct one for his individual requirements.

Constipation is not purely mechanical, nor is it merely a question of "roughage", of toxic absorption, or of a referred mental impression; a combination of these and other factors, particularly habit, makes the subject uneasy because the bowels have not acted at a certain time or because the call to stool fails. These patients often have morbid obsessions on the subject: they believe that their health depends on regular action of the bowels at a certain hour and so many times a day. Constipation gets on their minds. They take an unhealthy interest in lurid advertisements of patent remedies, develop the purgative habit, and become hypersensitive and apprehensive of any slight irregularity. They expect symptoms to develop. Moreover, there is always a tendency to depression and headache when symptoms are attributed to the large bowel. Osler is said to have declared that disease above the diaphragm tends to optimism and disease below the diaphragm to pessimism. The association of depression with constipation, real or fancied, and various colonic conditions lends support to his dictum.

In extreme cases obsession as to the action of the large bowel may become frank psychosis. One lady who complained of intractable constipation, for which she had taken purgatives and enemata for years, was with difficulty dissuaded from taking purgatives even for the one day of the examination. I was able to convince her that there was not a trace of the barium meal left in any part of the tract after 24 hours, in spite of her statement that the bowels had not acted or had only acted very ineffectively. After confirming my observations and convincing myself, I thought I had entirely relieved her mind, for it was clear that something was preying on her nerves, and both she and her husband, a doctor, imagined it was her bowel condition. We were all mistaken for, being relieved of this obsession, another, which had apparently been displaced by it, returned, and she committed suicide the following day. From the evidence at the inquest it seemed to be reasonably clear that it was the horrors and terrors of her flight from Russia in the revolution that were the real underlying trouble, and these had been masked for some years by the obsession of constipation; during these years she had lived in England, had married and had borne a child.

From his observations on students, Hurst (168) suggested that the average normal times in which food should reach various points were:

Caecum	$4\frac{1}{2}$ hours	
Hepatic flexure ...	$6\frac{1}{2}$	,,
Splenic flexure ...	9	,,
Brim of pelvis ...	11	,,

He is insistent on the fact that these are only average times, and that wide differences are possible even in perfectly normal subjects. If a mass movement some three or four times a day is normal, wide variations are likely.

Alvarez and Freedlander (14) carried out some experiments with small glass beads and came to the conclusion that food was retained in the bowel very much longer than had previously been supposed. They gave fifty very small—2 mm. diameter or less—chemically inert glass beads in a gelatine capsule; they found that these beads mixed intimately with the food and did not appear to have any influence on intestinal motility, certainly no more than that of seeds from berries or figs. The subjects were healthy young male medical students and some patients convalescing from minor operations. The striking fact emerged that the normal individual with a good digestion and a daily bowel movement did not pass anything like 100 per cent. of the beads in 24 hours; the majority of the subjects took four days to get rid of 75 per cent. and some had only passed half the beads at the end of the ninth day. Average percentages worked out as follows: 15 per cent. of the beads were passed by the end of the first day; 40 per cent. on the second day; 15 per cent. on the third, and from 5 to 10 per cent. on the fourth and fifth days. One constipated subject passed the last bead on the 40th day. On the second day the beads always came through a little faster than on the first day, and on the third day even faster than on the second. The rate of progress was found to vary widely in normal persons, but fast rates were associated with the passage of soft, badly-digested stools. A barium meal was found to have a purgative effect, so that X-ray experiments invariably indicated a faster rate of progress than that found to be normal with the beads by themselves. Usually the greater part of the barium was expelled within 24 hours, but from 15 to 50 per cent. might be left in the bowel after the preliminary extrusion, and would be slowly passed during the next four or five days (cf. p. 56).

Constipation has been defined by Hurst and others, but I would rather avoid doing so, for any definition leads not only medical men but also their patients into a fundamentally false conception. Each case is an individual, and this fact must not be lost sight of merely for the sake of making a definition. Some patients are always out of health if a daily action is not obtained; while others may regain health when they cease to worry their intestines into daily actions and establish a habit of twice a week. It is for the patient and his medical man to find out what Nature designed for that individual. Every engine has an optimum speed at which it is not only most efficient but at which it works most smoothly and lasts longest.

My own experience indicates that there are three types of constipation:

(1) an absence of mass movement, inertia of the colon; (2) stagnation in the caecum and (3) stagnation in the rectum.

Of these, the colonic inertia is the most frequent; the shadow of the food in the colon is unchanged for days on end. Some observers have suggested that the colon is hypertonic, but I do not think that the tonic state of the colon is in any way responsible for the delay; this is due to the absence of mass movement.

In the second type of constipation the delay is in the caecum and ascending colon; these portions remain filled for days at a time, in spite of the fact that some of the contents may have moved on to various portions of the colon. In other words, the mass movement takes place but is defective, the defect being not of a part of the colon, but of the mechanism. The constipation is probably due to inability to obtain a more or less fixed point, a *point d'appui* or temporary sphincter from which to work, rather than to a defect in the movement itself. If the *point d'appui* fails to act effectively when the mass movement occurs, the faeces can be propelled in either direction. Hence the food passes backwards as well as forwards, leaving the caecum always filled and distended, the "sloppy" caecum recognised as a "cause" of constipation; moreover, in time this condition might well lead to incompetence of the ileo-caecal valve. Because the food lodges in and perhaps distends the caecum (the "cesspool caecum") it does not follow that there is a mechanical fault in the caecal movement.

If the mass movement is not effective there is nothing but the comparatively feeble movement of the caecum to propel the faeces onward; i.e. the mass in the caecum has itself to act as the *point d'appui*. I have only once seen mass movement take place in the caecum, though I have often seen movements of a peristaltic nature in its lower part; these may possibly be sufficient to raise the food to a position in the ascending colon in which the mass contraction can catch hold of it and carry it along. As a result of his researches in comparative anatomy, Keith believed that there was some form of sphincter between the caecum and the ascending colon. Hirsch (154) maintains that there is radiographic, anatomical and physiological support for the existence of the remains of a sphincter an inch or so above the ileo-caecal valve. Although there are no radiographic indications of it to be seen in the ordinary course of events, there is possibly some such sphincter, and its function may be to prevent regurgitation when the mass movement is in progress. Several observations support this hypothesis: I have never seen the caecum empty suddenly between two observations, and have only once observed the mass movement of the shadow clear out the caecum. On the other hand, I have frequently noted large shadows left in the caecum while the contents of the hepatic flexure and transverse colon have passed far on towards the pelvic colon. Moreover, although the large intestine is always swept clean (except possibly for definite scybalae), traces of the opaque meal are often left in the caecum for days.

Since this mass movement is unparalleled in the human body, I hesitate to go any farther than this brief suggestion of the normal. Widely ballooned colons and greatly narrowed colons—that is, apparently atonic and hypertonic types—are seen, and have been described as the causes of constipation, but I doubt whether this is so. Rather, I would suggest, they indicate the condition of the colon between the movements, for I happen to have seen the mass movement sweep the shadow along both types of colon, and in both it was perfectly effective in displacing the contents. The part played by the caecum is not clear but, if my deductions are correct, this portion of the large gut has

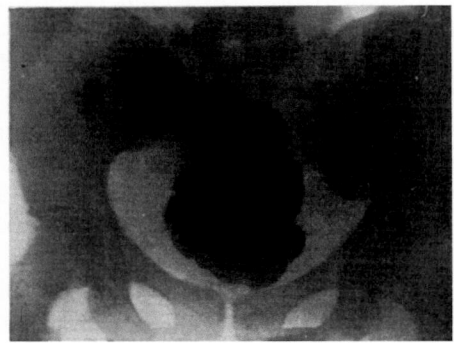

Fig. 146. Dilated rectal ampulla in a case of dyschezia.

a separate mechanism or peristalsis for mixing the contents and feeding them into the ascending colon, preparatory to the mass movement.

To the third type of constipation—rectal stagnation—Hurst has given the name of dyschezia. It is in reality a fault of defaecation, often acquired through persistent neglect of the call to stool, rather than a true constipation. In these subjects it is extraordinary to see the way in which the shadows accumulate and form great masses in the rectal ampulla without causing any call to stool (Fig. 146). The rectum is sometimes ballooned out to a great size, and is presumably atonic. When the bowels have been moved, only a part of this shadow disappears.

PART III
PATHOLOGY

INTRODUCTION

The division of pathology from disordered physiology is entirely arbitrary, but for purposes of convenience I have adopted this useful if misleading convention.

Before the advent of the opaque meal the diagnosis of abdominal conditions by clinical methods was so vague and uncertain that every abdominal section was an exploratory operation. To-day the surgeon usually knows fairly accurately the condition with which he will have to deal before he embarks on the operation, and can make his plans accordingly. But no matter how confident he may feel in the thoroughness and accuracy of the radiological examination and report, every abdominal operation should still be an exploration. There may be conditions present which the X-ray examination has not shown.

There are numerous cases in which abnormal anatomical relationships may lead to undue strains on various parts. These conditions can only be studied by means of the X rays and there is still a great deal to learn about them, for the possible variations and compensatory adaptations within the limits of normality are very wide. Because the stomach happens to be atonic, or merely exceptionally long, it is not necessarily the source of the symptoms, any more than a hypertonic and tightly contracted stomach can be acquitted of association with a pathological lesion. There are no standards. The most amazing anomalies of disposition are found in perfectly functioning abdomens. In fact, our knowledge of the physiology of the alimentary tract is exceedingly imperfect even in those conditions which can be studied by means of the opaque meal, and when we come to the secretory functions of the mucous membrane, which also undoubtedly give rise to symptoms, radiology is as yet of very little if any assistance. It is fortunate, however, that the radiologist gets his most accurate and definite diagnoses in just those cases where they will be of the greatest value, i.e. those in which surgical measures are indicated.

In the early days we were just guessing at the meaning of the things we saw by the faltering and oft-failing illumination of the fluorescent screen, and we followed cases to the operating theatre in trepidation. Plates were only sometimes successful, even with exposures that rendered movement inevitable. We did not even know, with any degree of certainty, that a dose of bismuth sub-nitrate many times greater than that stated as the maximum in the pharma-copœia could be given with safety. Disquieting reports of occasional deaths—possibly due to impurities—came through, and we were compelled to use very much smaller quantities than we employ to-day. At least two cases of poisoning occurred in America. Bennecke and Hoffman recorded a fatal case, the symptoms being suggestive of nitrite poisoning; nitrites were found in both the blood and the pericardial fluid. Later, Boehme proved that the administration of bismuth sub-nitrate was followed by the appearance of nitrites in the faeces and urine, but not in the blood.

Much of the evidence on which the early diagnoses were made would now be regarded as flimsy in the extreme, while direct and unequivocal evidence of ulceration was the dream of the visionary. The surgeons were always most helpful; they gave us facilities to follow our cases in the theatres and encouraged us even when we made bad mistakes in interpretation. The attitude of the clinicians, at first one of benevolent incredulity, gradually became one of helpful co-operation as results showed that our reports were becoming more accurate.

The whole alimentary canal, and especially the stomach, being an exceedingly sensitive muscular organ, and the opaque food then used being lumpy, spasmodic conditions were often found and, after a time, recognised as such. These spasmodic contractions were a source of much trouble in diagnosis, and their importance was not appreciated until the radiologist realised that, although they might be purely reflex, they complicated almost every active lesion involving the mucous membrane. They were then recognised to be important not only in diagnosis but in their interference with the gastric functions; in many cases they caused complete functional biloculations, of which no suggestion was found at the operation. The extent and severity of complications produced by spasm due to organic lesions did not appear to bear any definite relation to the size or appearance of the ulcerations, but seemed to depend rather upon the irritability of the ulcer than upon any other factor. Sometimes a large ulcerated surface gave rise to practically no spasmodic contraction, whereas even small ulcers—especially on the greater curvature—might cause such powerful and persistent spasm that the radiologist was confident that the surgeon would find a typical cicatricial hour-glass contraction. However, since the advent of the liquid opaque meal in place of the bread and milk or porridge mixture, far less evidence of spasm has been seen, and the spasmodic hour-glass stomach, once common, is now relatively rare. Whether this decrease is due to the type of meal or to the use of barium instead of bismuth I do not know, but I am strongly inclined to suspect the former. It seems likely, however, that spasm occurs with ordinary food more often than routine opaque meal examinations suggest, and that it is very largely responsible for symptoms.

To-day, thanks very largely to radiology, checked by surgery, the much maligned stomach is realised to be the organ that may have to make known the ills of any of the others. To it the disquietudes and disturbances of other parts are referred for expression, and in the past it bore an evil reputation as the centre and source of many diseases and humours of which it was entirely innocent. So the recognition of a normal stomach and the tracking down of the source of irritation that refers its grievance to the stomach to make its presence known become, radiologically, the problem of every case in which there is no obvious local cause of the symptoms in the stomach or duodenum.

CHAPTER XIII

THE OESOPHAGUS

METHODS OF INVESTIGATION AND THEIR LIMITATIONS

Oesophageal Bougie

Of the bougie it is difficult to write with patience. If other and less dangerous methods are available, it is an act of crude barbarity to pass such an instrument for diagnostic purposes into a tube the walls of which may be the seat of simple or malignant ulceration or may even be eroded by an aneurysm. The bougie is a most useful surgical instrument, ... but for diagnosis there is no other such savage relic in the whole of medicine or surgery.

I wrote this passage[31] many years ago and the warning is still needed. The bougie should never be used for diagnosis or dilatation without previous X-ray examination. It may wander far from its intended path. Force must never be used, for even with the gentlest manipulation a round-nosed bougie may pass into an ulcer and down between the mucous and muscular coats, without giving the surgeon any sense of resistance. In a case that came to my notice in the very early days this mishap led to the death of the patient from direct septic extension to the pleura. The post-mortem examination showed that the bougie had perforated the base of an ulcer and travelled in the sub-mucous layer almost to the cardiac orifice. In view of the fact that I saw four very similar cases in that one year (1907), I suggest that no patient with oesophageal obstruction, whether due to aneurysm or any other cause, should be examined by means of a bougie until an opaque meal examination has been made.

Oesophagoscope

The oesophagoscope reveals the whole of the track down which it travels, but nothing else. It is blind to conditions around the oesophagus and may be passed, all unsuspectingly, within a fraction of an inch of an aneurysm or growth that by its pressure is causing difficulty in swallowing.

X ray

The X-ray method shows the shadow of the food in the oesophagus. It does not show the oesophagus itself, but it reveals the presence of aneurysm and large new growths, and from the shape and behaviour of the food-shadow much may be learned of the nature of the lesion that gives rise to the symptoms. Moreover, it has two very great advantages: it is entirely free from danger and it involves no distressing manipulative procedures. It is obviously, therefore, the method of choice.

For the examination of the oesophagus the patient should stand in the semi-lateral position with the right shoulder forward (the right oblique position), so that the shadow of the heart is thrown away from that of the vertebrae. There is no definite angle, but the whole course of the oesophagus as it passes down through the mediastinum should be clearly seen. Schatzki(290) recommends the use of atropin which, he says, enables the barium cream to spread more evenly over the mucosa and to remain in place for a longer time.

Watch should be kept for the following points:

(1) Is there any obstruction to the passage of the type of food that causes the symptoms of which the patient complains? If so, is the outlet sharply pointed, or does it narrow down gradually?

(2) Is there persistent narrowing at any point? If so, what is the character of the passage; e.g. tortuous, as if running through a growth?

(3) Is there any indication of a growth or a mass of glands in the posterior mediastinum in the region of the obstruction?

(4) Is there any displacement of the oesophagus?

(5) Do the movements of the diaphragm give any indication of phrenic nerve paralysis?

OESOPHAGEAL DIVERTICULA

Pouches and diverticula have been described throughout the whole length of the alimentary canal. They are more common in some regions than in others and are probably best known in the colon, where they may be present in large numbers (cf. p. 312). They are also sometimes found in the small intestine, where they seldom give rise to symptoms, and in the duodenum,

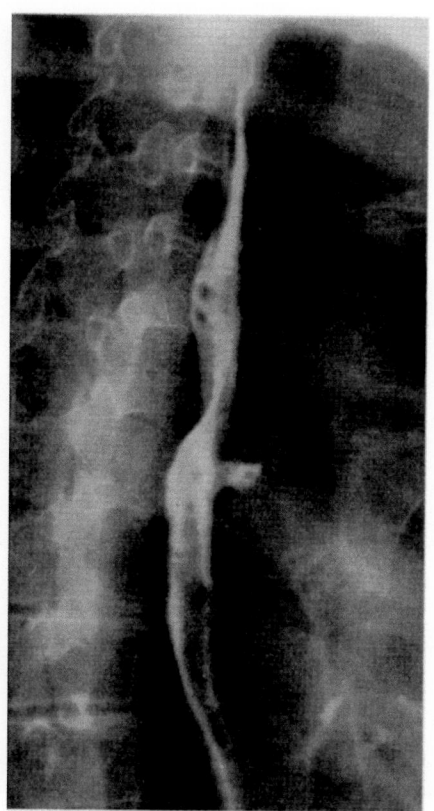

Fig. 147. Oesophageal diverticulum which gave rise to no symptoms.

where they not uncommonly do cause symptoms. They are much less often found in the stomach and are very rare indeed in the oesophagus. The origin of pouches is presumably the same in all regions, but none of the various theories advanced to explain them has proved convincing.

The very few cases of true diverticula of the oesophagus, as distinct from pharyngeal pouch (cf. p. 190), that I have seen have been small well-rounded pockets in the middle section of the gullet; they do not retain the opaque food

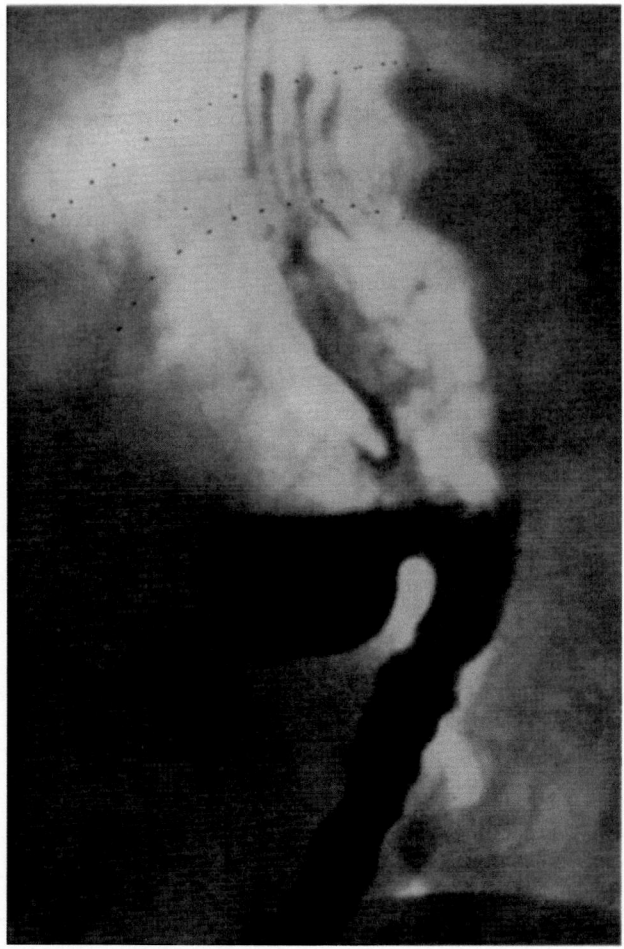

Fig. 148. Very large oesophageal diverticulum with dilatation above it. Diverticula of such size are very rare. The radiograph is taken in the left lateral position and the shadow of the aortic arch (dotted line) can be seen on the original film. There is well-marked spondylitis of the vertebrae. (Contributed by N. S. Finzi.)

for any length of time. They have all been discovered accidentally and have never been associated with any symptoms (Figs. 147 and 148). I do not know whether they may be sources of perforation or of cancer, but I have never seen a case of cancer in which the appearances suggested an origin from a diverticulum.

Another type of diverticulum is due to traction. In fibroid conditions affecting the bronchial glands or lungs, the oesophagus may be dragged and displaced to one side as a whole, but if an adhesion drags on an oesophagus that is already fixed, a tent-like projection of the wall will be produced. I have never seen a diverticulum of this kind grow to any size, but imagine that it might easily do so if the adhesions produced some obstruction.

Vestigial remains of the second branchial cleft have been described just below the tonsils:* "No traces of the second, third and fourth branchial grooves persist. The dorsal angle of the second pharyngeal pouch is nearest the sinus tonsillaris; in it the tonsil is developed, and above the tonsil a trace of the sinus persists as the supra-tonsillar fossa". I do not know of any pouches in this region that have been examined radiographically, and they must be very rare.

THORACIC OR OESOPHAGEAL STOMACH

This is an exceedingly rare congenital deformity which has usually been mistaken for diaphragmatic hernia. Le Wald (324) points out that in the latter the stomach develops above the diaphragm and remains above it, as there is no structural defect of the muscle. Very few cases have been recorded. The condition can only be diagnosed radiographically and depends on finding that the whole of the stomach, usually a very small organ, is an off-shoot from the oesophagus and placed entirely above the diaphragm. The condition does not appear to give rise to any symptoms.

DISPLACEMENTS OF THE OESOPHAGUS

The oesophagus, starting to the left of the middle line where it enters the thorax, returns to the mid-line in the region of the aortic arch and runs an almost straight course down through the posterior mediastinum, bearing to the left again as it reaches the cardiac orifice, which it joins at a varying angle that may be as acute as 45° in achalasia of the cardia; it may even attain an S-curve before entering the stomach, for when the oesophagus is markedly dilated it is also lengthened. In the lower two-thirds of its course it has no attachments, but lies more or less free in areolar tissue, and is easily displaced by any force to which it may be subjected.

Together with the other mediastinal contents, it may be displaced by fluid or by growth in the lungs, or may be drawn across by a contracted lung. It may be pushed aside by aneurysm, enlarged glands, substernal thyroid, persistent thymus, new growths, spinal abscess or, in fact, by any abnormal condition in this region. Displacement of the oesophagus may be a very important clue in the diagnosis of intrathoracic conditions. Tumours in the upper part of the

* Gray's *Anatomy*, 1926, p. 80.

thorax are apt to cause pressure symptoms, but in the lower part there may be gross displacement of the oesophagus without symptoms of any kind.

G. A. Pirie (270), at the 17th International Congress of Medicine, recorded a very interesting case of displacement: the oesophagus apparently wandered away

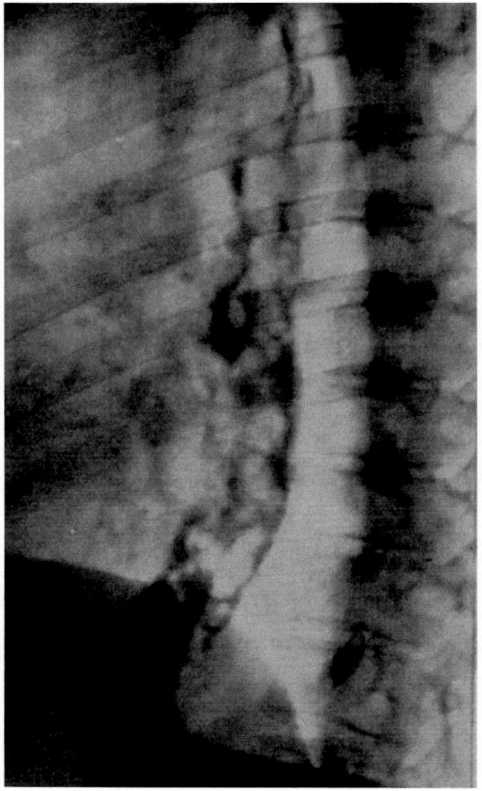

Fig. 149. Very marked oesophageal varix, giving distorted and blotchy picture of the mucous membrane. (Contributed by H. Berg.)

through the right lung, but unfortunately its course could not be traced all the way to the stomach. The condition was of twenty-five years' standing and was said to have been due to ulceration.

OESOPHAGEAL VARIX

When a detailed examination of stomach and duodenum fails to reveal the source of bleeding from the upper part of the alimentary tract, a careful study of the oesophageal mucosa may show an irregularity caused by tortuous anastomotic varices. Normally the mucosal folds form parallel lines, but if the varices are large and numerous the displacement of the opaque salt will give a patchy and grossly mottled appearance (Fig. 149) in which the course of the channels between the varices can be traced. Moreover, the width of the oesophagus seems to be definitely increased—due, presumably, to the presence of the varices in the lumen. The investigation is best carried out with the patient in the recumbent position and rotated into either the right or left oblique position. The first case was reported by Wolf(341) in 1928 and there are now numerous records in the literature. The principal references are Wolf(341), Hjelm(155), Berg(59) and Schatzki(290). This last author has now seen no less than 58 cases. About half of these have been confirmed either by oesophagoscopy or by autopsy.

OESOPHAGEAL OBSTRUCTION

The oesophagus, unlike the rest of the alimentary tract, has one function only: to act as a highway from the mouth to the stomach, and anything that interferes with this function causes the symptoms of oesophageal obstruction. A dogmatic positive or negative diagnosis is expected, is freely given by the radiologist and is usually accepted by the physician, for it is a general axiom that the oesophagus is either "guilty" or "not guilty", and that if the opaque food passes freely down there cannot be any obstruction. This is not true, for "obstruction" is a relative term and depends on three distinct factors: (1) the consistency of the food, in relation to (2) the degree of obstruction and (3) the power of the oesophageal peristalsis that is evoked to overcome the difficulty.

Moreover, an obstruction is not necessarily present continuously. Spasmodic contractions are just as frequent in the oesophagus as in other parts of the alimentary tract. Wherever the mucous membrane is inflamed or ulcerated there is likely to be a considerable spasmodic contraction. At one examination the opaque food allays the irritation and no obstruction is observed; at the next a hard particle may set up the irritation and produce spasm (cf. p. 200). It is therefore essential to go into the history of every case carefully and to be prepared to adapt the technique to any indications suggested.

In the investigation of early or intermittent cases of dysphagia, it is most important to know the nature of the food that causes trouble, and the history on this point should be carefully taken. Most patients will speak of difficulty with solids but of an easy passage with smooth liquids and well-masticated food. Some, for instance, will say that bacon always gives trouble, that they cannot eat fruit, or that they must avoid salad-dressing. If, with the ordinary type of opaque food mixed to a suitable consistency, the radiologist does not find anything abnormal, he should give some of the particular type of food that induces the symptoms; or, if it is not available, a mouthful of toasted bread crumbs, which the patient is instructed to swallow with as little mastication as possible, in order to irritate the suspected surface and so to induce spasm.

THE CAUSES OF OESOPHAGEAL OBSTRUCTION

(1) Pressure from without.
(2) Changes in the walls themselves.
(3) Foreign bodies.
(4) Reflex causes.

(1) *SOURCES OF EXTERNAL PRESSURE (OESOPHAGEAL COMPRESSION)*

(*a*) Aneurysm.
(*b*) New growth in the neck, mediastinum or lungs.
(*c*) Enlarged glands.
(*d*) Spinal abscess and new growths arising from the vertebral column.
(*e*) Bronchocele and pharyngeal pouches.

It should be noted that in this class of case the difficulty in swallowing is entirely due to mechanical pressure and steadily progressive. There is no element of spasm. Clinically, therefore, there will be no intermissions, and radiologically the appearance is also constant. The diagnosis of these conditions, except pharyngeal pouch, does not fall within the scope of this book.

PHARYNGEAL POUCH

By a confusion of terms, this is sometimes incorrectly referred to as an oeso-phageal condition because, extending downwards, it lies behind and obstructs the upper part of the gullet. It was fully described by Zenker and is often called a Zenker pouch. A very early account was given by Ogle [260] in 1866.

Symptoms

The earliest symptom of pharyngeal pouch is a sensation as if something had lodged in the throat; the patient makes many and persistent efforts to get rid of it. As the pouch increases in size, there is a sense of fullness in the neck and he has increasing difficulty in emptying the residue, and from time to time brings up mouthfuls of unaltered foodstuff. He is often conscious of noisy deglutition and suffers from distressing attacks of choking and coughing when he lies down. The symptoms may persist for years with little if any increase in severity. At one time I had the opportunity of watching the development of a case radiographically. At first there was merely a fleck of opaque food per-sistently sticking behind the larynx; it appeared to be in the sinus pyriformis although it was practically in the middle line. About six weeks later it was a definite pouch, half an inch in depth. Within three months it was larger than a walnut and very soon after that it had nearly doubled in size. In the early stages it was obviously posterior, with the opening in front and at the top, but as it increased in size these relations became obscured. The pouch tended to remain in the middle line and to displace the oesophagus so that the opening was to one side and increasingly difficult to demonstrate. I imagine that the rate of growth was in this case unusually rapid.

Sometimes the pouches attain a capacity of as much as half a pint, and there is considerable difficulty in dealing with the contents. To empty the pouch,

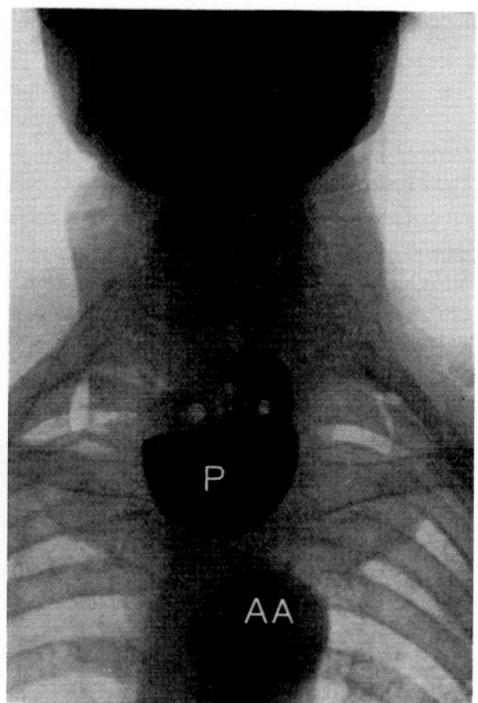

Fig. 150. Large pharyngeal pouch, *P.* *AA*, Aortic arch.

patients evolve various techniques, all more or less ineffective, for the walls are always so deficient in muscle that the pouch cannot empty itself. One patient used to lie down on his side, press his thumbs into his supra-clavicular fossae and make violent respiratory and swallowing efforts; some of the food was brought out of the pouch in this way and passed down the oesophagus, but the pouch was never completely emptied.

Diagnosis

The radiological diagnosis of this condition presents little difficulty. The typical appearance of a pouch is illustrated in Fig. 150. The swallowed opaque material has been arrested in a well-rounded sac in the lower part of the neck. The shape of the barium shadow is semi-circular: there is a smooth convex border below and a horizontal fluid level above. On screen examination such a sac is found to be completely inert, indicating the absence of muscle fibres; it is raised with each swallow and gradually becomes more and more filled. Eventually some barium will be seen in the oesophagus, and examination in the oblique and lateral directions may show that the entrance to the oesophagus lies in front of the upper part of the sac. This emptying from above is the distinguishing feature from all other obstructive lesions, which invariably empty from below. With the smaller pouches the mode of emptying is readily seen, as there is little obstruction, and considerable quantities of the barium pass over the pouch and straight down the oesophagus.

In addition to establishing the diagnosis of a pouch with certainty, X-ray examination can afford information on such points as the following: size, thickness of fibrous coat, position in relation to neighbouring structures, degree of oesophageal obstruction, tracheal displacement or compression, coincident lesions, adhesions to thoracic contents, effect of patient's attempt at emptying.

For the following abstract of a paper, not yet published, I am indebted to Dr E. D. Gray of Manchester:

It is difficult to estimate the frequency of pharyngeal pouch, but one may say that in a large general hospital about one case is seen each year. The condition occurs much more commonly in males than females, and is usually first recognised about the age of 60.

In order to appreciate the significance of the X-ray appearances one must consider the pathological anatomy of this condition. A pharyngeal pouch is a herniation of the mucous membrane through the muscular coat of the pharynx. The site of the herniation is constant—namely, between the transverse and oblique fibres of the cricopharyngeus, this being the special name given to the lowest part of the inferior constrictor muscle which takes origin from the cricoid cartilage. Dissections by the late Prof. Killian (198) indicate clearly the two sets of fibres which make up the cricopharyngeus, and the relation of these parts of the muscle to the neck of a diverticulum. The transverse fibres are below and the oblique above (Fig. 151). The wall of the pouch consists of the mucous and submucous layers of the pharynx, some loose areolar tissue and a fibrous coat.

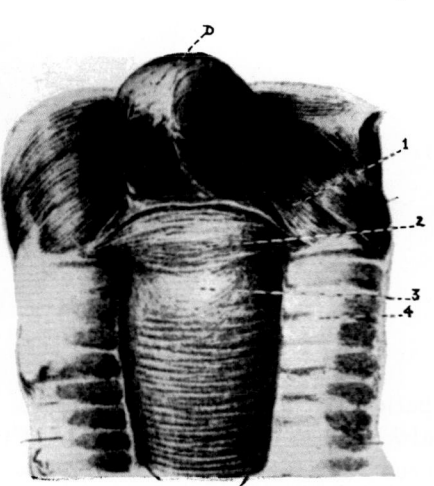

Fig. 151. Dissection showing the posterior wall of the hypopharynx and the relation of the pharyngeal pouch, D, to the cricopharyngeus, 2. 1, Oblique fibres. 2, Transverse fibres. 3, Oesophagus. 4, Trachea. (From G. Killian, "La bouche de l'oesophage"; *Annales des maladies de l'oreille et du larynx*, 1908, XXXIV (2), 1.)

In large pouches the fibrous covering may be

as much as 1 cm. in thickness and may become adherent to neighbouring structures. The pouch is usually of considerable size when first discovered. Because they seldom cause noteworthy symptoms small pouches are rarely observed, and I would suggest routine examination of the pharynx as part of the opaque meal investigation to disclose the earlier stages of pouch formation.

Another finding, which is far more frequent than that of a fully developed pouch, is illustrated in Plate fig. 153. This shows a small, pointed, barium-filled projection from the posterior pharyngeal wall which I consider represents a potential pouch. The shape and position of the projection suggest that it is due to a protrusion of the mucous membrane between the fibres of the cricopharyngeus. A small pouch usually lies directly behind the oesophagus and, in the resting phase, its neck is at right angles to the line of the pharynx. The alignment of the pharynx and oesophagus is not disturbed. One might suppose that food would pass the entrance to the pouch without subjecting it to any considerable pressure, but screen examination shows that the angle between the neck of the pouch and the pharynx disappears during swallowing and the pouch

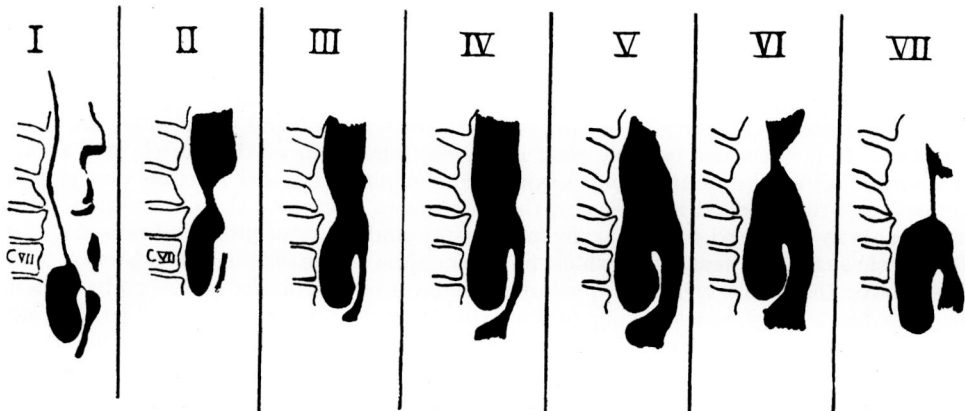

Fig. 152. To show alteration in the direction of the neck of pouch during swallowing. I, Resting phase. II–VII, Successive phases during first second after swallowing. (After Laurell.)

is therefore distended by each bolus. This alteration of direction is recorded in a series of radiograms published by Laurell (215) (Fig. 152). I consider that the right-angle seen in the resting phase is caused by tonic contraction of the oblique fibres of the cricopharyngeus, and that when these fibres relax during swallowing, the pouch comes into line with the pharynx.

As the pouch grows it descends and tends to deviate to one side, more commonly to the left. Its enlargement is not always symmetrical and one sees in some cases a localised protrusion from the lower convex border. In time, the pouch causes pressure on the oesophagus and trachea, but the important effect of its increase in size is the alteration in the alignment of the pharynx and oesophagus. Comparison of Fig. 152 and Plate figs. 154 and 155 will show that the pharynx is permanently in line with the larger pouch and the entrance to the oesophagus is oblique and consists of a narrow slit on the anterior border of the neck of the sac. Distension of the pouch with food increases the obliquity of the entrance to the oesophagus: it is this effect and not pressure of the fundus of the sac on the oesophagus which causes the dysphagia. The growth of a pouch is, as a rule, extremely slow. I observed one case over a period of three years without detecting any increase in size, and it is clear, from the length of history, that many pouches have been present for ten or more years.

Gray (140) holds that there is no foundation for the congenital theory of origin of these pouches. Zenker also believed that they were due to mechanical factors, and classified these as (1) pulsion, due to pressure from within, and (2) traction, due to adhesions from without. Gray denies that traction can play an important rôle, and says that, since the pouch moves up freely on swallowing, there can be no adhesions between it and the neck; the adhesions found in large pouches are secondary developments. He adopts the orthodox view that pharyngeal pouch is entirely due to pulsion, the result of some spasmodic obstruction. He says:

Killian (198) showed that the function of the transverse part of this muscle was that of a sphincter and that it remained tonically contracted throughout life except for momentary relaxations during the acts of swallowing and vomiting. The site of the sphincter is clearly visible on X-ray examination and it can be seen to relax for between a quarter and half a second to allow each bolus to pass into the oesophagus. After this brief interval it contracts again and lets through nothing more until the next swallow. It is therefore possible that imperfect relaxation of the muscle will result in part or all of the bolus being retained in the pharynx, and forcible pharyngeal peristalsis will be called into play in the attempt to overcome the obstruction. This will result in increased intrapharyngeal pressure and the mucous membrane may be forced through the weak area which has been shown to exist on the posterior wall just above the sphincter. The cause of the failure of relaxation is uncertain, but it is probable that the swallowing of imperfectly masticated portions of food is an important factor. It is often stated that X-ray examination in pouch cases shows no evidence of spasm at the entrance to the oesophagus, but I do not think enough attention has been paid to the nature of the bolus. We are accustomed to use creamy suspensions of barium for examination of this point; the findings might well be otherwise if a more solid bolus were used.

Laurell (215) has recently postulated a traction force as favouring the production of pouch. He considers that coincident with the negative pressure which develops in the pharynx during the earlier stages of the act of swallowing there is a negative pressure in the space between the pharynx and the cervical spine. He believes that this negative pressure outside the pharynx is maintained even when the intrapharyngeal pressure has become positive and that the two forces, therefore, act together.

Raven (279) believes in congenital pouch and describes several varieties of congenital and acquired pouches. He also mentions the natural pouches of the sloth bear, the pig and the great anteater, and gives an extensive bibliography.

A great deal of work is necessary before the aetiology of pharyngeal pouch can be established with certainty, and careful radiological examination of the pharynx in a large number of cases may possibly throw some light on the

PLATE V

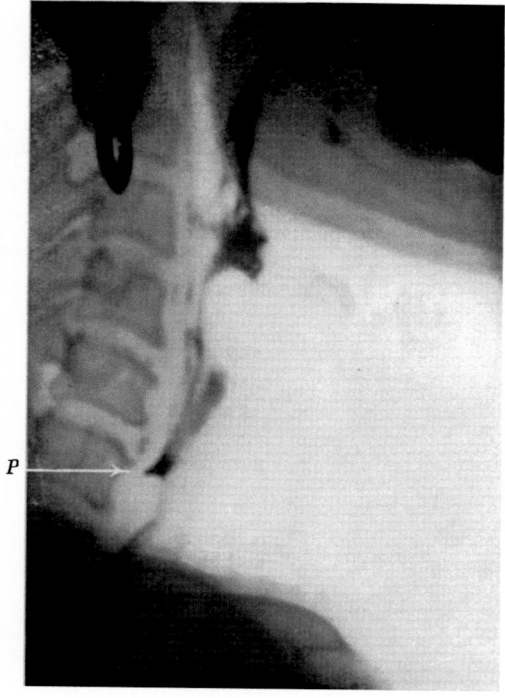

Fig. 153

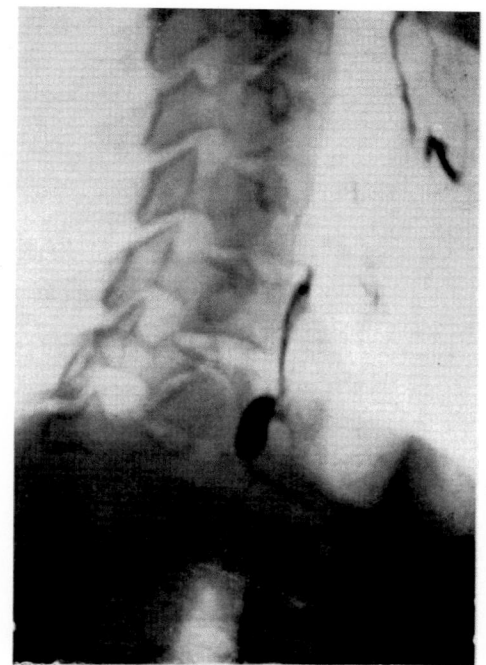

Fig. 154

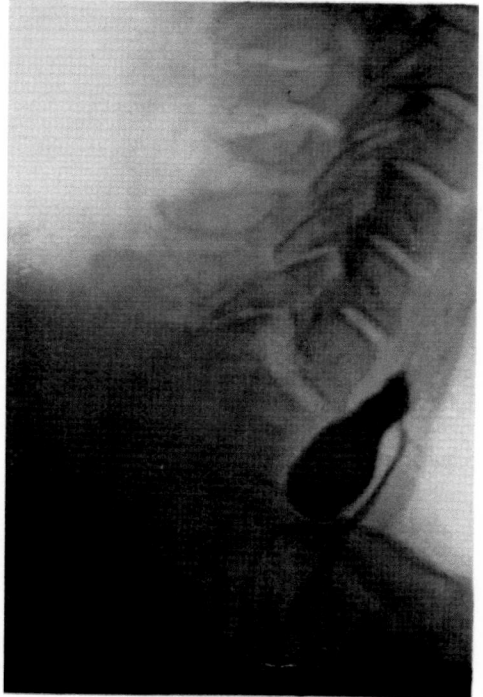

Fig. 155

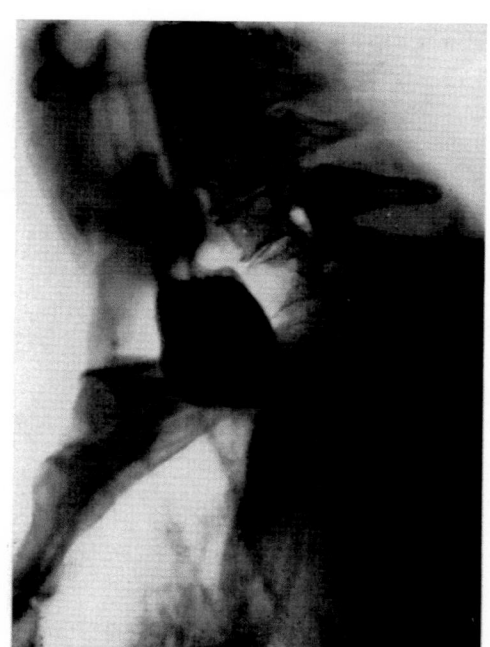

Fig. 156

Fig. 153. Potential pharyngeal pouch, *P*.

Fig. 154. Small pharyngeal pouch. This, like the potential pouch in Fig. 152, seems to originate lower than the cricothyroideus, the site of origin indicated by Killian.

Fig. 155. Lateral view of pharyngeal pouch, showing that the pouch is posterior and that it empties forwards. (Contributed by N. S. Finzi.)

Fig. 156. Lateral view of a large pharyngeal pouch. The opening, which is not seen, is probably to one side. (Contributed by H. K. Pancoast.)

problem. Believing as I do that there is normally negative pressure in the pharynx during swallowing, I think it likely that pulsion plays little or no part in determining the formation of a pouch. When the movements of the lower part of the posterior wall of the pharynx are watched during normal swallowing, two things impress the observer: first, that it slides up the anterior surface of the vertebrae by perhaps as much as an inch, with no evidence of being pulled forwards and away from the vertebrae; and secondly, that, when viewed from the front, it is obviously widened out (cf. Laurell). Both these observations

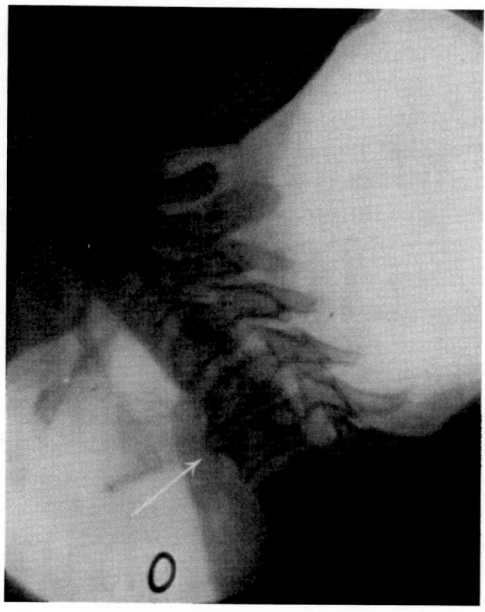

Fig. 157. Localised spondylitis affecting the 5th–6th intervertebral disc. This type of bony change seems to be very frequently associated with pharyngeal pouch. The patient, a man of 62, had a large pouch. The spine was radiographed to see if there were any bony changes in the vertebrae to suggest the formation of adhesions as a possible cause for the formation of the pouch.

suggest very strongly that the orthodox views of the function of the constrictor muscles need revision; they suggest further that the origin of pouches might very well be the formation of adhesions to the vertebrae. If the posterior pharyngeal wall were adherent, the lifting of the laryngo-pharynx at every swallow would drag it out, and thus form a pocket which would tend to increase in size by its repeated distension with food and by forcible swallowing efforts to dislodge its contents (cf. Plate fig. 156). The fact that the pouch moves up with each act of swallowing does not exclude the possibility of adhesions *at the site of origin*, and it is possible that the pouch, once started, extends downwards and that the adhesions remain. Mosher has actually found adhesions in some of these cases and has operated on them successfully.

Since adhesions indicate old injury or disease, I decided to look out for any evidence of pathological changes in the spine. Only one case of pharyngeal pouch was available at the time, and I sent for the patient and examined him. I found marked lipping of the vertebrae and a localised spondylitis just behind the site where a pouch would originate (Fig. 157), and it is interesting to note that in the two cases illustrated by Laurell there are also definite and well-developed spondylitic changes. These appearances seem to support my contention that traction is probably the originating cause and that intrapharyngeal pressures may not be important, but I admit that Gray's demonstrations have shaken my conviction. Laurell cites these two cases in support of his belief that the pouches are formed by pulsion, but he does not mention the changes in the spine. He states that he sees definite evidence of propulsive peristalsis above the pouches, and this I can well believe, but the mechanism is not normal; it is a reserve force brought into play to overcome the oesophageal obstruction resulting from the pressure of the pouch. Such appearances can always be seen above any obstruction high up in the oesophagus. Here, as elsewhere in the alimentary tract, peristalsis is a reserve force that exerts little or no propulsive effort unless called upon to overcome difficulty. It is not the primary motive power in unobstructed conditions.

(2) *CHANGES IN THE WALLS*

(*a*) New growths.
(*b*) Ulceration, with spasmodic contraction.
(*c*) Cicatrisation, following ulceration from caustics and acids, syphilis, etc.
(*d*) Abscess.
(*e*) Syphilis and tuberculosis. (Exceedingly rare.)

The various cases in this group can often be separated from one another only on clinical grounds. The growths are usually too small to cause any distinct shadow, while cicatrisation, ulceration and spasmodic contractions may give exactly similar appearances.

In this group of causes there are nearly always two factors to consider, viz. the organic and the spasmodic, and I cannot too strongly insist on the importance of spasm, which may be responsible for almost the whole of the symptomatic disturbance. A history that the degree of obstruction varies with the same type of food, or that it actually disappears from time to time, always points to an intrinsic cause and an element of spasm.

Oesophageal Spasm

Whenever the mucous membrane is involved there is likely to be spasm, and whenever there is spasm the obstruction may change, from day to day and hour to hour. Belladonna has some value in relaxing the spasmodic element, but is not sufficiently reliable in its action to be of much use in diagnosis. Because the oesophagus, like the rest of the alimentary tract, is highly sensitive, a small abrasion or ulceration may set up a spasm of such severity and persistence that complete temporary obstruction may result. The severity of the spasm appears to depend not upon the size of the ulcer but upon its irritability.

Spasm may also occur without any demonstrable lesion. A particularly interesting and severe case is recorded by Grier[141].

A blacksmith aged 55, previously a very strong and healthy man, was referred for X-ray examination on November 14th 1923. He gave a history of great difficulty in swallowing and constant regurgitation of food for the last two months, during which time he had lost 60 pounds in weight. Friends who were with the patient said that he had been indulging very freely in moonshine liquor for the past month or more. About four days before admission the obstruction in the oesophagus had become so acute that he was unable to swallow liquid foods or even water, everything he took being regurgitated. The man appeared to be in desperate circumstances; his emaciation was extreme and he was barely able to stand on his feet. When given a liquid barium meal, he swallowed about half a glassful, which went down the oesophagus to a point about the middle, where there was an absolute obstruction. The barium meal stayed at this point for some time, radiographs were made, and it was regurgitated while he was dressing after the examination. An absolute obstruction at the middle of the oesophagus was reported, with the belief that it was due either to carcinoma or to syphilis. The Wassermann reaction was negative. He was placed in a hospital and immediately put on belladonna. He was allowed only liquid foods, a spoonful or two at a time. He did not vomit after admission, and as soon as proper arrangements could be made, an oesophagoscope was passed and an absolutely normal oesophagus was found. Not only was there no constriction, obstruction, or any evidence of lesion, but the mucous membrane in the oesophagus was normal for its entire length and the oesophagoscope passed into the stomach without any difficulty. A second X-ray examination made at this time showed an absolutely normal oesophagus.

This was undoubtedly a case of spasm in the middle of the oesophagus which had become so violent and constant as actually to threaten the man's life. He would certainly have succumbed in a few days if he had not been relieved. The fact that these spasmodic conditions may occur in any part of the oesophagus and exactly simulate carcinoma argues that in every case in which the outline or shadow of a growth cannot be detected, the patient should be put on belladonna and the oesophagoscope should be used. The Wassermann being negative, the only reasonable diagnosis of this case from the X-ray examination alone would have been carcinoma of the oesophagus.

A. New Growths of the Oesophagus

New growths involving the oesophagus itself may be divided into two classes: (i) those that primarily involve the mucous membrane, and (ii) those which occur in the walls themselves. Vinson (319) reports a thousand cases, approximately 84 per cent. of which were men and 16 per cent. women. In 4 per cent. of these cases the X-ray examination failed to reveal the condition. There seemed to be a curious disproportion of Jews in the series, i.e. about 10 per cent., suggesting that they showed a definite idiosyncrasy to the disease. In about 5 per cent. of the cases there was a history of long-standing trouble extending from two-and-a-half to thirty years, suggesting that in these cases the malignant disease was superimposed on some non-malignant condition.

(i) Epithelioma of the oesophagus occurs most frequently during the fifth decade of life. Three common sites are mentioned, viz. the upper end just below the thyroid level; the middle portion, rather lower down than the aortic arch; and the neighbourhood of the cardiac orifice. It used to be taught that these were sites of election because they were subject to irritation, e.g. where the oesophagus crosses the bifurcation of the trachea. It is doubtful, however, if this distribution of the disease would be borne out by the systematic investigation of a large number of cases. In my experience the disease is found in any situation.

The symptoms are those of progressive obstruction, with intermittent symptoms due to spasm, and if the spasm is not present the growth is apt to be missed. The lower down in the oesophagus it is, the more gradual will be the onset of the symptoms, for the lower oesophagus dilates readily and the food is retained without discomfort after a time. In some of these cases, just as in achalasia, the food is retained in the lower end of the oesophagus and the observer must wait until the opaque mixture has percolated through the retained food.

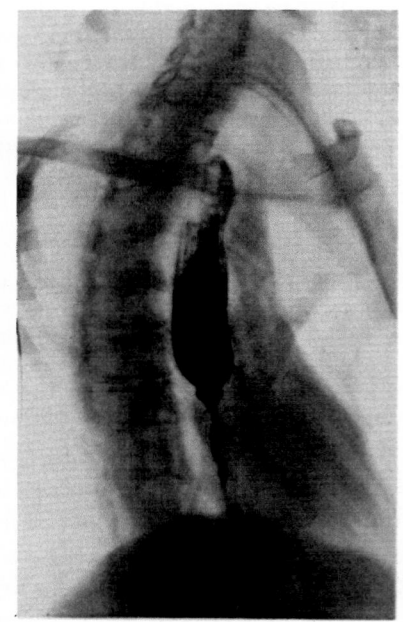

Fig. 158. Oesophageal obstruction due to growth. Note the tortuous course of the opaque food, without displacement. The faint outline of the growth itself can be traced.

The two points on which the differential diagnosis from achalasia of the cardia is made are: (1) the relatively short history, and (2) the detail of the outline of the lower end of the shadow, in which there is usually some persistent irregularity of outline in neoplasm, while in achalasia the outline is regular, except perhaps for little angular bends that may not be seen when the patient is re-examined.

Whenever the history points to intermissions and no abnormality is found, some toasted breadcrumbs or other irritant matter should be given before the opaque food. As non-malignant ulceration is exceedingly rare and is likely to be found only in younger subjects, the diagnosis of malignancy will most probably be correct. The posterior mediastinum is viewed to see if there is any abnormal opacity. A relatively small growth may give the impression of doubtful enlargement of bronchial glands, for the shadow is seldom definite. Mediastinal growths involving the oesophagus are, on the other hand, easily detected on the screen. The course of the opaque salt as it passes down is watched carefully, particular attention being paid to any point where it seems to be delayed or where the channel is persistently narrowed. Thicker foodstuffs or gelatine-barium suppositories may be useful in diagnosis, but it is quite possible for the observer to miss early neoplasm if he does not realise the part that spasm plays in the causation of symptoms. The diaphragm should be observed for phrenic paralysis, although this is usually a late symptom.

If the growth has developed, there is seldom any difficulty in the diagnosis, for all types of food will be definitely delayed, if not actually obstructed. The lower end of the shadow converges to a point and a trickle passes through, often in a tortuous course. A radiograph will sometimes show the actual outline of the growth (Fig. 158).

(ii) When the growth occurs in the walls themselves, the clinical history is one of a gradually and persistently increasing obstruction and a progressive inability to swallow more solid foods. The food should be mixed to a consistency which is likely to be held up, or alternatively a bolus of some food that the patient knows he cannot swallow may be given first. As the food passes through the obstructed area, the stream will be narrow and tortuous. A radiogram will sometimes show the faint shadow of the growth itself.

B. Peptic ulcer of the oesophagus

Oesophageal ulcers are not common, but a number are on record; Chevalier Jackson [182], in his unique experience with the oesophagoscope, has seen twenty-one cases. Cantieri [78], who described six cases, collected records of sixty-one from the literature. Their pathogenesis has been attributed to a reflux of gastric juice through the cardiac orifice. Islands of cylindrical-celled, gastric mucous membrane are to be found in the lower end of the oesophagus, and these may be the site of the ulceration. The ulcer is usually on the posterior wall, and is rounded and from half an inch to an inch and a half in diameter. The symptoms are pain in the epigastrium and over the xiphoid, often radiating to the back. The pain is often felt for as long as half an hour after eating. Vomiting and haematemesis are sometimes present; the loss of blood may be sudden, copious and fatal. Cases of perforation into the pleural cavity causing acute abdominal symptoms are on record. The following case is an example of this condition and illustrates very dramatically the inter-relationship of ulcer, spasm and pain.

A girl of 18 complained of intermittent difficulty in swallowing, and in the routine X-ray examination no abnormality was seen to account for the trouble. Clinically, she was of a neurotic type and it was thought that the trouble was a neurosis, although she gave a history of having brought up some blood on one occasion. In consequence of careful questioning I gave her some crumbled toast and made her swallow it rapidly, and she at once said that this had produced the pain. On giving a mouthful of bismuth food I now found that there was

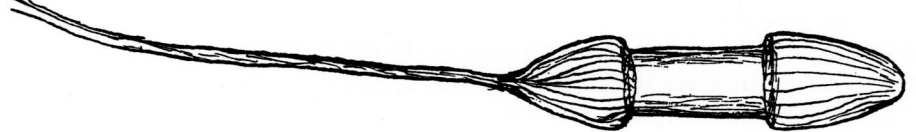

Fig. 159. Bougie electrode used for the ionisation of a peptic ulcer. It is made of solid zinc. The neck is bare but the ends are insulated with shellac and the connecting wire is encased in a rubber tube.

complete obstruction at the level of the sixth dorsal vertebra. A diagnosis of simple peptic ulcer was made, and the oesophagoscope revealed the ulcer, about $\frac{1}{4}$ in. in diameter. It was unsuccessfully treated with silver nitrate through the oesophagoscope, and was eventually passed on to me to try ionisation [36]. This did not seem possible through the metal oesophagoscope, and I decided to attempt to make use of the spasm to place a bare zinc electrode in direct contact with the ulcer. An olivary-pointed and bobbin-shaped zinc electrode was made and insulated with shellac, except the neck which was left bare and attached to a rather stiff copper wire covered with rubber (Fig. 159). This electrode was easily passed into the stomach and encountered no obstruction, and then the patient swallowed crumbled toast. When she declared that the pain had come on, the electrode was pulled up until the resistance of the obstruction was felt. A little extra pull brought the upper half of the bobbin through the spasmodic contraction, and the neck of the electrode was felt to be firmly gripped by the spasm so that, without force, it could not be displaced. The ionisation was then attempted, but the spasm relaxed and the bougie was felt, and seen, to slip. (The procedure was carried out with the patient standing in the screening stand.) Another and deeper-necked electrode was made and the same procedure was quite successfully carried out, the contact with the ulcer being shown on the neck of the electrode by a black mark where the electrolysis had taken place through this part of the metal. A complete cure was effected and, apart from one slight recurrence treated in the same way, the patient has had no further trouble of any sort in the last twenty years.

The same treatment was used in a few cases of malignant ulceration. There seemed to be some relief of symptoms for a time.

ABSCESS

The formation of an abscess about the base of an oesophageal ulcer is not unknown, and such abscesses may perforate and discharge through the oesophagus. High up, they may cause displacement and pressure symptoms; lower down, they give rise to shadows that, apart from the clinical picture, would be mistaken for glandular enlargements. A number of cases have been encountered in which the ulceration of new growths or foreign bodies has perforated the walls and led to the formation of an abscess that has discharged into the pleural cavity and even into the lungs themselves.

(3) *FOREIGN BODIES IN THE OESOPHAGUS*

Children are apt to swallow coins, toys, pins, pebbles—in fact, anything they can lay hold of—and so to cause great anxiety. With very few exceptions, however, these cases are not really urgent. It has been suggested that a copper coin left in the oesophagus for even a few hours may cause ulceration. Personally, I do not believe it, for I have seen a penny brought up in an attack of whooping-cough after it had lain more than six months in the lower half of the oesophagus. It was eroded to a thin wafer.

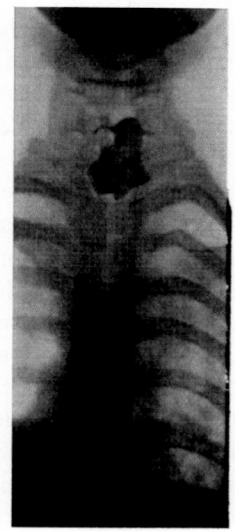

Surprisingly large objects can stick in the oesophagus without causing urgent symptoms and, still more surprisingly, most of them eventually pass through the cardiac orifice. My experience of foreign bodies is that, once they have entered the stomach, they will pass on without assistance. I have seen many startling objects pass through without mishap (Fig. 160). In adults the objects most frequently swallowed are pins, coins and tooth-plates; perhaps the strangest case in my experience was that of a man who had swallowed his week's wages: four sovereigns, two half-sovereigns and a few shillings.

Fig. 160. Small swallowed tooth-plate.

The whole hoard was found lying together in an intestinal coil and was all passed out together on the following day. Once I watched a large open safety-pin progress day by day through the gastro-intestinal tract of an infant only a few days old, and eventually delivered it successfully per rectum. Ordinary pins nearly always go down head-first and hardly ever lodge in the oesophagus. On the whole, Nature deals very kindly with these little indiscretions of diet; nevertheless, the radiologist should always take a radiograph in self-defence.

A lady, under observation in a nursing-home, decided to commit suicide by swallowing her false teeth. I was called in and found a complete upper set lodged at about the level of the clavicle. An unsuccessful attempt was made to extract them by use of the oesophagoscope, and it was decided to operate. I again examined just before operation and the teeth were in the same position. She went straight to the operating-theatre and the teeth were not found; probably they had moved during the administration of the anaesthetic, for next day they were found at the cardiac orifice, where they remained for two or three days before they passed on into the stomach. The patient was examined periodically and the progress of the teeth was watched until, in ten days' time, they had reached the anus, from which they were passed without assistance.

Open safety-pins are exceedingly difficult to extract, especially from the lower end of the oesophagus, and the best way of dealing with them is to help them downwards into the stomach. In fact, in my experience, it is much easier and less dangerous to assist foreign bodies on into the stomach than to attempt to pull them up. On one occasion a penny had been lodged for some time in the lower third of the oesophagus, and the surgeon, in attempting to extract it with an oesophagoscope, had to use some force. The operation was being done under X-ray observation, and the coin was seen to slip suddenly out of the jaws of the forceps and to pass into the pleural cavity, and almost at once a pneumothorax developed. Sepsis set in, and the patient died.

Fortunately, most foreign bodies found in the oesophagus are opaque to the X rays and do not need the opaque food method for their detection. Fortunately, also, most of them are well-rounded and do not cause serious trouble. They are apt to lodge—for a time at any rate—at about the level of the clavicle, and coins and flat objects lie in the coronal plane. They are therefore very readily seen on the screen and were easily removed in the old days by the coin catcher. If, however, they pass below the clavicular level they are more difficult to extract, because of the lax attachments of the oesophagus in its lower part; when traction is made on the foreign body the mucous membrane tends to ruck up and obstruct its withdrawal. Force in attempted extraction may induce spasm; I remember one case in which the coin catcher itself was caught by the induced spasm and could not be moved until anaesthesia had been pushed to the full extent.

Opaque food is necessary to detect certain objects, such as plum-stones, fish-bones and some tooth-plates, which throw no distinguishable shadow. Sometimes it seems incredible that a plum-stone should have been invisible to radioscopy when in the oesophagus, while the same stone viewed outside the body casts a heavy shadow.

Tooth-plates are often very difficult to see, as vulcanite and porcelain cast only faint shadows, although metal fittings are easily seen. It is quite impossible to say for certain that a small tooth-plate is not in the oesophagus; in cases that are at all doubtful the patient should be oesophagoscoped or examined again on the following day.

It is essential to examine in the semi-lateral or oblique position, as the following case illustrates:

The patient, a young woman, was shot by her lover, and the bullet entered just below the nose. After a stay of about two months she went out of the local hospital, convalescent, but became short of breath. It was then suggested that the bullet had lodged in the back of the pharynx and had dropped down into the air passages. Three times she was examined by X rays at the hospital where she had been treated, and no foreign body was found, and it was not until ten months after the accident that she was brought to the Manchester Royal Infirmary. Her condition was pitiable. She could hardly crawl along for shortness of breath. Her eyes were starting out of her head and she was distinctly cyanosed. A rapid examination showed a foreign body, not in the lungs, but in the upper end of the trachea, and it was a fragment of tooth-plate. The fragment was no thicker than a pin and could not be seen against the vertebral column in the direct antero-posterior position, but was discovered at once on turning the patient into the oblique position for examining the mediastinum. The bullet was easily located, embedded at the base of the skull. Tracheotomy was performed at once, and the foreign body was removed later. The patient made a perfect recovery, but the ignorance of the use of the oblique position very nearly cost her her life.

In exactly the same way Dr Thurstan Holland discovered a set of false teeth half-way down the oesophagus in a patient in whom previous examinations had failed to reveal their presence. She had been treated as a neurotic until, too late, she went to another hospital where, although the teeth were located and removed, she died from ulceration.

In some cases the radiologist can demonstrate the presence of tooth-plates by observing the behaviour of the opaque food as it finds its way past them. In some the stream is divided; in others portions of bismuth are left adherent to, or in pockets about, the foreign body. A small fleck of opaque food persistently held up at one point is strong presumptive evidence of the presence of a foreign body if the history also points in this direction. The oesophagoscope often shows that this appearance is due to retention of the food between the wall and a lodged foreign body. Sometimes the opaque food can be seen dividing around the foreign body, which appears momentarily as a clear area in the dark shadow.

From the radiological point of view the technique of using pledgets of cotton wool impregnated with opaque salt gives very satisfactory results. A number of small balls of cotton wool, not much larger than peas, are soaked in a suspension of barium sulphate and placed on the back of the patient's tongue so as to be swallowed with as little mastication as possible. The delay of one of these pledgets is almost if not quite certain evidence that a foreign body is present and that the cotton wool has caught on it. Some of the surgeons who oesophagoscope cases after this procedure complain that the retained barium obstructs their view and makes the recognition of the foreign body difficult. I have little experience of the method, but I should think that the accuracy of diagnosis by this means would be far higher than by the oesophagoscope except in the hands of one of the few absolute masters of its technique.

The only possible error in the diagnosis of foreign bodies is one of localisation; the radiologist must be quite sure that the foreign body does not lie in the trachea or bronchi. This point is easily settled by observing the relationship of the shadow to that of a mouthful of opaque food.

(4) *REFLEX CAUSES*

(*a*) New growths and inflammatory lesions of the larynx and in the neck.

(*b*) Ulceration and new growths of the cardiac end of the stomach.

(*c*) Neurotic and hysterical obstructions due to nervous lesions.

New growths and inflammatory lesions of the larynx and in the neck are readily diagnosed by other methods, and the X-ray examination is very rarely of any value except in demonstrating that the food, although it enters the pharynx, does not readily enter the oesophagus.

Ulceration and new growths of the cardiac end of the stomach, when situated close to the cardiac orifice, may give rise to marked obstruction simulating achalasia of the cardia. For instance, in one case an ulcer on the lesser curvature, two inches from the orifice, was the only pathological condition noted post mortem in a patient who had shown all the signs of extreme dilatation of the oesophagus—a typical achalasia. This had led to such weakness from starvation that he had died from the shock of the operation of gastrostomy. In another case, where marked dilatation had taken place and no food appeared to enter the stomach, advanced carcinoma of the stomach was found, but it did not involve the orifice, which appeared to be quite patent and normal in all respects. In both these cases, although marked dilatation of the oesophagus had been noted in life, there was no dilatation nor any indication of hypertrophy or thickening of the cardia at the autopsies.

NEUROTIC AND HYSTERICAL OBSTRUCTIONS

I have seen no cases in which this diagnosis was confirmed, but neurotic patients have frequently given me trouble by stating that they could not swallow. Persuasion and distraction of the attention, however, usually overcome this difficulty and demonstrate the nature of the case.

Globus Hystericus

Globus hystericus is probably not a definite entity. In some cases in which it has been diagnosed I have, however, found a rather marked calcification of the thyroid cartilage, and it is quite possible that this is the cause of the trouble, the thyroid being less flexible and more subject to injury. The first case that I saw was in a woman who said that she had suddenly developed difficulty in swallowing when eating calves' feet. When seen, she was considerably wasted. On examination I found an indefinite shadow in the region of the larynx, and thought it was that of a partially ossified swallowed tarsal bone, but the oesophagoscope failed to demonstrate any foreign body. Further examination showed that the shadow was due to calcification of the thyroid; this was the first time that I had seen it.

Since those early days I have noticed this calcification of the thyroid in association with dysphagia fairly frequently, and I have little doubt of its relationship with the symptoms. In fact, in a recent case I explained the nature of the trouble to a patient who had lost a considerable amount of weight; within three days she had lost all symptoms and ceased to be conscious of what was in reality a very minor discomfort. She has had no return of the symptoms.

Vallecular Dysphagia

Recently Woods (342) and McGibbon and Mather (226) have described a condition under this name. The patient suffers from difficulty in swallowing which results from the filling of the valleculae with food so that the epiglottis is forced backwards against the postpharyngeal wall. The diagnosis can only be made by careful local and general examination combined with X rays. McGibbon and Mather suggest that the phenomenon may be secondary to some disturbance of the neuromuscular mechanism of swallowing or may be a primary entity of unknown pathology. In most cases symptoms are relieved when they are explained to the patient. I think myself that the exciting cause probably lies in some minor and unrecognised injury that disturbs the balance of the swallowing mechanism, just as calcification of the cartilage may be the starting-point of a disorder of deglutition.

PARALYSIS OF THE OESOPHAGUS

Paralysis of the oesophagus is not uncommon. I have seen many cases, and in each of them there was a propulsive act of deglutition which seemed to be the only force at work (Figs. 161 and 162). The food was propelled into the oesophagus and remained there, gradually sliding down in the course of many minutes with the help of drinks of water. In the first of these cases it was obvious that the patient had to push each mouthful down the oesophagus by sheer force as far as the level of the clavicle—mainly, it appeared, by the action of the tongue. There was evidently no obstruction beyond this point; the food passed down quite freely and easily and not a trace was left adhering to the walls, whereas in the upper third there were traces of the food for a long time. It was quite clear that there was paralysis in the upper third while the lower two-thirds were quite normal. This is an interesting finding in view of the dual nerve supply (see p. 65).

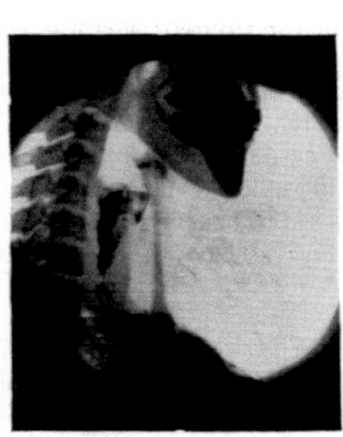
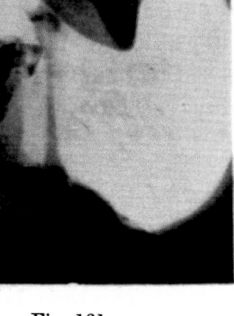
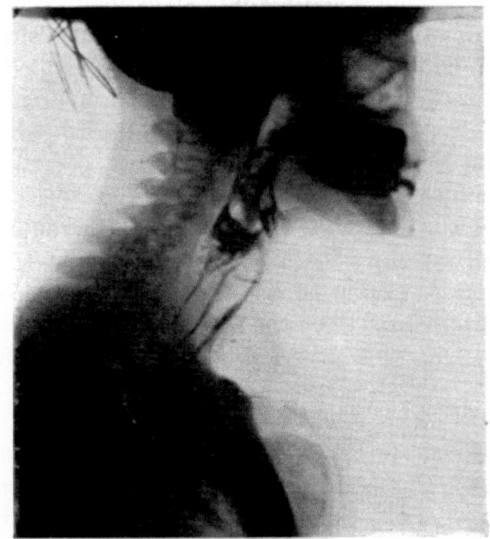

Fig. 161   Fig. 162

Fig. 161. Paralysis of the oesophagus. The food remains inert in the upper end of the oesophagus. It is only displaced by forceful propulsive swallowing.

Fig. 162. Paralysis of the oesophagus. Some of the food has passed down the trachea.

THE STAGES OF OESOPHAGEAL OBSTRUCTION

Whatever the cause of obstruction the result is the same, and there seem to be three definite stages, not only in the X-ray appearances but also in the clinical history.

Stage 1: Difficulty in Swallowing

This is most marked in the upper part of the oesophagus.

The patient has not lost weight but gives a history of some difficulty in swallowing, especially when he tries to eat his food fast and without mastication. Usually there is little or no pain, provided that he masticates carefully and eats slowly, but he often states that he has to force each mouthful down separately.

On examination with the ordinary type of opaque food it is probable that, at the most, a little delay is noted at one particular part. If, on the other hand, the patient eats lumpy bread and milk quickly, it may show definite delay at this point, and occasionally a violent peristaltic wave squeezes the food almost into a ball and forces it through the obstruction.

Stage 2: Pain after Swallowing

This is not so marked in the lower as in the upper part of the oesophagus because the lower two-thirds is more mobile and adaptable. This is the stage of painful deglutition and the patient has begun to lose flesh. He probably states that he cannot swallow solids at all and that even gruel sometimes regurgitates into his mouth, but he seldom actually brings the food back. The pain *after* swallowing is the main feature, and it is his dread of eating, far more than the actual obstruction, that leads to the wasting for, although the food he eats is eventually forced through, yet the pain is so great that he prefers starvation. The patient's sensations are no sure guide to the position of the obstruction.

On examination there is a definite delay at the point of obstruction. There is seldom any mistake in the diagnosis unless a thin mixture is used; this may pass through unobstructed. The food is held up, it cannot pass on; the oesophageal walls bring all their peristaltic power to bear on the obstruction and, as the powerful waves move downwards, the food, being unable to pass through the obstruction, escapes upwards in a narrow stream through the descending contraction. When one sees the picture one is not surprised that this is the stage in which pain is the marked feature—sometimes so marked that it suggests a life-and-death struggle.

The waves are not a continuous succession of contractions of equal strength; a series of great efforts is followed by a period of comparative rest while the muscle braces itself up for another effort. These intermittent contractions are, I believe, characteristic of failing compensation, not only in the oesophagus but also in the stomach, in certain stages of pyloric obstruction. In this stage the compensation is failing and the muscle wall is about to relax, give up the struggle and become dilated.

Stage 3: Dilatation

Naturally, in cases where the obstruction is high up and the oesophagus has little room to dilate, this stage is not so well marked as when the obstruction is in the lower two-thirds of its course.

Clinically, this is the stage of starvation and the patient is rapidly losing flesh, but the pain and difficulty in and after swallowing are comparatively slight, so that he feels and often becomes better for a time. He no longer has any actual difficulty in making the food pass down, but sooner or later it is brought up again. The lower down the obstruction and the greater the degree of dilatation the longer is the food likely to be retained, so much so that in marked cases a clinical diagnosis of pyloric obstruction is not at all infrequently made. In one of these cases quite considerable quantities of opaque salt were found, two days after the meal had been given, in the dilated pouch that extended above the diaphragm, and the patient gave a history of having seen in his vomit food that he had taken some days before. Indeed, in a few cases it is very difficult to recognise clinically whether the trouble is oesophageal or gastric, for the food returned from such a pouch has the same acid smell as gastric vomit, and fermentation takes place just as readily in a dilated oesophagus as it does in the stomach. Moreover, the stomach tube is apt to give most misleading information for, instead of canalising the obstruction, it may either stretch the thinned-out oesophageal wall before it, giving little sense of resistance, or may coil up in the oesophageal dilatation. I have seen a diverticulum, one and a half inches long, pushed out over the dome of the diaphragm by the sheer weight of the tube, in a case where an entry in the notes stated that bougies had been passed into the stomach! On more than one occasion I have found very marked oesophageal obstruction in cases diagnosed as carcinoma of the stomach on the evidence of the chemical examination of a test meal that could not possibly ever have been in the stomach.

It might be expected that this state of affairs could not last long, but when the cause is in part spasmodic the complete relaxation of tone that allows the dilatation also relaxes the spasm, which is often the most important element in the obstruction. When the cause is not rapidly progressive, a cycle may be established oscillating between the second and third stages: a spasmodic obstruction passes through the usual three stages until dilatation results; after a time the oesophagus is too worn out to keep up its spasmodic contraction and relaxation takes place, so that food passes through; as the patient regains strength the muscle recovers its power, and again the spasm is produced. In the larger number of cases, however, a compromise is effected and there is no definite cycle but a more or less permanent condition of dilatation with intermittent leakage, so that the patient lives in comparative comfort but in a state of semi-starvation.

In advanced cases, no matter what the consistency of the opaque food, it simply flows into the oesophagus and lies in the dilated tube, for there are no peristaltic waves of sufficient force to disturb it. Peristaltic waves are represented by mere ripples in the outline. If the sac is called upon to hold more than a certain quantity one of three things happens:

(1) The intra-oesophageal pressure is so raised that the obstruction is overcome and some of the contents pass on.

(2) The column of food rises so high in the oesophagus that the patient ejects some of it.

(3) The dilated oesophagus dilates still further, and sometimes dilatation is carried to an extreme, especially when the obstruction is in the lower part of the oesophagus. Not only does the oesophagus dilate laterally but it increases in length so greatly that its lower part curves out over the cupola of the diaphragm to the right of the middle line, displacing the mediastinal contents and the lungs.

Pathologically, this is the stage where compensation has failed. The fight in which the musculature has called up all its reserves has ended in defeat. The hypertrophied wall is dilated, thinned out, and incapable of effective contraction. It might reasonably be expected that the autopsy would show a thin-walled, dilated oesophagus, but this is in fact rarely recorded in the post-mortem notes. The only explanation I can suggest is that, although the oesophagus has been so distorted during life, in death the same conditions do not exist. Probably rigor mortis and the contraction of the elastic elements of the muscle restore the oesophagus to a semblance of the normal.

Like all involuntary muscle, the oesophagus in life has a wonderful power of recovery, and even a grossly dilated gullet may completely recover its activity and tone in a very short time if it can be rested, i.e. if the obstruction can be reduced or feeding carried on by some other method. In one woman in whom the oesophageal shadow was noted as two inches in diameter, the cause of the obstruction was never determined. It had been present for some months and yielded of its own accord. When I saw her a week later it was impossible, even with solid food, to note any abnormality.

BACK-PRESSURE DILATATION

In occasional cases of hour-glass contraction of the stomach with very small upper sacs, such as used to be seen, the back pressure is so marked that all the symptoms suggest oesophageal obstruction, and in one such case the actual lesion was at first missed, and was only discovered by accident on giving more food in order to demonstrate the patency of the oesophagus to a friend. On another occasion I watched the small upper sac fill up, yet the patient went on eating without any difficulty until the whole oesophagus was distended up to the level of the fourth dorsal vertebra. He had acquired the habit of using the oesophageal ampulla to supplement the capacity of the very small upper sac of a cicatricial hour-glass stomach.

ACHALASIA OF THE CARDIA

(Cardiospasm; Idiopathic Dilatation of the Oesophagus; Oesophagectasia)

This condition is found at all ages and is generally rather sudden in its onset and chronic in its duration. Langmead (214) has described a case in a baby of sixteen months.

Dilatation of the oesophagus without any organic obstruction has passed under the name of cardiospasm ever since it was first described by Purton (276) in 1821. Einhorn (112) in 1888 first made the suggestion that the condition was not in fact due to a spasm but to an absence of relaxation. Rolleston (282) in 1896, not knowing Einhorn's work, arrived at the same conception, but both these papers seem to have been overlooked, and the prevalent idea was that weakened musculature was at the root of the trouble. Hurst (170), not knowing Einhorn's and Rolleston's papers, came to the same conclusions as they had, and sought a new name, one that would be descriptive and accurate, for apparently cardiospasm was a terminological error. Oesophagectasia was first suggested, and later Sir Cooper Perry coined the name of achalasia (absence of relaxation) of the cardia. I am not entirely convinced by the arguments, for post-mortem conditions do not necessarily indicate correctly the conditions that have obtained in life. For instance, at two necropsies I have seen there was certainly no hypertrophy of the cardia, nor was there any indication of thinning of the oesophagus, and it appeared normal in every way. There was nothing to suggest the persistent dilatation that had been observed over a long period. Moreover, the onset of spasm was seen in two cases (cf. Fig. 164). Perhaps too much stress has been laid on the absence of any thickening of the cardiac orifice in these cases, but the name "achalasia of the cardia" has found general acceptance.

The pathology of the condition is still in dispute. It has been attributed to reflex action, to the unbalanced effect of the crura of the diaphragm on the oesophagus, and to various other causes. Hurst (174) in 1924 suggested that most cases are due to progressive organic disease involving Auerbach's plexus, and Hurst and Rake (180) quote illustrative cases. They compare the condition with Hirschsprung's disease and idiopathic dilatation of the ureter, which they ascribe to a similar cause: a loss of tone due to partial destruction of the nerve supply. The reader is referred to this extensive paper for further information. Recently, however, Knight and Adamson (207) reported experiments showing the existence of a true intrinsic sphincter at the cardia, relaxed by the vagus and contracted by the sympathetic. Excision of the vagus reproduced the radiological, pathological and clinical picture of achalasia of the cardia. Certainly in some of my own cases the presence of an actual sphincter seemed quite definite, particularly in the case of the boy aged 9 recorded below.

In the later stages, the oesophagus is dilated and so elongated that it forms a very definite angle as it passes towards the cardiac orifice. The dilatation always ends some distance from the cardia, usually at the level of the diaphragm. The appearance is that of an obstruction at the cardia, and may differ in no radiographic point from that of obstruction due to other causes (Figs. 163 and 164). As more food is given, the column fills from below right up into the neck and may be two inches or even three inches in width. In extreme cases the oesophagus will accommodate large quantities of food. A portion of this is usually vomited and the rest may pass on in time, whenever the orifice relaxes. Twenty-four hours' residue is, however, not uncommon. No definite peristaltic waves are usually seen, but small indentations occur to break the outline: little, futile attempts at peristalsis.

The history of the case often extends over years. The youngest patient in whom I have seen it was a boy who, at the age of 9, stole an unripe apple from an orchard on the way home from school. A piece of apple had apparently

L R

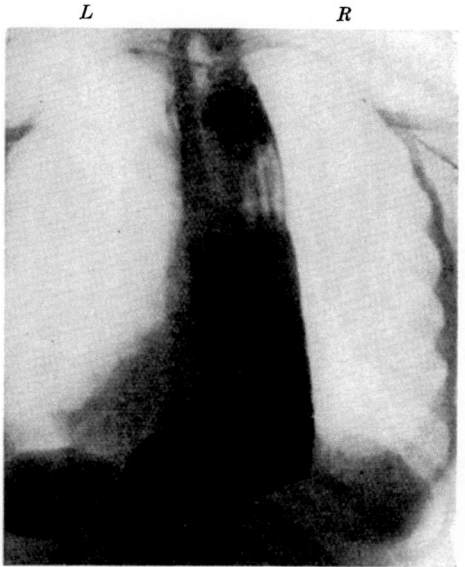 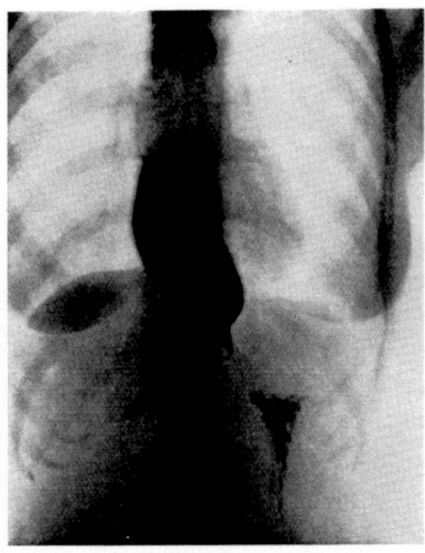

Fig. 163   Fig. 164

Fig. 163. Old-standing case of achalasia in which the oesophagus has become much dilated and tolerant to holding large quantities. The act of vomiting only partially emptied the cavity. A thin tail of the opaque food is passing through the cardiac orifice. The increase in width of the oesophagus is accompanied by increase in length, so that the last few inches lie nearly flat on the diaphragm, forming an angle around which it is practically impossible for a bougie to find its way.

Fig. 164. Achalasia of the cardia in a woman. The appearances are practically identical with those described in the case of the boy aged twelve; the spasm came on *after* the first food had passed through.

stuck in the oesophagus, and from that day onwards he had developed a typical achalasia. When I saw him at the age of 12, he was extremely emaciated. When I gave him liquid opaque food, the first two or three ounces flowed straight through into the stomach, but the cardia suddenly closed (cf. Fig. 164), and the whole of the rest of the mixture stayed in the oesophagus, which was much dilated. At examinations five and twenty-four hours later, no more of the opaque food in the oesophagus had passed through into the stomach. This case is more dramatic in its origin than most, but the ultimate appearance was very much the same as is seen in all these cases. I have only seen the onset of the "spasm" in two cases.

The condition is always very chronic, and the patient lives for years with a large, dilated oesophagus, which leaks intermittently when the spasm relaxes. There is, however, a most curious mechanism by which the whole oesophagus can be emptied by some patients. The following case, recorded twenty years ago (44) but not then explicable, is typical of the very few that I have seen.

The man, a well-nourished coachman, brought to me by Prof. Murray, stated that nine years before, while he was eating his tea, the food had suddenly been returned, although he had never previously had any trouble. For the whole of the nine years he had suffered from this obstruction without any intermission. On examination we found the oesophagus distended with air; a mouthful of opaque food fell, as if through space, from the pharynx to the cardiac orifice. The patient took half a pint of food without any difficulty and the picture was that of a generally dilated oesophagus about three inches in diameter, the bismuth food extending up to about the level of the fifth dorsal vertebra as a wide column. Above this the oesophagus was distended with air. The patient had found out that, when he had filled his oesophagus in this way, he could make the whole of the food pass into the stomach, but it was very painful. We watched the act on two occasions; it evidently demanded a very great effort and took him several minutes to accomplish. There was no thin stream of food passing through at any time; to our astonishment, the collected food was simply moved *en masse* from the oesophagus to the stomach without any narrowing whatever.

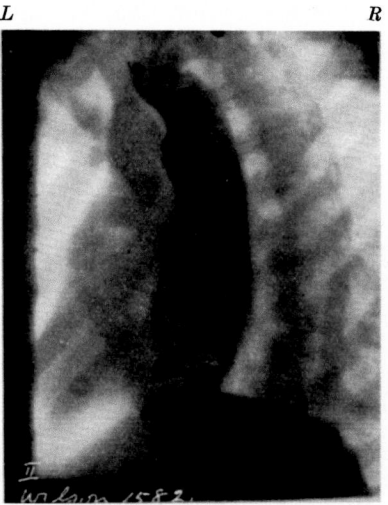

L   R

Fig. 165. Old-standing achalasia of the cardia. The filling defects in the lower part of the shadow are due to retained ordinary food. Note the bulging of the dilated oesophagus into the arch of the aorta.

I was entirely at a loss to interpret this extraordinary muscular effort. The pressure generated by the swallowing of large quantities of air into the oesophagus seemed to be a *vis a tergo*, but why the whole of the food (and of the air also) should pass bodily into the stomach in this way I could not understand. If, however, Payne and Poulton's (265) view of the mechanism of the cardia (cf. p. 145) is correct, then this appearance would be only an extreme manifestation of a normal alternative mechanism.

Operations have been performed to free the oesophagus from its attachments to the diaphragm, and many expedients have been tried to dilate the cardia, but no satisfactory treatment has as yet been devised, probably because the cause is not known. Sometimes the passage of a large bougie will give relief for some weeks or months. Plummer (272) collected many cases of this condition and treated them successfully by dilatation with a bougie. He modified Mixter's suggestion of allowing the patient to swallow a silk thread which finds its way through the obstruction and eventually into the small intestine. He found that considerable traction could be made on the free end, and the thread used to guide a bougie through the obstruction. Olivary-nosed bougies are employed, with holes through which the thread passes. In obstinate cases a dilator, an expansile bag, can be placed in position with this simple guide, and the orifice stretched as much as necessary. Hurst (170) in 1913 described mercury bougies, by means of which the sphincter could be dilated with the minimum of discomfort and danger. These are passed and directed by posturing under X-ray guidance. The condition, however, tends to recur and the procedure has to be repeated at intervals.

CHAPTER XIV

THE DIAPHRAGM

The position and movements of the diaphragm are affected by changes both in the chest and in the abdomen. Its general level may be raised by anything that increases the intra-abdominal pressure, e.g. lying on the abdomen, especially after a full meal, or by ascites and growths. Occasionally, when extensive fibroid changes have followed peritoneal adhesions, it has been found anchored down below its normal position. It may be pressed downwards by fluid or growth in the chest, or pulled upwards by fibroid changes in the lung.

In observing the diaphragm, very particular attention should always be paid to the costo-phrenic angle on both sides, and more especially behind, for it is in this space that the first accumulations of free fluid are seen and the results of old pleuritic adhesions most often found. It is, of course, essential to examine in the upright position, otherwise any small collection of free fluid in the pleural cavity will escape detection.

UNILATERAL ELEVATION OF THE DIAPHRAGM

Causes:

    (i) Physiological.
    (ii) Phrenic nerve paralysis.
    (iii) Eventratio diaphragmatica.
    (iv) Diaphragmatic hernia:
        (*a*) Congenital,
        (*b*) Traumatic.
    (v) Sub-phrenic abscess.
    (vi) Sub-hepatic abscess.

Physiological

Apart from upward displacement of the diaphragm as a whole, there are numerous cases of unilateral elevation, some of which are temporary, others permanent. Temporary elevation of the left side is frequently seen in the X-ray department and, in fact, it may be induced experimentally in some subjects by distending the stomach with carbon dioxide, especially if it already contains a fair quantity of food. The left side of the diaphragm may be raised in this way perhaps a couple of inches, but it quickly descends with eructation. There is no alteration in the rhythm of the movement of the diaphragm. These temporary elevations of the diaphragm are of no pathological significance, but they are always, in my experience, associated with rather large collections of air in the fundus of the stomach.

Paralysis of the Phrenic Nerve

This may be due to trauma, e.g. from operations on cervical glands, or to the invasion by malignant disease of any part of the course of the nerve. The nerve supply of the two sides of the diaphragm is independent, and the diaphragm on the affected side may be considerably elevated (Fig. 166). The point on which the diagnosis rests is that the movements of the affected side are *inverted*, i.e. the affected half of the diaphragm goes up with inspiration and down with expiration. This is known as paradoxical movement. After a time,

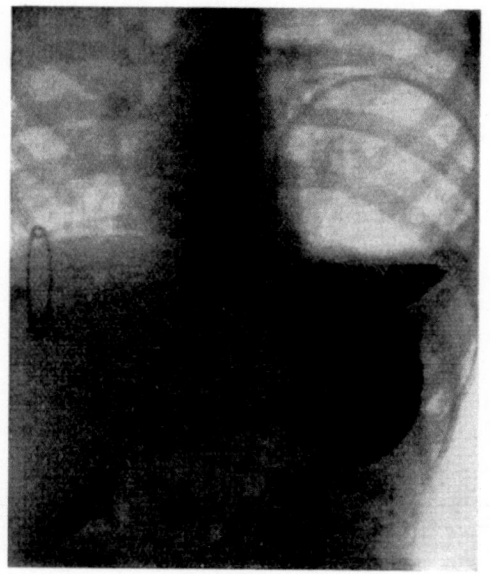
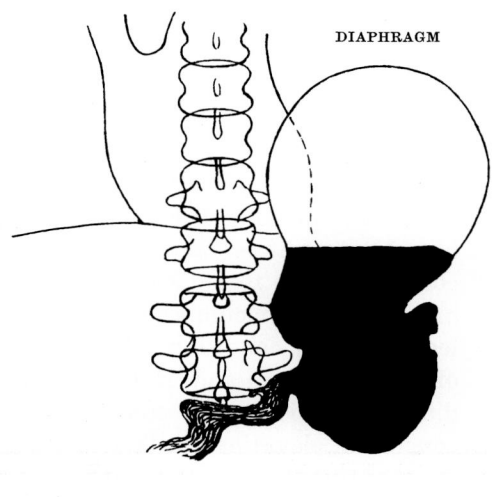

Fig. 166   Fig. 167

Fig. 166. Radiograph of the diaphragm in phrenic nerve paralysis.
(Contributed by J. M. Woodburn Morison.)

Fig. 167. Tracing of Fig. 166.

however, there is a tendency for the affected side to be fixed in its high position and to show very little movement at all. The mediastinal contents also are displaced from the affected side towards the sound side on inspiration, and vice versa. Except on the history, this condition is indistinguishable from eventratio diaphragmatica.

Eventratio Diaphragmatica (Petit's Congenital Elevation)

Congenital elevation of the diaphragm was first described by Petit (248), who died in 1750. He had himself seen two cases and recorded that others had been seen by his colleagues. He recognised it as a congenital defect. There is

considerable literature upon the subject, the most extensive papers being by
J. M. Woodburn Morison (248), H. Walton (329), R. D. Carman and S. Fineman (82),
T. R. Healy (151), A. E. Uspensky and M. O. Wichert (317), L. T. Le Wald (321),
F. W. O'Brien (259), and W. Altschul (10).

In the large majority of cases the elevation is on the left side. The diaphragm
may be as high as the second rib, and its movements inverted as in phrenic
paralysis. In fact, the only difference between these two conditions is that the
one is congenital and the other acquired. The bow-line of the diaphragm can
usually be made out, no matter what its position may be, but, as the lung
extends down both behind and in front of the dome, the bow-line is not always
obvious. The structure of the lung is seen through the dome of the diaphragm
for a considerable distance down the chest. The patients in whom this condition
is found are quite unaware of it and, to the best of my knowledge, it does not
give rise to any disability or predisposition to disease, although gastric symptoms are said to be prevalent.

Diaphragmatic Hernia

Strictly speaking, this is not an elevation of the diaphragm but it is included
here because it is very similar in appearance to the elevations. It may be
congenital, due to a defect in the diaphragm, or acquired, and it is commonly
mistaken for a pneumothorax. Dunhill (110) has devoted a recent Arris and Gale
lecture to this condition. Radiographically it is very like a congenital elevation
of the diaphragm and, in the absence of a history of trauma, it is exceedingly
difficult to distinguish congenital deficiencies of the diaphragm from Petit's
congenital elevation; in fact, the only point upon which the diagnosis can be
made is the demonstration of the remains of the diaphragm, i.e. the neck of the
hernia, cutting into the contour of the cavity (Fig. 168). The opaque meal is, of
course, necessary and the radiologist looks for the neck of the hernia by tilting
the patient into various positions and watching for the indentation in the outline.
In nearly all cases, however, the splenic flexure and the colon are also herniated
and the dual shadow of the stomach and colon make the demonstration of the
impression of the diaphragm exceedingly difficult if not impossible. Morison
maintains that in Petit's eventration the upper limit is an unbroken bow-line,
but that in diaphragmatic hernia some degree of irregularity will be detected.
He also states that in diaphragmatic hernia the horizontal level of the fluid in the
upright position lies above the normal level of the cardiac orifice. With this I do
not agree. In the cases I have seen, the upper limit of the hernial sac—the dome
of the stomach—was fixed, and did not move with respiration.

Traumatic Diaphragmatic Hernia

This is quite uncommon in civil life except after severe crushing. Ambroise Paré (248) recorded two cases in wounded men; in one the opening in the dia-

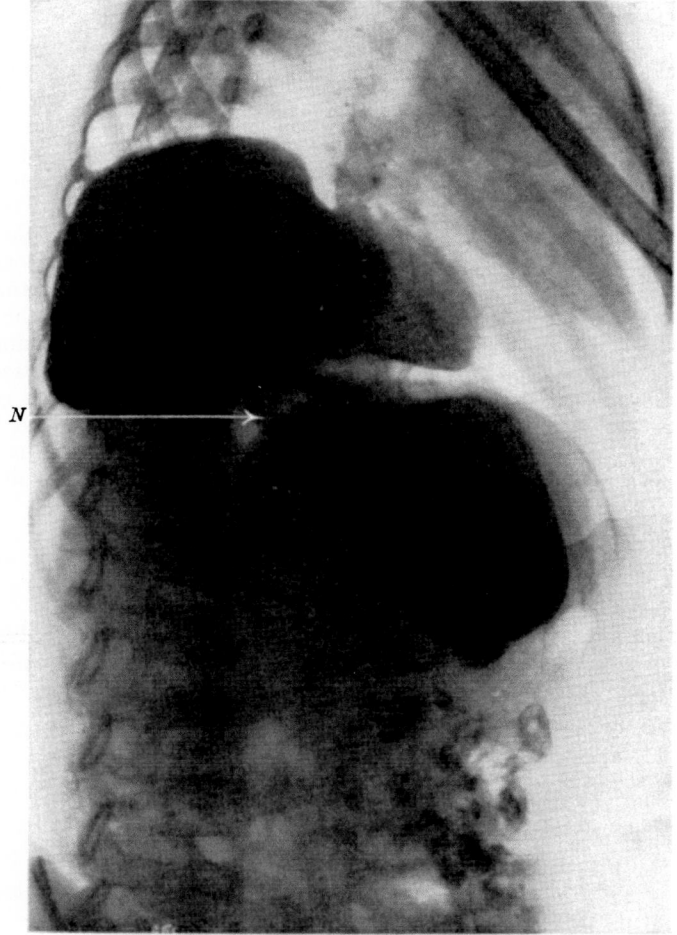

Fig. 168. Lateral view of a diaphragmatic hernia. Lateral supine position showing the neck, N, through which the cardiac end of the stomach has passed. It is unusual to find such a well-marked loculation. (Contributed by J. Currie McMillan.)

phragm would only admit his thumb, yet the whole of the stomach had passed up into the thorax. During the Great War and immediately after, a certain number were met with and studied in some detail.

A patient was sent to me for examination of the chest for pneumothorax, although the symptoms were gastric. He was a soldier who had been wounded two years previously, the bullet having emerged at the back, over the fifth rib on the left side. The wound of entry was not seen. The immediate shock had been considerable, but he had crawled in from No Man's Land and gradually recovered completely from what was regarded as a pneumothorax due to a penetrating wound of the chest. The pneumothorax had persisted, but only in the last few months had he had difficulty in keeping his food down and become markedly emaciated. There was no pain, and vomiting was the only symptom. It was the chest, not the abdomen, that the physician wished me to examine.

The fluorescent screen showed that the whole of the left chest was transradiant up to the second rib, like a pneumothorax, but the air extended below the usual diaphragm level and was bounded by fluid. The heart and mediastinum were somewhat displaced to the right. Opaque food showed that the whole of the left chest was occupied by a much distended stomach, the opaque food flowing right up into the chest when the patient lay on his back. The splenic flexure had accompanied the stomach through the diaphragm. This was quite clearly a case of traumatic hernia, although no trace of the indentation from the edges of the hole in the diaphragm could be detected. It was also clear that the reason for the patient's emaciation was marked pyloric obstruction, which must have been due to torsion; practically no food had passed out of the stomach in five hours and there was still a large residue after twenty-four hours. Operation showed that there was no organic lesion at the pylorus. The surgeon freed the stomach and splenic flexure from their adhesions in the apex of the chest and repaired the large rent in the diaphragm. The patient did not survive the operation, for he was in a very weak state.

I understand that in most of the cases that were operated on, the surgeon repaired the diaphragm and restored the anatomical position. In one subsequent similar case, however, no attempt was made to reduce the deformity and repair the damage, a simple gastro-enterostomy being performed with eminently satisfactory results; the patient regained complete health and strength in spite of the fact that the fundus of his stomach was in the region of his clavicle.

Looking back on these cases, it is fairly clear that the radiological appearances in these and other patients pointed definitely to traction on the pylorus as the cause of the symptoms. Why the patients should have been free from gastric symptoms for a long period after the injury is not easy to understand.

The outstanding impressions left on my mind are:

(1) That diaphragmatic hernia may simulate pneumothorax very closely; this was the clinical diagnosis in all the cases I saw.

(2) That the stomach may be displaced high up into the chest without causing definite gastric symptoms; it is not the displacement but the effects of displacement that give symptoms.

(3) That operation should, in the first place, aim at relieving mechanical disability rather than restoring anatomical position. Anatomical position does not seem to be necessarily of much importance in relation to function.

Congenital Absence of the left half of the Diaphragm

This has been recorded by Le Wald (322), who is of opinion that many of the cases recorded as hernia are in reality congenital absence which the radiologist has failed to recognise. A case was published by Harris and Clayton-Green (99), who drew attention to the fact that the diaphragm is not essential to life and that it is not present in animals below the mammal. One of the subjects described by Le Wald was so physically fit, in spite of the absence of part of his diaphragm, that he was known as a good athlete and had been selected to take part in a five-mile relay race.

Le Wald claims that the differential diagnosis between congenital elevation and partial absence of the diaphragm can be made by X-ray examination, especially in the lateral position. When part of the diaphragm is missing, repeated examination will show a change in the contour of the shadows thrown by the upper border of the stomach or the colon in this region, although at times they may appear dome-like.

In the course of anatomical demonstrations, a subject presented himself for the study of the large intestine, having taken opaque food the previous evening. He was a well-developed youth who played in his college football and other teams and had never suspected that the disposition of his viscera was other than normal. Figs. 169 and 170, traced from the radiographs, show the condition that was found, i.e. the whole colon disposed in almost normal form in the chest and the transverse colon running from somewhere in the region of the heart apex up towards the left scapular region, high up in the chest, while the descending colon came from this region right down to the sigmoid, which apparently had none of the usual sigmoid curves.

One would expect to find the stomach also in the chest, and I only know of one other case in which this has not been so. The extraordinary length suggested adhesions to the pelvis, but the stomach was perfectly free. I attempted to discover what viscera occupied the right flank by examining three hours after an opaque meal, but although half of the food had passed on and was found in the caecum, none of it was seen in the small intestine. The position of the liver was not determined. Air entry was perfect throughout both lungs and, apart from the displacements caused by the viscera, the lung would have been passed as normal. It was extraordinary to watch the air entry, the lungs expanding into and around the colon shadow. It would have been most instructive to investigate this case in detail, but unfortunately this would have made the subject too conscious that he was not built as other men. Few cases have impressed me so much with the way in which Nature can depart from normal anatomical lines and yet obtain perfect function. By a curious coincidence an almost similar case was reported by Hackwood (145) in the *British Medical Journal* almost on the day on which I discovered this case. It was not recognised until the abdomen was opened. Le Wald has also described an exactly comparable case. Other reports have been published by Hunter (164, 165, 166) and Anderson (21). Hunter's cases were found in the foetus.

Oesophageal Orifice Hernia

Some authorities believe that the cardiac portion of the stomach and the oesophagus can herniate through the oesophageal orifice of the diaphragm when the musculature becomes weakened by old age or some other cause. In 1925 Åkerlund classified the condition under three headings: (1) paroesophageal; (2) congenital, with shortening of the oesophagus, and (3) a hitherto unrecognised form which had not been confirmed anatomically and was difficult to demonstrate by X rays; it was distinguished from paroesophageal hernias by the fact that the whole cardiac section of the oesophagus, together with that of the

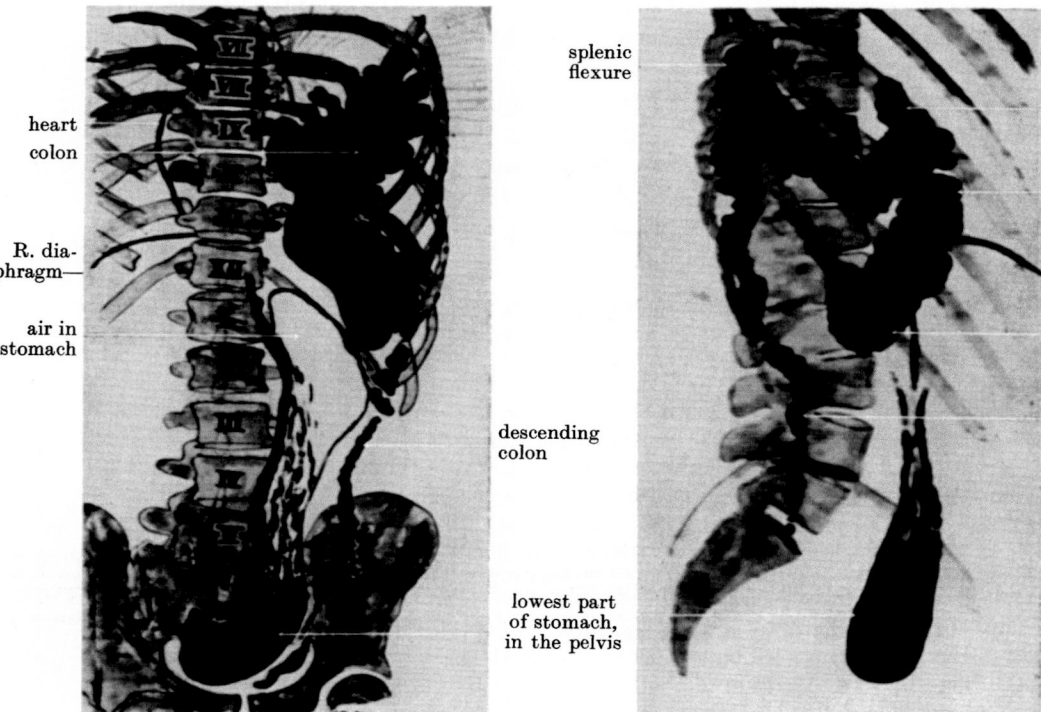

Fig. 169

Fig. 170

Fig. 169. Congenital absence of the diaphragm in a healthy athletic student. Postero-anterior view.

Fig. 170. Lateral view of congenital absence of the diaphragm.

stomach, was displaced upwards through the diaphragm. He said that if this third variety were included, hiatus hernia was six or seven times as frequent as all other forms of diaphragmatic hernia. Bársony (54a) in 1928 and Berg(59) in 1931 published confirmatory observations, and Knothe reported in 1932 that he had seen 300 cases in a single year. Sauerbruch, Chaoul and Adam (289a), however, doubt whether the syndrome exists at all and say that the description arises from a misinterpretation of radiographs which really show a dilated oesophageal ampulla. The controversy is still acute (348). Hurst (176) has recently published an article on recurrent cases of hernia of the stomach through the diaphragm, with a typical history. He points out that the routine radiological examination fails to reveal these hernias, which are not present when the patient stands up. Berg recommends that the patient should lie on his back and drink the barium in this position. If the patient is instructed to increase the intra-abdominal pressure by bearing down, the condition is more likely to be found.

Sub-phrenic Abscess

A sub-phrenic abscess is a collection of pus directly below the diaphragm. It is more common on the right than on the left side, and its origin may be traced to a number of abnormal conditions; the appendix is said to account for 36 per cent. of the cases but, now that patients with appendicitis are nursed in a reclining position and not flat, this percentage has probably been reduced. The other common causes are perforation of duodenal and gastric ulcers, perinephric infection and liver abscess. In the cases that owe their origin to perforation of ulcer, it is not at all uncommon to find gas in the abscess cavity, which, of course, makes the radiological detection straightforward.

The appearances produced by a sub-phrenic abscess may vary considerably. The diaphragm is *raised* and has limited movement or is *fixed* on the affected side. On screen examination the presence of a small quantity of fluid in the costophrenic angle, due to pleural reaction, is often noted and is almost pathognomonic if the diaphragm is raised and fixed. This fluid is sterile, but may become infected. Later on there may be considerable accumulations of fluid in the pleural cavity. If the abscess contains gas, the bow-line of the diaphragm is seen above it, with the fluid level of the pus below. The position of the abscess in relation to the peritoneum produces variations in the radiological picture:

(*a*) If the abscess is located in a peritoneum-covered area of the liver, the earliest signs are that the right side of the diaphragm is fixed in the expiratory phase, i.e. considerably higher than normal, and the liver looks as if it were pushed up. There may or may not be air in the abscess cavity. The lower edge of the liver is not as a rule displaced downwards because of the adhesions that occur around the abscess. There will probably be some fluid in the base of the chest.

(*b*) If the abscess occurs in a region which is not covered by peritoneum, i.e. between the bare area of the liver and the diaphragm, the same appearances are seen, but there is said to be a greater tendency for the liver to be pushed downwards.

(*c*) It is stated that if the abscess occurs behind the liver, it gives rise to rotation of the liver, which is then particularly easily palpated.

It is not always easy to distinguish with certainty between a sub-phrenic abscess and a diaphragm that is merely pushed up by any of the various causes of enlargement of the liver. As a rule the diaphragm is not fixed in these cases, and there is no fluid in the base of the pleural cavity. Moreover, the lower edge of the liver is displaced downwards.

Sub-hepatic Abscess

This is not diagnosed directly, but by the displacements it produces, e.g. the liver is probably pushed up and the diaphragm is not so definitely fixed as in sub-phrenic abscess. The appearance of something lying between a liver which is displaced upwards and a stomach which is also displaced suggests an abscess or other abnormality. If there are clinical signs suggesting sepsis, the displacement will probably be due to sub-hepatic abscess.

Hydatid Cyst

Hydatid cyst of the liver is rare in this country but relatively frequent in Iceland, Australia, New Zealand and some of the South American countries. There are many references to it in radiological literature, and Anderson[20] has given an account of the incidence and radiological diagnosis based on his experiences of the disease in New Zealand. But the most extensive and complete radiological account of the subject is by Claessen[98], whose work was aided by the Icelandic Government and published in 1928. He records 44 cases, 37 of which were in the liver, although many writers have held that the disease is more common in the lungs. Cysts in the liver give fairly typical appearances, pushing up the diaphragm to a varying extent into the pulmonary field as a smooth, well-rounded projection. The diaphragmatic movements are limited, but there is no fluid in the costo-phrenic angle, as there does not appear to be any pleural reaction. Daughter cysts may show as rounded projections from the mother cyst. Very often the cyst has a patchy appearance due to irregular calcareous degeneration of the walls. Cysts sometimes perforate the diaphragm and discharge through the lungs; before X-rays were introduced these cysts were probably diagnosed as pulmonary. Not infrequently, hydatid cysts are sub-hepatic and displace the stomach and other viscera.

Spasm of the Diaphragm

This gives rise to pseudo-tympanites with much abnormal distension. It is rare, and affects both men and women. It is referred to by A. F. Hurst[178] and by T. G. Moorhead[246]. Radiographically, although the abdomen is enormously distended, there is no apparent excess of air in the intestine, and on examination it is found that the diaphragm is in the position of full inspiration and more or less fixed in this position. Moreover, the domed appearance is much flattened, so that the muscle forms almost a straight line on the level of the twelfth dorsal vertebra.

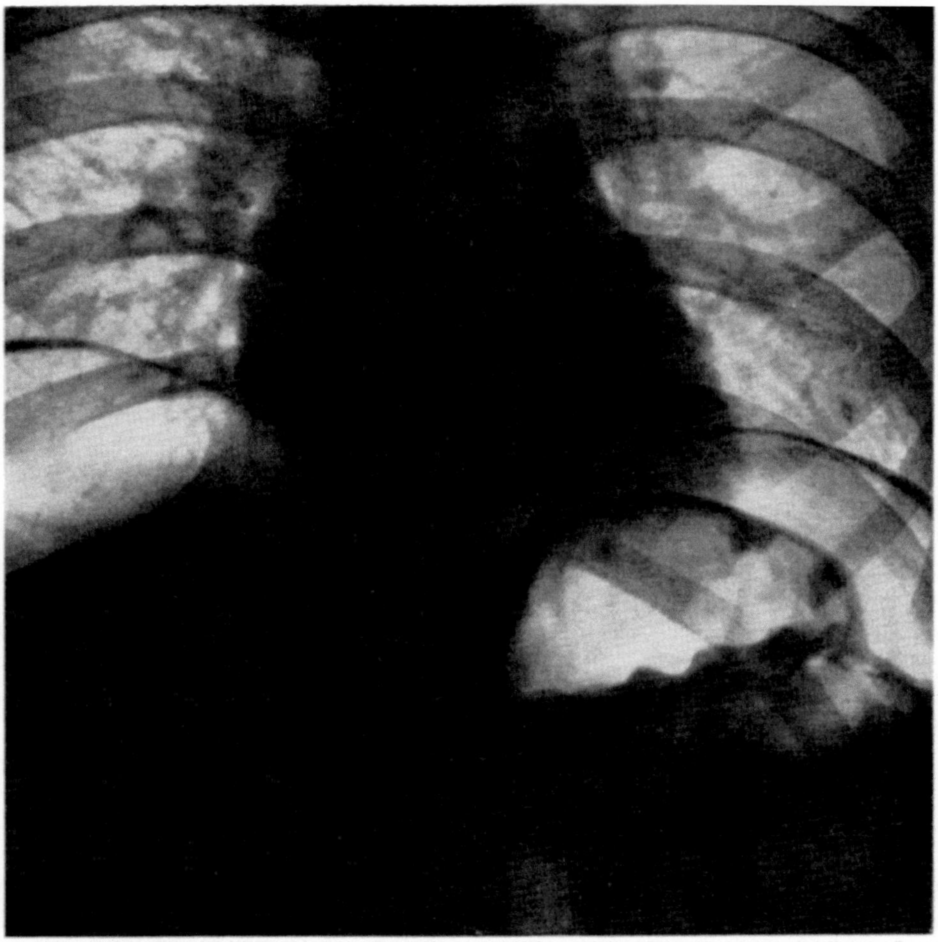

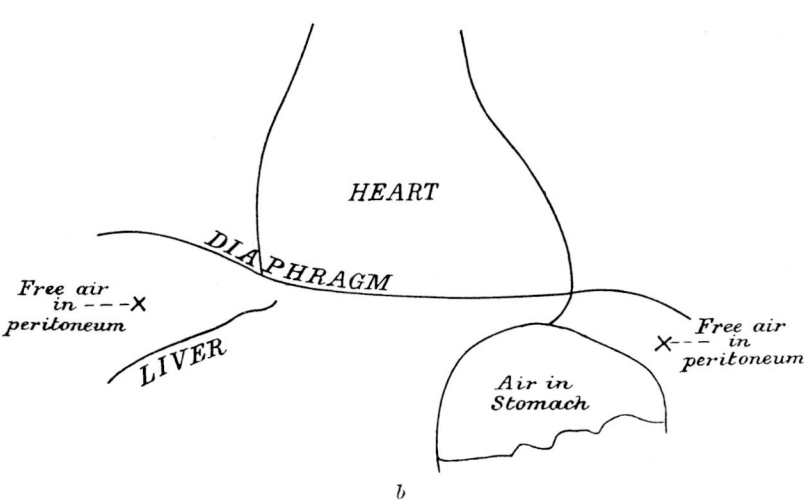

Fig. 171. *a, b.* Radiograph and tracing of free air in the peritoneal cavity. An extremely rare case in which it appears that an ulcer has perforated and formed a valvular opening into the peritoneum. The air persistently recurred although the patient exhibited no indication of peritoneal inflammation and, on posturing, it was freely movable within the peritoneal cavity. (Contributed by J. Duncan White.)

The condition is very distressing and difficult to treat unless the cause is understood. The patients improve, as a rule, in the recumbent position, and the distension can be reduced by manipulation, but is apt to return. The best treatment appears to be suggestion, the patient being told the nature of the condition and trained to overcome it. It seems possible, however, that air sucking (p. 280) may be associated with a similar trouble. Both conditions may be closely associated with hysteria, although the type of case described by several writers does not, on the face of it, look as if it could fall into any such category.

Free gas in the peritoneal cavity

This may arise from perforation of various parts of the alimentary tract, but it is very unusual to see it in the X-ray department, as such cases are almost invariably acutely ill. Dr Duncan White has, however, shown me radiographs (Fig. 171) of a case in which there was obviously access of air to the peritoneal cavity, for its presence was noted time and again while the patient remained in hospital. The re-accumulation of air was unaccompanied by severe symptoms and the patient went home. Subsequent examinations showed that the condition still persisted, and it was believed to be due to a gastric perforation that was sealed in some valvular manner.

On a few occasions I have diagnosed large localised abdominal abscesses containing fluid and gas; at operation these were found just beneath the abdominal wall and contained the most foul-smelling pus that I have ever encountered. I have not detected any abscess that did not contain gas, but presumably such localised abscesses occur. It is improbable, however, that they would be recognised radiographically, unless they produced displacements and the blood picture indicated sepsis.

Free gas may be found in the abdomen for some time after operation, as it takes a long time for air to be absorbed. In the days when the injection of air, oxygen or carbon dioxide into the peritoneal cavity was practised as a diagnostic radiographic method, the air and oxygen remained for weeks, but the carbon dioxide was absorbed fairly rapidly.

Air in the peritoneal cavity is also met with sometimes when the diaphragm has been injured in aspirating a pleurisy or performing artificial pneumothorax.

The diagnosis of free air, of course, depends on viewing the patient in various positions and seeing that the air moves about. Air in a distended coil of intestine is the only condition with which it is likely to be confused. It should not be forgotten, however, that coils of gas-filled intestine may wander into many positions that, anatomically, would seem to be impossible, e.g. between the liver and the diaphragm, and between the lesser curvature of the stomach and the liver. These coils are not duodenum, the only part of the intestine that it seems anatomically reasonable to find in this region.

CHAPTER XV

GASTRIC, DUODENAL AND JEJUNAL ULCERATION

Introductory

Thanks very largely to radiology and to the fact that surgery could prove or disprove the findings of the radiologist, ideas on the value of symptoms have been revolutionised in the last twenty years. Clinicians now realise how utterly unreliable were the signs and symptoms on which they had, perforce, to base their opinions. Dyspepsia was considered a *sine qua non* for a diagnosis of ulceration; haemorrhage was almost unequivocal evidence of it; pain, and especially the time relation of pain to the taking of food, was of the first importance. Now they know that haemorrhage is merely an accident or an incident, and that it may bear little relation to the size, the site, or even the presence of ulcer. Pain also appears to be a mere incident and may be entirely absent. The pain of duodenal ulcer is often felt about two hours after food, but this formula is quite unreliable and may also apply, as far as I can see, to ulcer in any part of the stomach. Extensive ulceration is sometimes seen not only without pain but actually without any sign of indigestion. It is difficult for those who have the old ideas of symptoms deeply rooted in their minds to realise how fallacious were the guides of those days—so difficult that, even in the presence of unequivocal radiological evidence of ulceration, radiologists may find it difficult to convince clinicians of the facts. Only by the persistent operative proof of X-ray diagnosis have the old prejudices been gradually broken down, and the report of the competent radiologist come to be regarded as of more value than all the traditional signs and chemical tests put together.

Although the radiologist should always go into the clinical history and obtain all the help he can from it, he should not allow himself to be prejudiced by it in an examination. He must report on the facts as revealed by his examination; it is for others to determine the line of treatment and, fortunately for the patient, the demonstration of an ulcer is no longer *ipso facto* the indication for an operation. When an ulcer has been reported it is no part of the radiologist's duty to say whether the clinical picture, of which the X-ray demonstration of the ulcer is a part, calls for operative or for medical measures.

With the increase in the efficiency of apparatus and the development of technique, deductive guess-work as to the presence of ulceration has given place to a certainty of diagnosis that, in the hands of a real expert, reaches a remarkable degree of accuracy. In fact, the radiologist's attitude towards the X-ray diagnosis of gastric ulcer has completely altered. He no longer takes great credit for the positive and unequivocal diagnosis of an ulcer, but worries very considerably if he misses one. But let it not be forgotten that ulcers heal, sometimes quite rapidly. Perhaps the radiologist should have a printed legend on all report sheets: "This report is only valid till...". A surgeon once upbraided me for failing to find an ulcer although it was then several years since I had examined the patient!

The accuracy of the diagnosis depends on the skill and persistence of the observer, but there are still two sites where accuracy is not certain in spite of painstaking technique, viz. the fundus, where palpation cannot be applied, and the pyloric end of the lesser curvature, where the wall of the stomach is thick. At any rate, these are the two sites in which my own failures have been most frequent.

In the early days of gastro-intestinal work diagnosis depended on the detection of gross appearances, such as the hour-glass contraction and evidence of cicatrisation. The detail of to-day was impossible, almost undreamed of. The detection of an ulcer crater was unknown, and the radiologist had to rely upon indirect evidence: spasm, delay in emptying, localised pain on deep pressure, and so forth. These things, although of interest, have now lost much of their diagnostic importance, for he now relies almost implicitly on the demonstration of the actual crater of the ulcer. Probably in the old days many ulcers were missed, for these indirect signs were far from trustworthy, but they paved the way for the present routine: a routine that, in the hands of an expert, is a tedious and meticulously careful analysis of the whole surface of the mucous membrane. The high percentage of accuracy can never be achieved by the labour-saving service of snapshot radiography, but only by a concentrated search in which sight and touch are co-ordinated to unravel the secrets of the ordered or disordered mucous membrane. Snapshot radiography plays a comparatively small part in the examination, and with few exceptions the films are merely records for reference or demonstration, the diagnosis being made on the screen observations. The radiologist who depends on radiography entirely will show quite a large number of ulcer craters as projections on the profile of the opaque shadow, but the observer who develops the technique of palpation (cf. p. 18), using the first mouthful of opaque food to visualise and unravel the folds of the mucous membrane, will discover many more ulcers, especially those which are not on the lesser curvature and which are almost certainly missed by pure radiographic methods.

INDIRECT SIGNS

Indirect signs were of more value in those early days than now, for the cases then were the chronic dyspeptics who went on year after year, from one physician to the next, in search of relief. Many of them showed evidence of long-standing cicatrisation, the typical hour-glass stomach that is almost a rarity to-day. It is worth reviewing these indirect signs of other days, because they do in some measure help us to understand a little more of the mechanism, and to show those who have only used the present methods something of what was seen when a bread-and-milk meal was given, and when the radiologist had to depend on secondary evidence for which to-day there is no need.

I believe that the present type of opaque food is misleading and that, under normal conditions with ordinary food-stuffs, there is probably a larger spasmodic element in most organic lesions involving the mucous membrane than the examination suggests. Probably the functional disturbance depends not so much on the lesion itself as upon the resulting spasmodic contraction. Because of the modern smooth, creamy opaque meal this spasmodic element is apt nowadays to be forgotten. The bread-and-milk food used in early years made spasm a prominent feature. At that time I thought that all ulcers must be in a more or less irritable condition; that I should find no ulceration unless there was some spasm to call attention to it, and that if the spasm were not present it would be induced by the bread-and-milk opaque food. In fact, in order to make certain of inducing spasm, I often gave toasted breadcrumbs before the opaque meal, and they did actually induce spasm in a number of cases where the bread-and-milk meal had failed, the diagnosis of ulcer being confirmed at operation. Often it was the spasm, and the spasm only, that gave the diagnosis, and whenever there was an hour-glass appearance one suspected ulceration.

If this contraction resolved under massage and manipulation, we held that it was merely due to spasm; if it did not, we gave large doses of tincture of belladonna which should, theoretically, relieve spasm but which in reality was very uncertain in action. If a contraction of hour-glass type persisted in spite of these measures, we held that it was due to an ulcer, and with the chronic cases of those days we were usually correct. But spasm complicated even the cicatricial type of hour-glass contraction, even the type in which the puckered scar and adhesions formed pockets in which the opaque food lodged. We attempted to assess the relative parts played by these two factors of spasm and scar tissue formation, usually with little success. The hour-glass deformity that we saw was nearly always due to spasm. In some of the cases where we thought that the contraction must be purely organic on account of its persistence (in some instances retained food had been seen in the upper sac after 24 hours), we found at operation relatively little organic narrowing. In fact, we failed to distinguish the cicatricial from the spasmodic hour-glass even in some of the extreme cases, and gained very little faith in our methods of differentiation.

Before the detection of the ulcer crater was possible, insistence was laid upon the importance of re-examining every case, if possible both when the patient was complaining of the symptoms and also when he was free from them, so that a comparison might be made and an opinion formed on whether the gastric contraction was or was not responsible. Quite frequently the re-examination showed a contraction that had not been present before, and led to a diagnosis of ulceration which would otherwise have been missed.

Spasm seemed to play such a large part that the suggestion was made that it might be the determining factor in the arrest of haemorrhage when once a vessel had been eroded by ulceration. If this is true, treatment directed to *increase* gastric spasm would seem to be indicated until all haemorrhage has ceased.

Spasm at the pylorus also, as shown by the retention of food, was not only more common with the bread-and-milk meal than it is to-day, but was relied upon to a great extent as evidence, for we still believed in the acid control of the pylorus, and did not know what varied stimuli and what widely separated impulses contribute to pyloric control. We were dealing mostly with cases which to-day would rightly be regarded as having been sadly neglected, and in whom we often found extreme delay in emptying; twenty-four, forty-eight or even seventy-two hours afterwards nearly all the food would still be found in the bottom of the great, flaccid, atonic stomach that sagged away down into the pelvis. These wretched "dyspeptics" had been going on year after year with this condition; most of them were treated symptomatically by gastro-enterostomy without any serious effort to determine whether or not ulceration was present, and many were greatly benefited. At operation some showed no external signs of ulceration, but a considerable proportion presented obvious evidence of old scarring, sometimes such a dense mass of cicatrisation that malignancy was not only suggested but considered probable.

One case in particular I recollect in which a surgeon of wide experience told me that he hardly thought he should have done a gastro-enterostomy, as there appeared to be no hope for the patient and it would only prolong her suffering. Yet twenty years later that patient is perfectly well and has never looked back. I take it that it was not only the cicatricial mass but the added spasm, which happened not to have subsided under the anaesthetic, that led the surgeon to his conclusion; the patient was only about 23 and had not suffered from prolonged indigestion, so that one would hardly expect a large cicatricial mass.

Pain

All my observations on spasm seem to support Hurst's view (167) that "tension is the only cause of true visceral pain". Poulton (274), as a result of a number of experiments, holds that visceral pain is due to stretching and consequent deformity of the nerve endings in the walls of the viscus. He believes that visceral pain is an affair of the whole visceral wall and not of any isolated lesion in it, and that peptic ulcer produces painful effects secondarily by causing reflex increase of tone. Morley (252), dealing with the pain of appendicitis, regards the initial pain as due to increased tension and the later localised pain as a result of irritation of the parietal peritoneum. He believes that true visceral or splanchnic pain exists but is characteristically ill-defined. It is usually a dull pain felt vaguely in the centre of the abdomen and is probably produced by tension in the muscular wall. It exhibits primitive features. The relatively insensitive viscera are protected by the highly sensitive wall of the cavity in which they lie. This wall responds to wounds from without or insults from within by inflammation. The viscera themselves are very slightly sensitive only, and the threshold for the stimuli which excite true visceral pain must be high. The importance of examining while symptoms are present is therefore obvious, for it may be possible to detect the tension and spasm that are causing them.

Pain on deep localised pressure over the site of a suspected ulcer was a point on which we were inclined to lay stress. However, we discovered fairly early that the absence of pain had no negative value whatever, but that the definite presence of a point of pain, especially when confirmed at a second examination, was almost diagnostic when it coincided with, or even approximated to, the site of a contraction of the stomach. This view of the diagnostic value of a painful spot has not altered since the early days.

Miller, Pendergrass and Andrews (237) give a table showing the time-relation of pain in gastric and duodenal ulcer and, although the numbers are small, it is of interest to note that gastric lesions tended to cause pain sooner after food than did duodenal ulcers, but that there was no evidence to support the idea that the higher the lesion the earlier the pain. Another table in their paper shows the factors relieving pain and the frequency of other symptoms: 57 per cent. of gastric and 38 per cent. of duodenal ulcers had definite spots of epigastric tenderness. I am not, however, at all certain of the meaning of a "point of pain on deep pressure". The arguments of Morley and Twining (253) are reasonable but do not, in my opinion, quite cover the ground. They say:

We are satisfied from these investigations that the correspondence between the point of deep tenderness and the position of the ulcer is a clinical fact....Our results, therefore, entirely confirm Hurst's recent statements as regards the facts, but our interpretation of them is diametrically opposed to his [i.e. that the stomach wall when ulcerated is not insensitive, but endowed with true visceral tenderness]....We believe that contact between the parietal peritoneum and the inflamed visceral peritoneum over the ulcer provides the adequate stimulus, though whether that stimulus is mechanical and due to roughening, or chemical and due to bacterial toxins, we can advance no opinion.

Hurst and Stewart (181) divide tenderness in gastric and duodenal ulcer into (1) visceral tenderness and (2) reflex tenderness and rigidity. The visceral tenderness is the localised deep tenderness which corresponds to the site of the ulcer.

THE FREQUENCY AND DISTRIBUTION OF ULCERS

The partnership of radiology and surgery has revolutionised our ideas on the frequency and distribution of abdominal disease. The figures that are given for the incidence of ulceration in the stomach and duodenum vary according to the opportunities of the investigator. As Albrecht (7) points out, the pathologist only sees those few cases of gastric ulcer that pass through the post-mortem room, and comparatively few dyspeptics die in institutions. The surgeon only sees those selected cases that come to operation.

The most striking feature of all recent figures is the relative frequency of duodenal ulcer. At the beginning of the century it was comparatively unknown and supposed to be associated with extensive burns, while gastric ulcer was regarded as one of the commonest abdominal conditions; indeed it was the fashion for any anaemic young lady to be suspected of a gastric ulcer.

Albrecht (7) has recently reviewed his radiological findings in a large series of dyspeptics sent to his department for investigation and examined by the elaborate and painstaking technique developed by Berg. His analysis, which shows a high proportion of duodenal ulcers, probably presents a much more accurate picture of the distribution than was formerly possible. Balfour (27) (in America), reviewing the work of the Mayo Clinic, and A. J. Walton (330) (in England), analysing his own material, both point out the extraordinary frequency of duodenal compared with gastric ulcer.

In an analysis of 1527 cases of dyspepsia, Albrecht found 363 ulcers, i.e. 23·77 per cent. of all the cases of dyspepsia referred to him. Of these, 305 (84 per cent.) were in the duodenum and 52 (14·3 per cent.) in the stomach. Six (1·7 per cent.) were gastro-peptic. The relation of duodenal to gastric ulcer was thus 5·86 to 1.

The figures given by Balfour from the Mayo Clinic for cases operated on in 1930 show 524 duodenal ulcers (78 per cent.); 85 gastric ulcers (12 per cent.) and 64 gastro-jejunal ulcers (9·5 per cent.). The relation of duodenal to gastric ulcer was practically 6 to 1. The proportion of duodenal ulcers becomes even more remarkable when one takes into account the fact that—as I was informed verbally—only 40 per cent. of duodenal ulcers diagnosed radiologically are treated by the surgeon in this clinic. I have no note of the proportion of gastric ulcers treated without surgery, but I gathered that it was not so high. The duodenal ulcers were very frequently multiple, and the most important from the clinical point of view were those on the posterior wall. Operation was successful in 88–90 per cent. of cases; in 3 per cent. the ulceration recurred, and about 3 per cent. developed gastro-jejunal ulcers. The mortality was about 1 per cent.

A. J. Walton analyses 1436 of his own operation cases, which he describes as "in greater part medical failures". The relation of pyloric and duodenal ulcer to gastric was 2¼ to 1. In England, therefore, the disparity between gastric and duodenal ulceration seems to be less than in Germany and America. My impression—for I have no statistics available—is that my figures in X-ray practice would have shown a considerably higher percentage of duodenal ulcers.

Sutherland (307), working in the X-ray service at the Mayo Clinic in 1927, found that the relative frequency of duodenal to gastric ulcer in his series was 9 to 1. Miller, Pendergrass and Andrews (237) give a ratio of 4 to 1, and Moynihan (256) in a series of 695 operated cases found approximately the same ratio.

There seems to be a geographical variation in incidence: at one time duodenal ulcers were common in Leeds (where Moynihan was doing his pioneer work on this condition), comparatively rare in Manchester, forty miles away, and almost unknown in Liverpool, eighty miles away—not only in the operating theatre but also in the post-mortem rooms. Moreover, the relative incidence of gastric and duodenal ulcer seems to differ definitely and markedly in different parts of the world. For the Mayo Clinic the two sets of figures I have seen give 1 : 6 and 1 : 9; in certain German clinics it is 1 : 6, while others give a figure as low as 1 : 1. Moreover, the type of ulceration appears to differ. In Germany it is more widespread and shows greater tendency to perforation; for this reason German surgeons tend to adopt radical treatment and excise large areas of the stomach wall. In the United States and Great Britain there is a relative absence of inflammatory changes in the mucous membrane, and operative procedures are almost always conservative, gastro-enterostomy or pyloroplasty yielding very satisfactory results. Walters (327) of the Mayo Clinic, who worked in Schmieden's clinic in Frankfurt, is much impressed with the difference in the type of ulceration; he has confirmed it by examining excised specimens from both clinics. He found that ulceration of the stomach and duodenum in Germany is generally associated with extensive inflammation of the mucous membrane, whereas in America it tends to be localised, with healthy mucous membrane extending right up to the affected area.

The geographical incidence of disease is emphasised by the experience of some of my old students in Cairo. At the Kasr-el-Aini Hospital there are approximately 500 gastro-intestinal examinations a year, and yet only 2 gastric and 6 duodenal ulcers were found during 1931. Clinically these conditions appear to be very common, but the extreme rarity of actual pathological lesions is confirmed both in the operating theatre and in the post-mortem room. On the other hand, polyposis of the large intestine, seldom seen in Europe and America, is so common in Cairo that it is almost regarded as constant. This, however, is readily explained by the fact that, in the country districts, the Nile water is used for all purposes and intestinal parasites are the rule rather than the exception.

Church and Walters (96) have published a study of twenty-five cases in which partial gastrectomy was performed for duodenal ulceration. In three of these, i.e. 12 per cent., there was gross gastritis and in three more there was some microscopic evidence of gastritis. Aschner and Grossman (24) found gastritis in 64 per cent. of 124 cases of duodenal ulcer which they record, and regard it as a usual predisposing condition, the ulcer being merely a phase of the process of inflammation. These findings are in striking contrast with the figures of German and Austrian observers and offer yet another illustration of the geographical variations encountered.

Other Statistics

Some other interesting data given by Miller, Pendergrass and Andrews [237] show that many of the figures quoted in text-books are unreliable. For instance, they found the peak period for both gastric and duodenal ulcer at about 45 years of age, whereas text-books usually cite 35 for duodenal and 25 for gastric ulcer. They also found that, of all ulcers, seven occurred in men to every one in a woman. The ratio of gastric ulcer was 9 male to 1 female, and of duodenal ulcer 8·5 male to 1·5 female. Walton found that gastric ulcer was twice as common, and pyloric and duodenal ulcers three times as common in men as in women.

Albrecht's analysis of the location of the ulcers showed that 52 per cent. were on the lesser curvature, 17 per cent. on the posterior wall, 3·3 per cent. on the greater curvature, 24·6 per cent. in the pyloric end, and 1·8 per cent. in the cardia.

At the Mayo Clinic 50 per cent. of all cases of malignant disease occurring in the clinic were gastric, and carcinoma was found to be three times as common as gastric ulcer. I doubt whether similar figures would be found in this country; my impression is that gastric ulcer and carcinoma are about equal in incidence here.

In quite a considerable number of cases two or even more separate lesions may be present at the same time, e.g. an ulcer of the body of the stomach and one at the pylorus or in the duodenum. Once I had a patient who had spasmodic obstruction of the oesophagus—probably due to a peptic ulcer—a cicatricial hour-glass contraction with ulcer, and a thickened pylorus with well-marked obstruction.

THE ULCER CRATER

Haudek [149] of Vienna (whose early death in 1931 is so deeply deplored) was the first to demonstrate the pocket formed by an ulcer crater. Before that, various people had talked of the bismuth sticking to the floor of an ulcer but had not radiographed what they described, nor had they described what other observers could confirm. My impression at the time, knowing the apparatus in use, was that imagination played no little part in the radiographic detection of ulcers which had really been diagnosed clinically. Many observers had seen the bismuth sticking in the folds of cicatricial scarring, but Haudek first demonstrated the niche, the actual crater of the ulcer, and we rightly give him the credit for this discovery by applying his name to these niches. It was, however, many years before radiologists, thanks largely to the detailed study of the mucous membrane initiated by Forssell (121) and elaborated by Berg (58), realised the true character of the niches that they filled with opaque food.

The detection of the ulcer crater is the one unequivocal sign of an ulcer (Figs. 172–177). The method of palpation by which these pockets are detected is described on p. 18. The pocket may be on the profile of the shadow, and then it is at once seen when the stomach is filled, and there is no difficulty in making

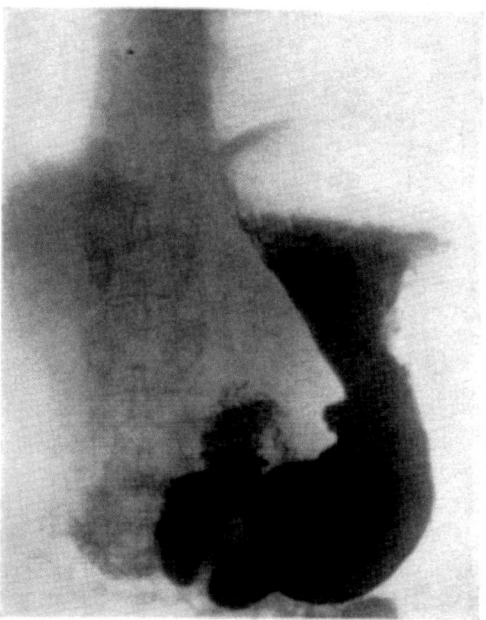

Fig. 172. Typical "penetrating" ulcer on the lesser curvature.

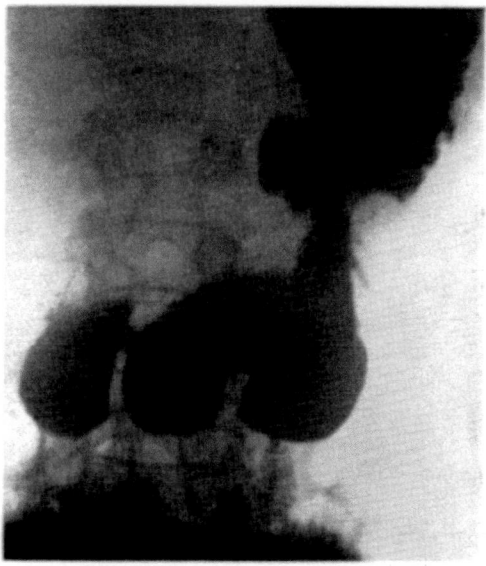

Fig. 173. Large "penetrating" ulcer on the lesser curvature, possibly malignant. The irregular lower margin, apart from the demonstration of the course of the rugae in this area, is the only point on which the diagnosis of malignancy rests.

the diagnosis and obtaining a film record. But the smaller craters on the anterior and posterior walls can only be detected by the manipulation of the first mouthful as it canalises the stomach. The radiologist has to "paint" the walls of the stomach by manipulating the small quantity of opaque food up and down between the rugae, looking for a constant pocket of shadow that cannot be displaced and that indicates ulcer, or else for the convergence of the folds of the rugae towards a point—a very suggestive sign which calls for detailed examination and repeated search.

If a pocket is found, the radiologist attempts to keep it filled by constant pressure while he exposes a film, rotating the patient, if necessary, to show it

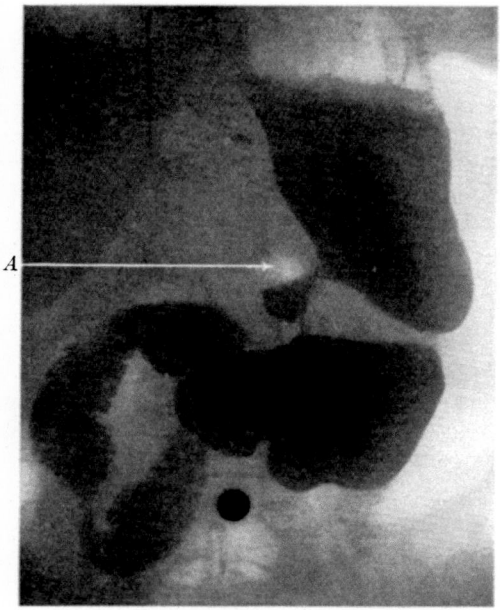

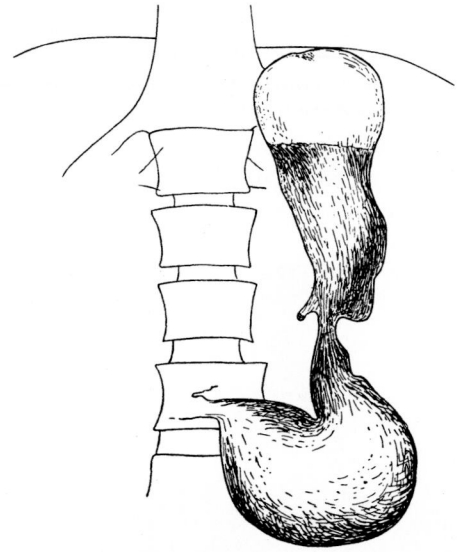

Fig. 174. Large old-standing ulcer on the lesser curvature with air cap (*A*) above the food in the pocket. (Contributed by F. Haenisch.)

Fig. 175. Small "penetrating" ulcer on the lesser curvature with spasmodic contraction.

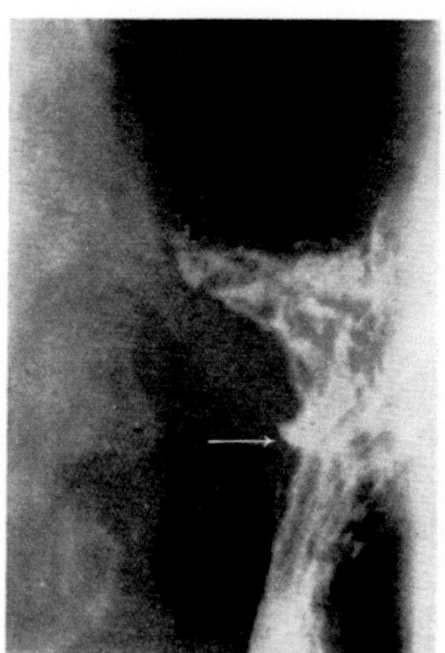

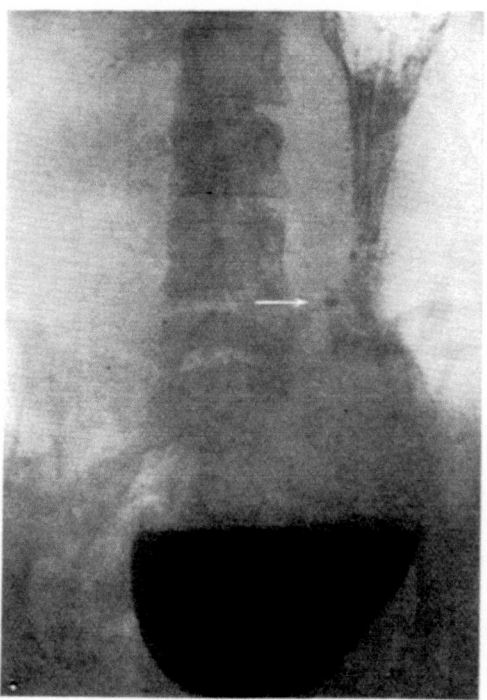

Fig. 176. Small ulcer on the posterior wall close to the lesser curvature, retaining the food after palpation. The arrow points to the ulcer niche.

Fig. 177. Small ulcer on the posterior wall detected by palpation and only demonstrated radiographically with great difficulty. The arrow points to a fleck in the ulcer crater.

better or to get it on the profile. In some cases, however, he has to make certain of the diagnosis on the screen, and is lucky if he can get a film to show the fleck satisfactorily. After the stomach is filled with, say, half a pint or less, he returns to the suspected area and, turning the patient this way and that, he may perhaps be able to see on the profile the little crater that he had detected with much greater certainty and precision by his manipulation of the first mouthful. When once such an ulcer has been detected in this way, palpation takes on a new meaning and the radiologist realises that without it many ulcers would be missed.

The "Penetrating" Ulcer*

When the radiologist detects a projection on the outline of the opaque food in the stomach, he makes a positive diagnosis of ulcer, and when the apparent pocket is deep he describes it as a "penetrating ulcer". The question arises whether or not he is justified in this description. All radiologists have seen "penetrating" ulcers—ulcers that seem to go right through the stomach wall and sometimes even show a small bubble of occluded air above the opaque food in the niche. When a pocket like this is found, on palpation, to be fixed there seems little reason to doubt the diagnosis. Yet I have seen these radiographic appearances when operation has shown merely a flat ulcer that hardly penetrated the muscular coat at all and had no overhanging edges whatever. It is difficult to reconcile the X-ray appearances with the pathological specimen and to imagine how an ulcer of this kind could have given rise to such a definite X-ray picture of a pocket. The only reasonable explanation of the discrepancy is that, in conscious life, the mucous membrane is heaped up to such an extent that it actually overlaps the ulcerated surface and forms a crater (Fig. 179). Konjetzny (210) has now published beautiful drawings of sections of the mucous membrane treated in such a way that oedema and other changes are preserved in the specimen.

For many years I have relied on radioscopic palpation to convince myself of the presence of quite minute ulcers by watching the residue left in such pockets when the opaque food has been manipulated up and down the rugae. The smallest of these ulcers was no more than an eighth of an inch in diameter and did not even penetrate the whole thickness of the mucous membrane. The crater in this specimen was far too shallow to account for the definite and quite

---

* When I first wrote the substance of these pages (49), I did not know that Forssell had already reached the same conclusions concerning the X-ray appearances presented by an ulcer (Fig. 178), and I therefore failed to acknowledge his priority. The conical shape of the healing ulcer that I then described, and had taught for many years previously, is published in Berg's book on the mucous membrane, but obviously he also had recognised the appearance long before. Both these observations were original to me, but the credit for explaining the formation of the ulcer crater should certainly go elsewhere. I mention this because one writer has already ascribed the credit to me.

heavy shadow of food residue that was constantly retained on palpation. I am certain, therefore, that when radiologists diagnose a "penetrating" ulcer they are often picturing a far more extensive pathological condition than actually exists. If I am right, we may—and actually do—get an appearance of penetration from a mere erosion of mucous membrane, the heaped-up mucosa being almost entirely responsible for the depth of the apparent crater (Figs. 180 and 182).

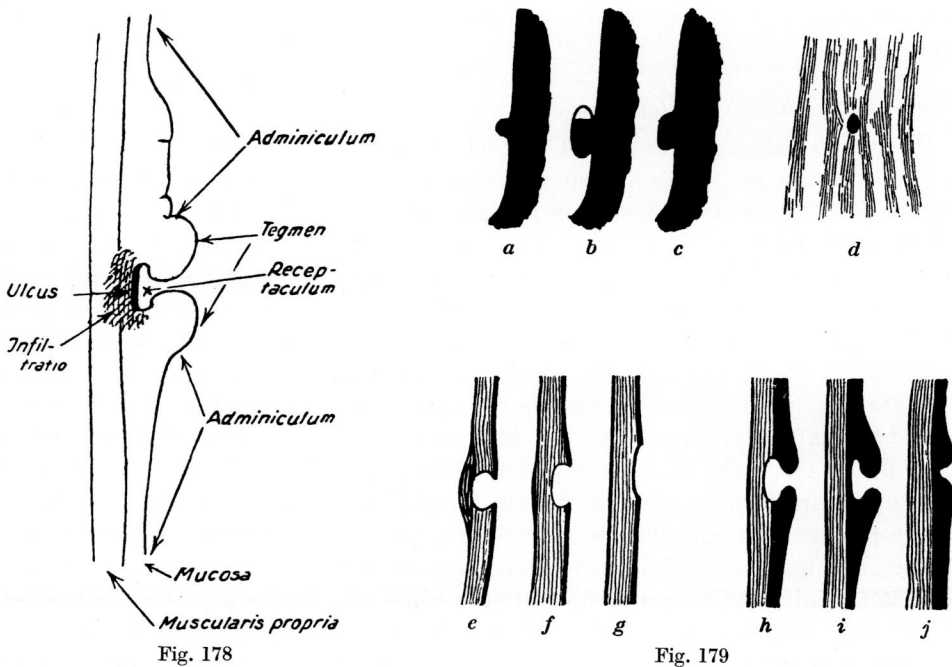

Fig. 178   Fig. 179

Fig. 178. Diagram showing the way in which the mucous membrane is heaped up around an ulcer, giving a false impression of perforation. (Contributed by G. Forssell.)

Fig. 179. *a, b, c,* Typical X-ray appearances of gastric ulcer on the margin near the lesser curvature. *d,* Crater of ulcer hidden among the folds of the mucous membrane on the anterior or posterior wall. *e, f, g,* Diagrams of pathological specimens of perforating, penetrating, and mucous membrane erosion ulcers. *h, i,* Suggested interpretation of the X-ray appearances, the pocket being due to overfolding of the heaped-up mucous membrane. *j,* Diagram of suggested conditions of healing of ulcer. The mucous membrane loses its heaped-up condition; the ulcer becomes shallow and conical or V-shaped before it disappears.

If this explanation is correct, it is not difficult to understand how even apparently large ulcers can disappear in a comparatively short time, a sequence that radiologists frequently have the opportunity of observing. It would obviously be impossible for a true chronic penetrating ulcer to heal in a few weeks, but far from improbable that an erosion might heal in that time. Moreover, the way in which the ulcers close in, radiographically, seems to support

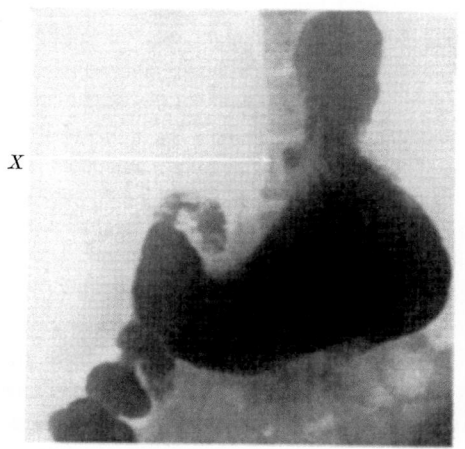

X

Fig. 180. Ulcer crater (X) showing the mucous membrane heaped up around the ulcer and displacing the opaque food. (Recumbent posture.)

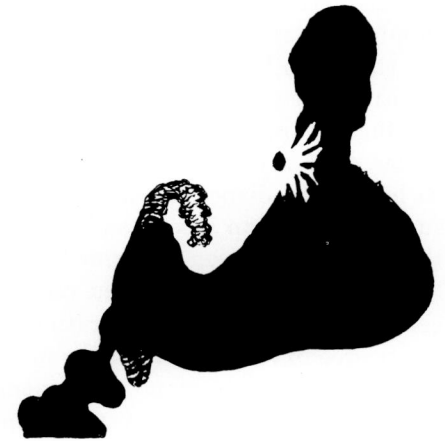

Fig. 181. Diagram of Fig. 180.

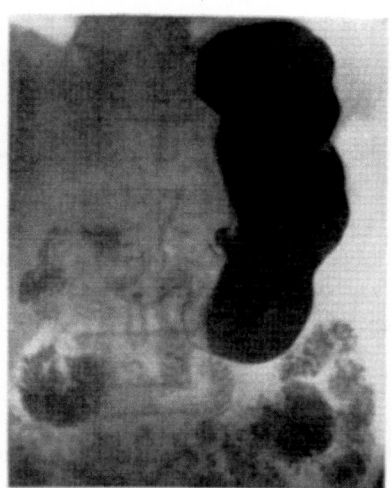

Fig. 182. Similar appearance to that shown in Fig. 180. (Recumbent posture.)

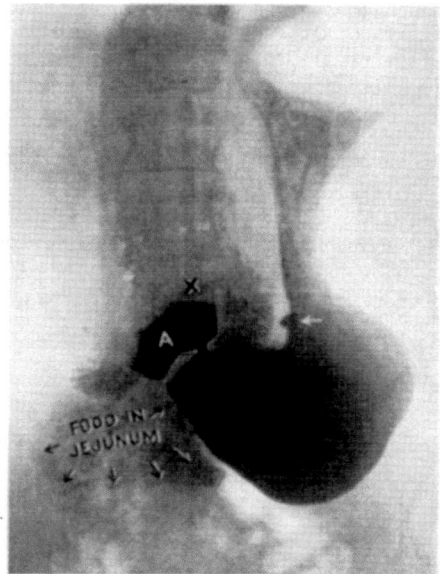

Fig. 183. Healing ulcer (shown by dart) on the lesser curvature. The cone-shape of the crater suggests that the ulcer is healing. A, Duodenal cap. $\times$, Umbilicus.

this deduction: they do not heal over the crater and tend to enclose the pocket, as might be expected if the neck of the niche represented the ulcerated margin, but the crater becomes shallower and V-shaped (Fig. 183), until, just before it disappears, it is no more than a pencil point. It then seems to flatten out suddenly, leaving no apparent trace, even in the contour of the rugae. This appearance indicates to my mind that, as healing progresses, the surrounding mucosa loses its heaped-up disposition and assumes its normal level. In practice I have often suggested that an ulcer was healing, judging by the V-shape of the crater, and the opinion has been confirmed both clinically and radiologically.

An ulcer can be diagnosed radiographically, but it is not yet possible to be certain whether it is a perforating ulcer, a penetrating ulcer or a mere erosion; the degree of local spasm of the muscularis mucosae that causes the heaping-up of the mucous membrane will depend on the intensity of the irritation from the ulcerated surface. As this surface heals and becomes less sensitive, so the local spasm will subside, with the result that the crater becomes less pocket-shaped and more V-shaped. The mucous membrane pattern shows no deformity after healing.

I suggest, therefore, that the nomenclature of the radiologist is at fault and that, whatever he sees, he is not justified in diagnosing "penetrating" ulcer. He has no definite means of determining whether this ulcer crater is in fact due to penetration of the muscular coat, or to actual perforation into a dense mass of surrounding reaction, or whether it is merely formed by heaped-up mucous membrane. If the ulcer moves freely on manipulation, he may be certain that the appearance of penetration is false.

ULCERS IN SPECIAL REGIONS

(1) FUNDUS AND UPPER STOMACH

Ulcers in any part of the fundus and upper stomach are rare, and often escape detection, especially if the patient is only examined in the upright position. Palpation is not possible because of the costal margin, and the technique of investigation of the mucous membrane in this area is unsatisfactory. The radiologist has to depend on the observation of the first mouthful and on gravity, posturing the patient as best he can on the couch, so as to allow the heavy food to run over the mucous membrane of the fundus. One procedure I have found of some value is to fill the fundus and then to get the patient to sit up for a minute, so as to allow the food to fall towards the pylorus; then he lies down and is quickly examined before the main body of the food falls back into the fundus. It is sometimes possible to demonstrate disorders of the mucous membrane pattern and to diagnose ulcer or growth by this method. If the procedure shows a shadow suggesting a niche, the patient is so turned that it comes on the profile and a radiograph showing the projection may be obtained. In the section on achalasia of the cardia (cf. p. 210) I mentioned two cases of oesophageal obstruction, occurring at the cardiac orifice, which came to the post-mortem room in early days. One was a small cicatrised ulcer about two inches from the cardiac orifice on the anterior wall, the other a malignant ulceration of the fundus which did not involve the cardiac orifice. In both cases the only symptom noted at examination was oesophageal obstruction, and both showed very marked distension of the lower end of the oesophagus. On the strength of these two cases I think it reasonable to suggest that at least some cases of achalasia of the cardia owe their origin to gastric causes.

(2) BODY OF THE STOMACH

Ulcers of the body of the stomach may or may not be associated with spasm leading to hour-glass deformity. An hour-glass contraction, even if only transitory, should make the radiologist search the mucous membrane with meticulous care for a pocket hidden away in its folds, or for any suggestion of convergence in the rugae. If a pocket is suspected, the patient should be rotated until it comes on the outline, and an attempt should be made to obtain a radiographic record. There is usually little difficulty with fairly large ulcers in or near the lesser curvature.

The first case in which I discovered and reported on an ulcer, after reading Haudek's paper, was disconcerting, but very instructive. I found a very large and conspicuous pocket on the lesser curvature (Fig. 184), and had no doubt that it was due to a

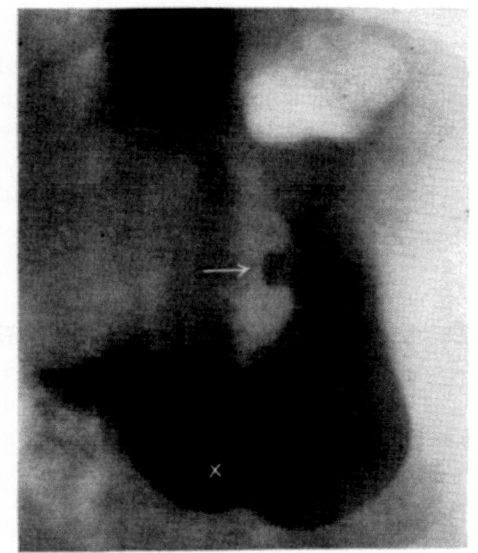

Fig. 184. The first "penetrating" ulcer reported by the author. It was not found at the operation.

chronic penetrating ulcer, such as Haudek had described. I therefore made my first definite and absolutely unequivocal report of the presence of a large ulcer, although the symptoms were vague and there was no associated spasm. The surgeon failed to find the ulcer, which must have been penetrating into the pancreas; apparently he did not search the posterior wall thoroughly and therefore missed it. After this lesson I haunted the theatres when my cases were being operated on and gradually gained implicit confidence in the interpretation of such craters.

At first, "penetrating" ulcers were only found on or close to the lesser curvature. With improved technique they are now found in other sites. The symptoms are not as a rule so prominent as might be expected from what are apparently gross changes. On p. 30 a fairly recent case is mentioned in which a physician refused to accept the radiologist's diagnosis of an obvious chronic ulcer solely on the ground of absence of symptoms. In fact, the greatest pain, as far as it is possible to judge, seems to be caused by the smaller ulcers, away from the lesser curvature, that are frequently associated with intense spasm whenever the symptoms are severe.

A girl, with indefinite subacute symptoms and very severe pain after food, could only force a few ounces of opaque food into her stomach, where it formed a small funnel-shaped shadow, and after twenty-four hours it was all still in the same position. When she was operated on, the surgeon found, high up on the greater curvature, an ulcer threatening to perforate. There was no cicatrisation. Spasm was the obvious feature in this case, and the apparent cause of her symptoms.

The absence of spasm in some ulcers of the lesser curvature is quite definite; operation records show that in my original tabulation in 1914 I had failed to detect only four ulcers that were discovered at operation, and that these were all on the lesser curvature near the pylorus. Whether this absence of spasm is or is not responsible for the special tendency of ulcers of this type to sudden profuse haemorrhage I do not know, but the coincidence is certainly suggestive.

Hour-glass Contraction

The characteristic shape of the ordinary upper sac of an hour-glass stomach (Figs. 185–187) is rather puzzling at first, but is explained by the arrangement of the muscles (cf. p. 65). It is due to contraction of the circular fibres which draw the greater towards the lesser (and thicker) curvature. Radiologists see this typical shape caused by ulcerations on the lesser or the greater curvature, on the anterior or the posterior surface. It indicates either that no adhesions have formed, in which case the niche is quite mobile to palpation, or that the contraction has taken place before the development of any tendency to perforation and the formation of adhesions. If an ulcer tends to perforate and form adhesions, its site becomes a more fixed point than the lesser curvature, and consequently the passage between the two sacs is contracted towards this point. In a few instances I have seen the channel passing out apparently along the greater curvature, while in others it follows the posterior wall, and is sometimes firmly adherent to the pancreas (Figs. 188 and 189).

Even a small ulcer may cause an hour-glass contraction that prevents the food passing into the lower part of the stomach for hours. In three of my early cases

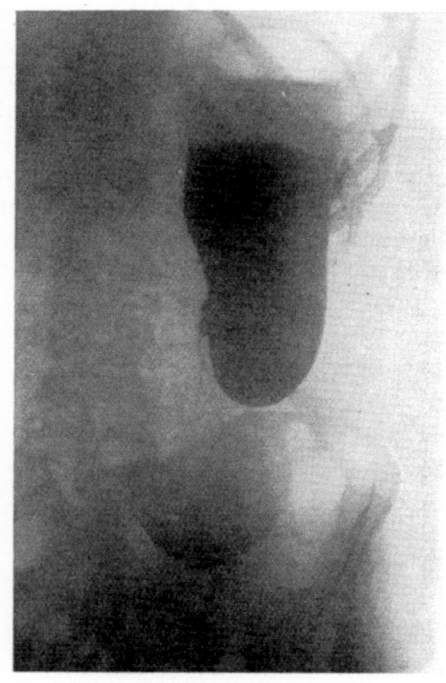
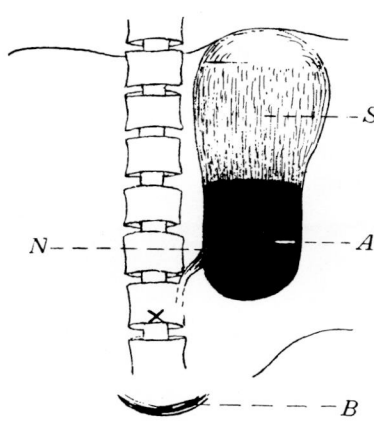

Fig. 185   Fig. 186

Fig. 185. Typical old-standing cicatricial hour-glass stomach. Note the retained food or secretion in the upper sac. (Contributed by C. Thurstan Holland.)

Fig. 186. Old-standing cicatricial hour-glass stomach. Note the very large quantity of secretion, S, most of which collected during the examination. The hypersecretion suggested a pyloric ulcer, which was in fact found at operation. The neck, N, of the hour-glass was not very narrow; in fact it would admit three or four fingers. A, Upper sac. B, Lower sac.

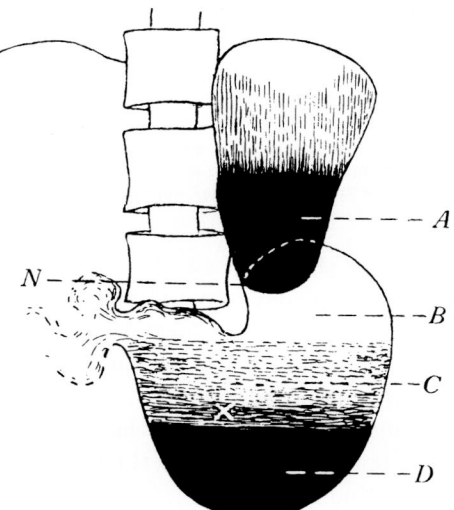

Fig. 187. Old-standing cicatricial hour-glass stomach associated with marked pyloric obstruction. The food in the lower sac is what remains of the meal given 24 hours previously. A, Upper sac. N, Neck of the hour-glass. B, Gas from fermentation in lower sac. C, Retained non-opaque food. D, Opaque food.

of pyloric obstruction, in which I had also noted hour-glass contraction, gastro-jejunostomy failed to relieve the symptoms. At the operation, evidence of ulceration of the body of the stomach was also noted, and healing was expected to result from the gastro-enterostomy—as indeed often happened. The symptoms were all ascribed to the thickening of the pylorus that was present, but to judge from the patients' descriptions of their symptoms, and also from the fact that they were all cured by subsequent operations, the real cause was probably the insignificant-looking ulcer of the body of the stomach and the spasm it set up.

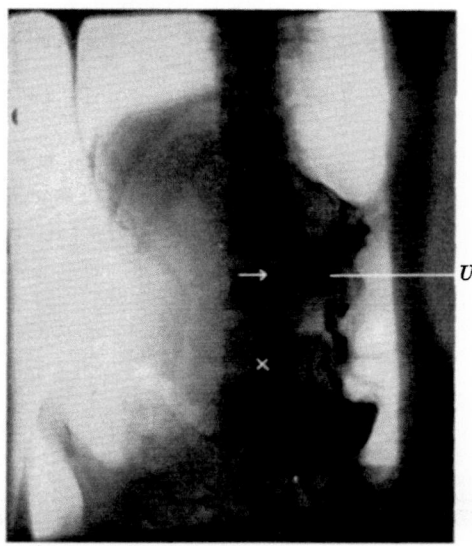 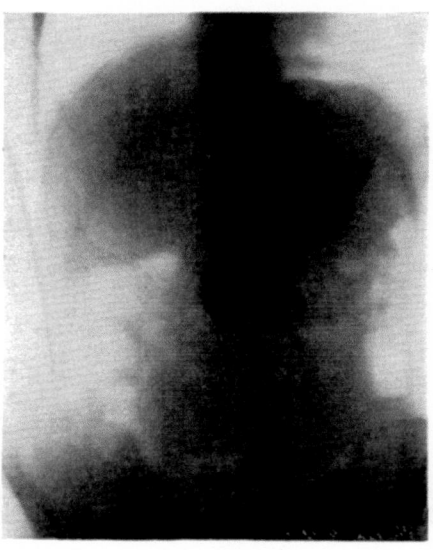

Fig. 188   Fig. 189

Fig. 188. Old-standing ulcer with cicatrisation, forming an hour-glass that opens on the posterior wall. Cicatricial pyloric obstruction was also present. On palpation the ulcer pocket, *U*, was fixed and induration could be felt. This cicatrisation was adherent to the pancreas.

Fig. 189. Hour-glass stomach due to an adherent ulcer on the greater curvature. The adhesions have formed a fixed point, and the stomach has contracted from the lesser to the greater curvature so that the opening of the hour-glass is on the greater curvature. Pyloric ulceration was also present and there was a large residue of the five-hour meal.

There is a natural delay in the progress of thick food as it passes down the stomach and forward over the kidney. In an atonic stomach this delay may be exaggerated and may readily be mistaken for the sign of a spasmodic contraction such as may occur about the junction of the middle and upper thirds. As the food descends to this point it assumes a conical shape. The apparent spasm may relax with comparative suddenness, because the food slips over the brim and passes on into the lower portion, often in a thick stream, giving a somewhat bilocular appearance for a time.

As early as 1913, Case noted a very marked spastic indentation, forming an hour-glass contraction of the stomach, in sixteen cases of duodenal ulcer. I myself saw this appearance fairly frequently, and it was nearly always associated with duodenal ulcers. As a sign it is of no great importance, for it is also associated with cholecystitis and possibly other conditions. Electrical stimulation over the site of a duodenal ulcer has been found to give rise to a contraction in the body of the stomach such as would give the appearance of an hour-glass (cf. p. 69).

Belladonna exerts a marked influence on some spasmodic contractions and produces no apparent effect on others which nevertheless may relax under massage. Relaxation may be startlingly sudden. In one very marked hour-glass contraction which was thought to be partly organic, I found that belladonna practically removed the obstruction between the upper and lower parts of the stomach. Acting on this suggestion, the patient lived in perfect comfort for three years, taking small doses of Tr. belladonnae from time to time. Subsequently, however, and without any warning, a duodenal ulcer perforated. At the operation the hour-glass condition was found to be due to a cicatrised ulcer that was probably still active and was surrounded by adhesions. Belladonna, therefore, may relax spasm even in the presence of active ulceration and give rise to a false sense of security by relieving symptoms that might otherwise be absolutely definite indications for surgical interference.

(3) PYLORUS

Pyloric ulcers tend to give rise to spasmodic contraction of the pylorus. This spasm is frequently intermittent and probably accounts for the intermissions in the symptoms. The obstruction, largely spasmodic in the earlier stages, is so extreme and so persistent that the stomach may become completely atonic, extending to four or five inches below the umbilicus, while only a very small quantity of the food is passed out in twenty-four hours. Later on, the ulceration leads to cicatrisation, but there is no reliable information on the relative importance of the two factors. In most cases of active ulceration close to the pylorus, I have noted very copious and rapid secretion of gastric juice.

The pars pylorica contains comparatively little opaque food at any one time, and the shadow is therefore not so easy to see as that of the large mass in the body of the stomach. Moreover, the opacity of the vertebral column is superimposed in the direct postero-anterior position, and renders it almost impossible to make certain of details. Detection of the crater is, however, the one diagnostic sign. In the old days, the appearance of the pars pylorica itself seldom gave any definite evidence of ulceration, but there are several signs that point towards the presence of an active ulcer in this region (cf. p. 245).

Ulcers in and about the pyloric canal seldom, if ever, appear like the large "penetrating" type of ulcer seen on the lesser curvature. Why this should be so, I do not know, but I suspect that the mucous membrane may be less lax in this region and therefore less easily heaped up to form the appearance of a deep pocket. Whatever the cause, even large pyloric ulcers may give little suggestion of the niche, and the most painstaking manipulation may be required to discover an irregularity in the mucous membrane holding the opaque food (Figs. 190 and Plate fig. 191). These are, in my opinion, the most difficult of all ulcers to detect definitely. Often, when an ulcer is suspected from indirect evidence, the radiologist's opinion at the end of a long search is based on the momentary filling of the floor of the ulcer. As often as not, especially with small ulcers actually in the pyloric canal, he may be quite unable to obtain a film to show the fleeting

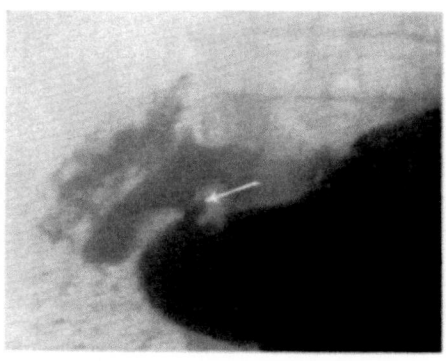

Fig. 190. Pyloric ulcer. The crater of the ulcer (shown by dart) is actually in the pyloric canal. (Contributed by A. Köhler.)

appearance on which he bases his diagnosis. By far the most difficult diagnosis to make is one of "no ulcer found" when indirect evidence suggests a pyloric lesion.

Spasm plays a fairly large part in the symptomatology and also in the X-ray appearances of these ulcers. Quite a slight degree of spasm will often cause delay in emptying and such closure of the pyloric canal that the radiologist has to exercise all his patience before he can get sufficient relaxation to allow the opaque food to enter; even so the spasm only too often returns before he is convinced. He tries posturing, massage, manipulation and, above all, waiting, and sometimes by one or other method he succeeds in observing the channel while the spasm is relaxed.

Sometimes it is of great assistance to re-examine after Tr. belladonnae has been pushed to the limit for twelve hours. I particularly remember one case of this type in which I eventually detected a minute ulcer in the pyloric canal that had escaped recognition at repeated examinations both by myself and by other observers. From the delay in emptying and the history, I was convinced that there must be an ulcer close to the pylorus, causing intermittent spasm. At the operation, the tiny ulcer gave no indication on the peritoneal surface, and was not obvious even when, at my request, the pyloric canal was laid open. This patient has had no suggestion of recurrence, and his periods of intermittent pain and semi-invalidism have disappeared. It was a very minute lesion to have had such a crippling influence on a man's life.

PLATE VI

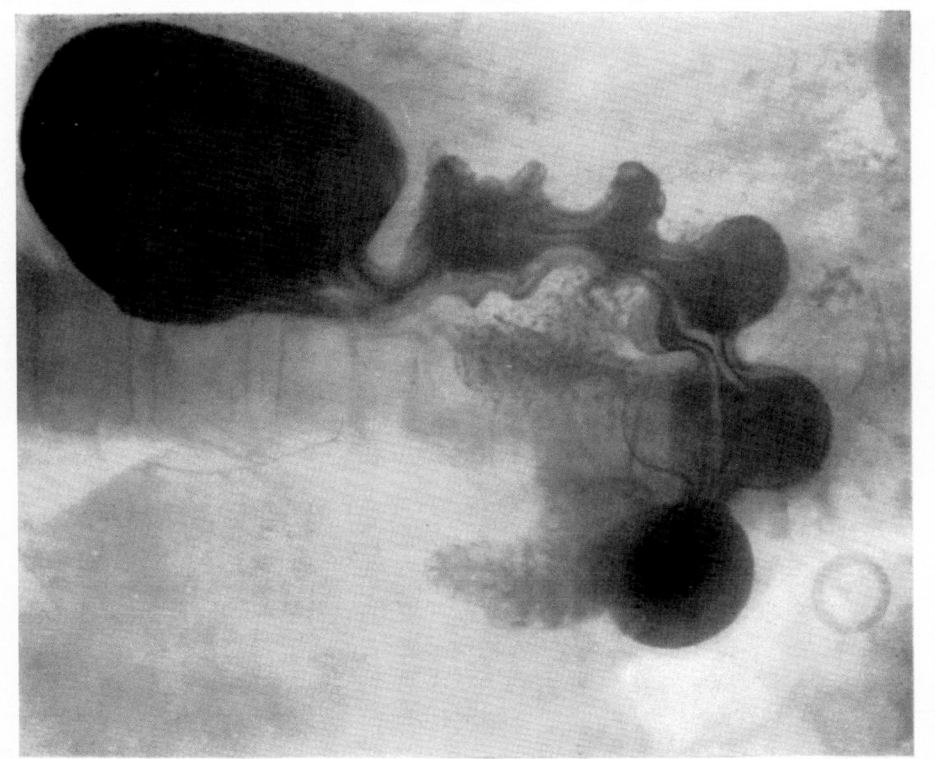

Fig. 192. Case of ulceration at the pylorus with extremely active peristalsis. Radiograph taken in the recumbent position. Note the contours of the mucous membrane pattern following the indentations of the peristalsis.

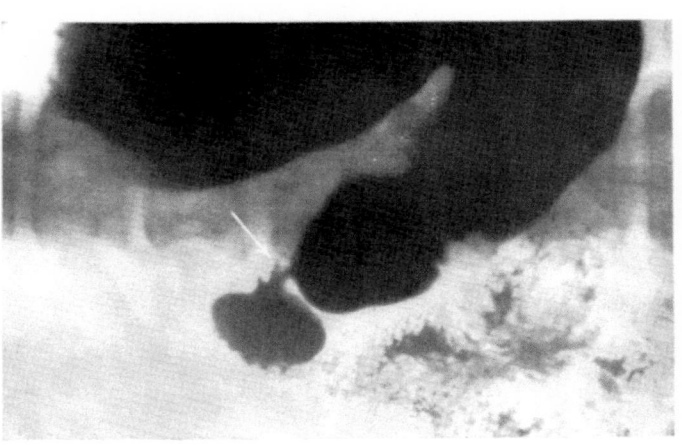

Fig. 191. Ulcer crater on the duodenal side of the pyloric canal. Pyloric spasm was a marked feature. (Contributed by H. M. Tovell.)

PLATE VII

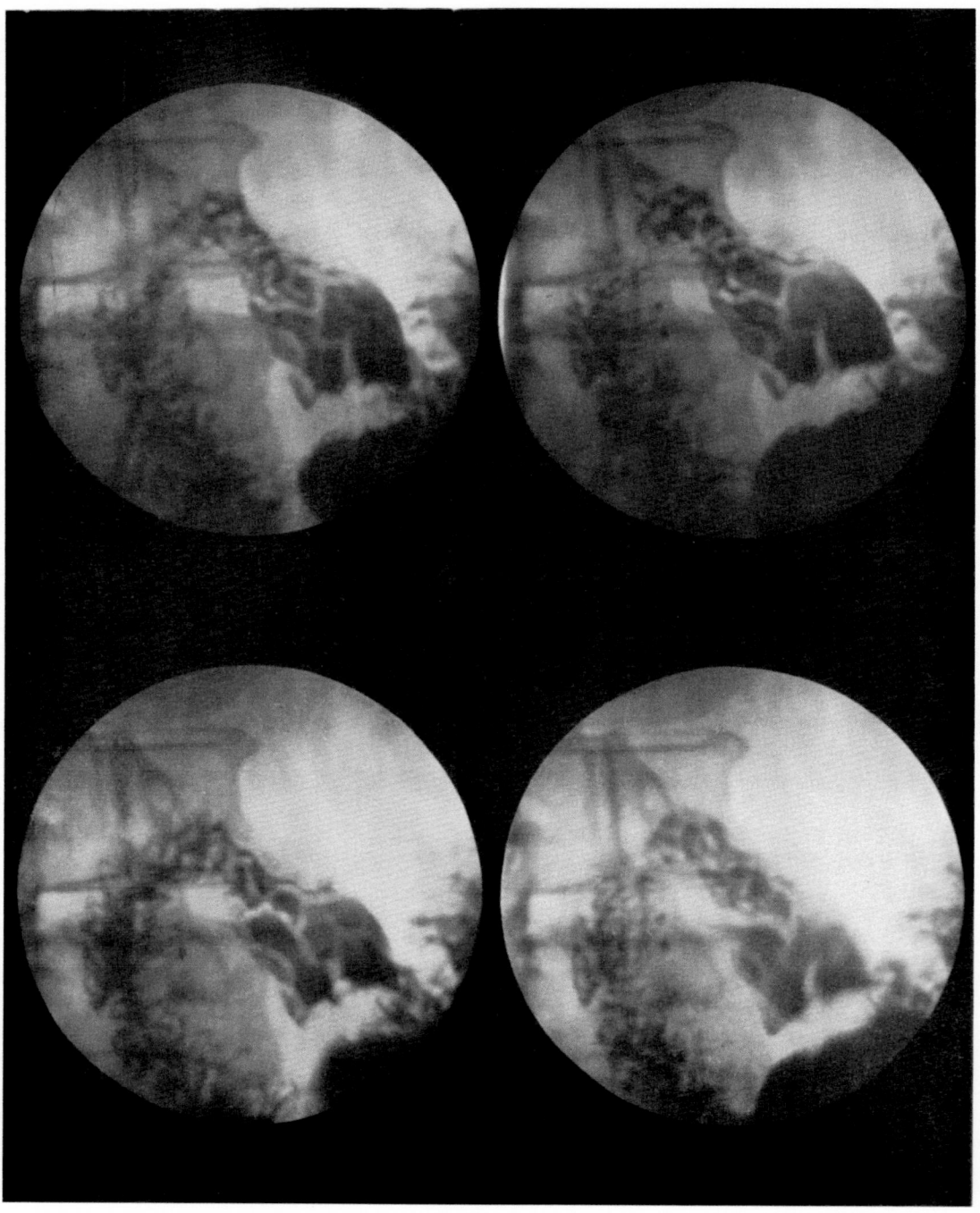

Fig. 193. Serial views showing the normal duodenal mucous membrane pattern.
(Contributed by Å. Åkerlund.)

Indirect Signs of Pyloric Ulcer

Any clue is of value when the detection of the crater is often so extremely difficult. The presence of pyloric spasm should be taken as a warning to examine with the utmost care. If some of the food is seen in the duodenal cap, an undue length of the pyloric canal has very considerable significance. Asymmetry of the pyloric canal in relation to the duodenal cap, an appearance of entering it at one side or the other, may be due to the extension of the spasm to the duodenum, and is more often associated with duodenal ulcer than with an ulcer in the pylorus. The type of peristalsis may form a clue. Plate fig. 192 shows excessive peristalsis which indicated a closure of the pylorus due to a small ulcer in the canal.

Excessive outpouring of secretion, showing as a fluid level above the opaque food, is of some significance (Fig. 186). In some cases an inch or more may collect in five minutes. Of course, the observer must make sure that this appearance is not due to the settling out of the opaque material in the food, which should be adequately suspended. He can form a rough idea of the free-acid content by giving an ounce of saturated solution of sodium bicarbonate. After giving the solution, the stomach contents are shaken, either by manipulation or by instructing the patient to draw in and push out his abdomen rapidly. The increase in the air space in the fundus indicates the amount of carbonic acid gas given off. This test is very rough and ready; an air space about two inches wide may be increased by an inch when there is abundance of free acid, whereas if the acidity is normal it is not likely to be increased by as much as half an inch. The *absence* of free acid is not significant, but its *presence* in large quantities in secretion that has been rapidly poured out strongly suggests an ulcer or a marked irritation of the pylorus. In my opinion it almost, if not quite, rules out malignancy. The test may be of some value in the differential diagnosis of carcinoma and ulcer.

Sometimes there is a definite tender spot on deep pressure over the site of the ulcer, whereas in cases of irritation the tenderness is not so localised.

Such are the indirect signs of pyloric ulcer. We place comparatively little reliance on them nowadays, but they will quite often be of great assistance in leading to the one and only definite sign of ulceration, the detection of the irregularity in the surface of the mucous membrane that indicates a break in continuity. With patient and persistent manipulation it should be possible to demonstrate the crater on the screen in almost every case.

(4) DUODENAL ULCER

Before the introduction of liquid opaque food made it possible to detect deformity of the duodenal cap, the X-ray diagnosis of duodenal ulcer was speculative and was based on indirect signs which are no longer of any importance. They were entirely unreliable, and no useful purpose would be served by reviewing them, except to state definitely that duodenal ulcer is found in association with any type of stomach.

The first radiograph illustrating duodenal bulb deformity and the food filling a crater was, I believe, that published in 1910 (29). At that time fine detail in fluoroscopy and radiography was not available, and I held that it was not possible to be certain whether the fleck of food retained in the duodenum was in the pocket of an ulcer or in the fold of a cicatrix or other cause of puckering. The names particularly associated with the diagnosis of duodenal ulcer are Haudek (149), Cole (101), and George and Gerber (130), who published an excellent atlas. The classical work of Åkerlund (4, 5, 6) and Berg (60), with modern technique at their disposal, has advanced the diagnosis of duodenal ulcer to little short of mathematical certainty in the hands of expert workers.

The duodenal cap usually fills satisfactorily if the radiologist waits patiently (Plate fig. 194). If, however, there is irritation, it is sometimes extremely difficult to get the cap outlined. With patience, in both the upright and horizontal positions, it is usually possible to hold some opaque food in the cap and to manipulate it sufficiently to demonstrate that the outline is not persistently deformed. (For details of technique see p. 24.) Palpation and manipulation also play a very large part in the satisfactory filling and visualisation of the cap, and especially in the demonstration of the crater. To compress and hold the duodenum in the requisite position while a film is exposed may be extremely difficult; moreover, the appearance has often changed by the time the exposure is made. In fact, even a radiologist of long experience very frequently cannot obtain radiographic proof of what he has seen on the screen. To overcome this difficulty the compression devices of Åkerlund, Berg and Chaoul are of great assistance (cf. p. 22).

Ulceration of the duodenum is almost entirely confined to the first part (probably at least 95 per cent.). Out of 496 cases collected by Jefferson (186), 491 (99·2 per cent.) were in the suprapapillary section. Whenever there is ulceration there is *persistent* deformity of the cap. If the cap is normal, even for a moment, there is no ulceration. In the early days of the positive diagnosis the deformity was assumed to be directly due to the ulcer, but in fact it is a compound of spasm of the muscular coat and heaping up of the mucous membrane, and the resulting picture varies so widely according to the site of the ulcer and the degree of spasm that the best way of describing the conditions is to let Plate figs. 195 to 202 tell their own tale.

Unfortunately, similar deformities may be produced by adhesions, either from the ulcers themselves or from the gall-bladder, so that, although the positive diagnosis is usually correct when deduced from the deformity, it cannot be upheld as definite unless the actual crater of the ulcer is detected. Deformities of the duodenum should always be confirmed, for spasm may be transient.

It is not by any means possible to demonstrate the niche in every case.

PLATE VIII

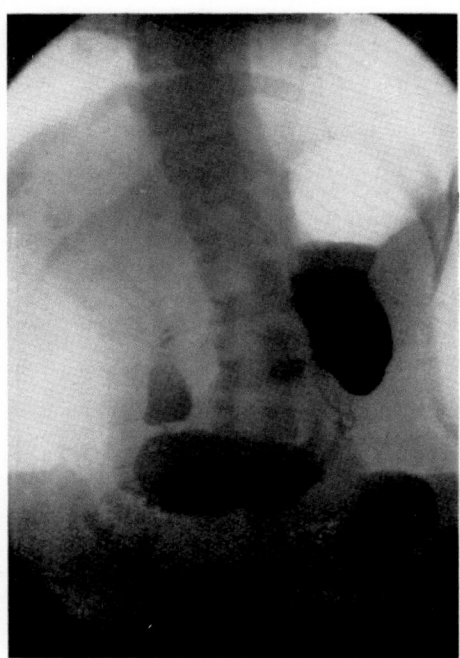

Fig. 194. Normal duodenal cap. There is also a very large "penetrating" ulcer on the lesser curvature with cicatricial contraction.

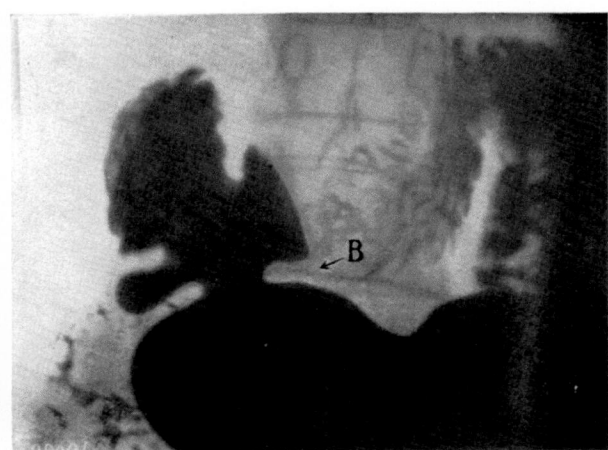

Fig. 195. Deformity of the duodenum due to an ulcer. The crater was not located but is probably on the anterior or posterior wall. The pylorus, *B*, is unusually patent.

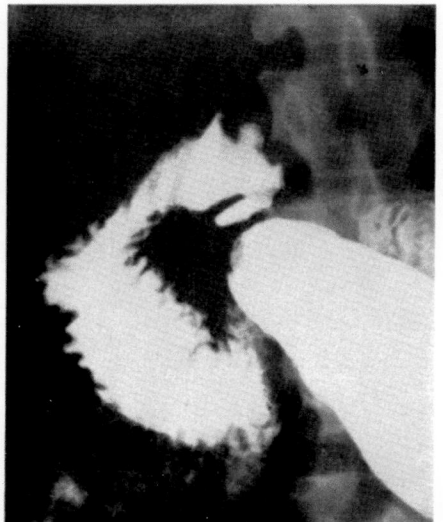

Fig. 196. Chronic indurated ulcer of the first portion of the duodenum. (Contributed by Arial W. George.)

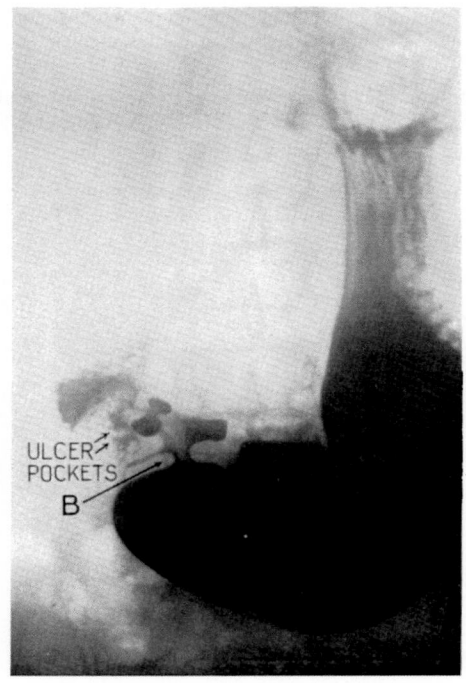

Fig. 197. Two ulcer craters (touched up) in the distal end of the duodenal cap. *B*, Pylorus.

PLATE IX

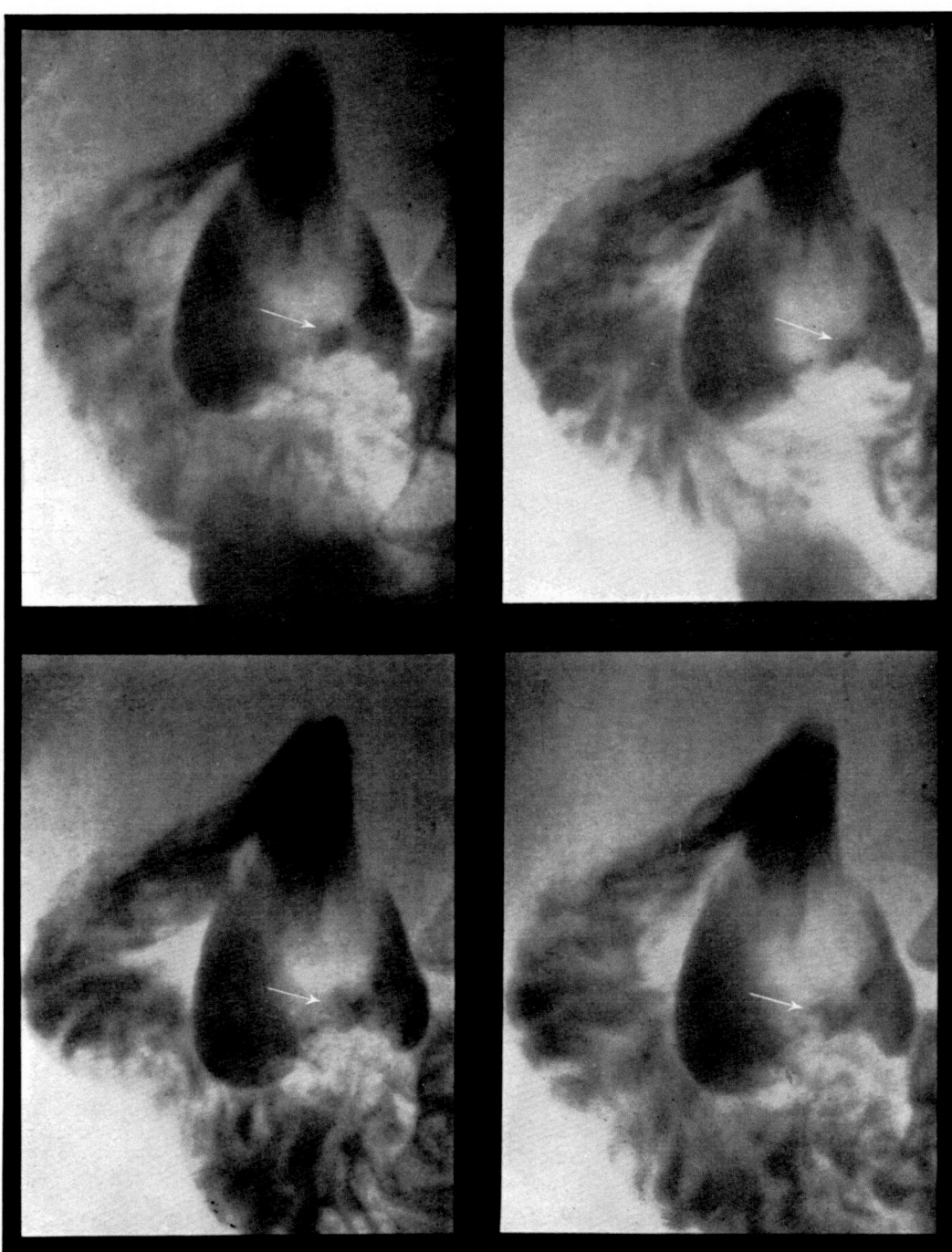

Fig. 198. Duodenal cap which appeared to be normal until compression was applied, i.e. no spasm was present. Compression, however, showed the presence of the crater, which is seen in the four serial pictures. (Contributed by Å. Åkerlund.)

PLATE X

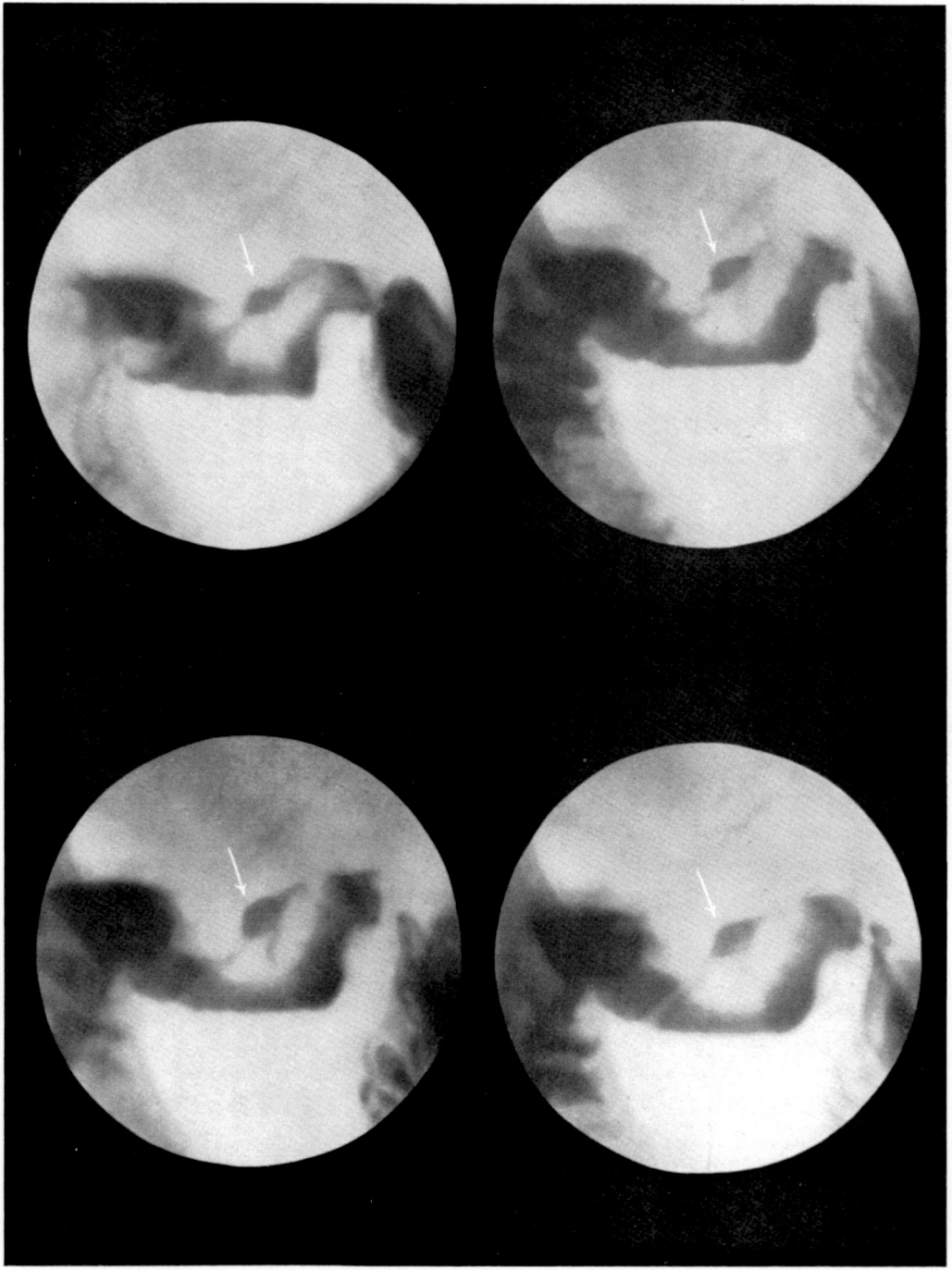

Fig. 199. Serial views under compression, showing the crater of an ulcer *en face*. Note the converging folds of mucous membrane. (Contributed by Å. Åkerlund.)

PLATE XI

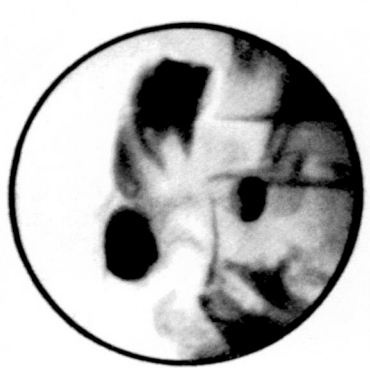

Fig. 200. Small ulcer crater on the anterior wall of the bulb, showing radiating folds. (Contributed by H. Berg.)

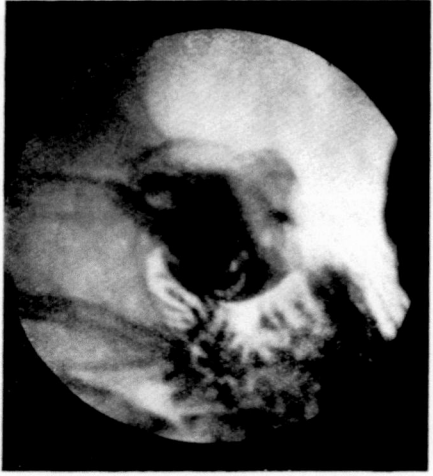

Fig. 201. Ulcer crater close to the pylorus demonstrated by compression in semi-lateral position. Note the radiating folds of the mucous membrane. (Contributed by Å. Åkerlund.)

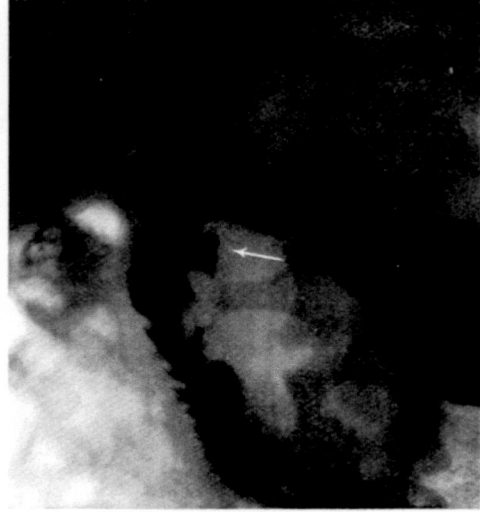

Fig. 202. Radiograph showing an ulcer of the second part of the duodenum. The case had been radiographed previously and no deformity noted. On the strength of this previous examination the diagnosis of ulceration, as against a diverticulum at the site of the ampulla of Vater, was made, and this was confirmed at operation. (Contributed by H. Graham Hodgson.)

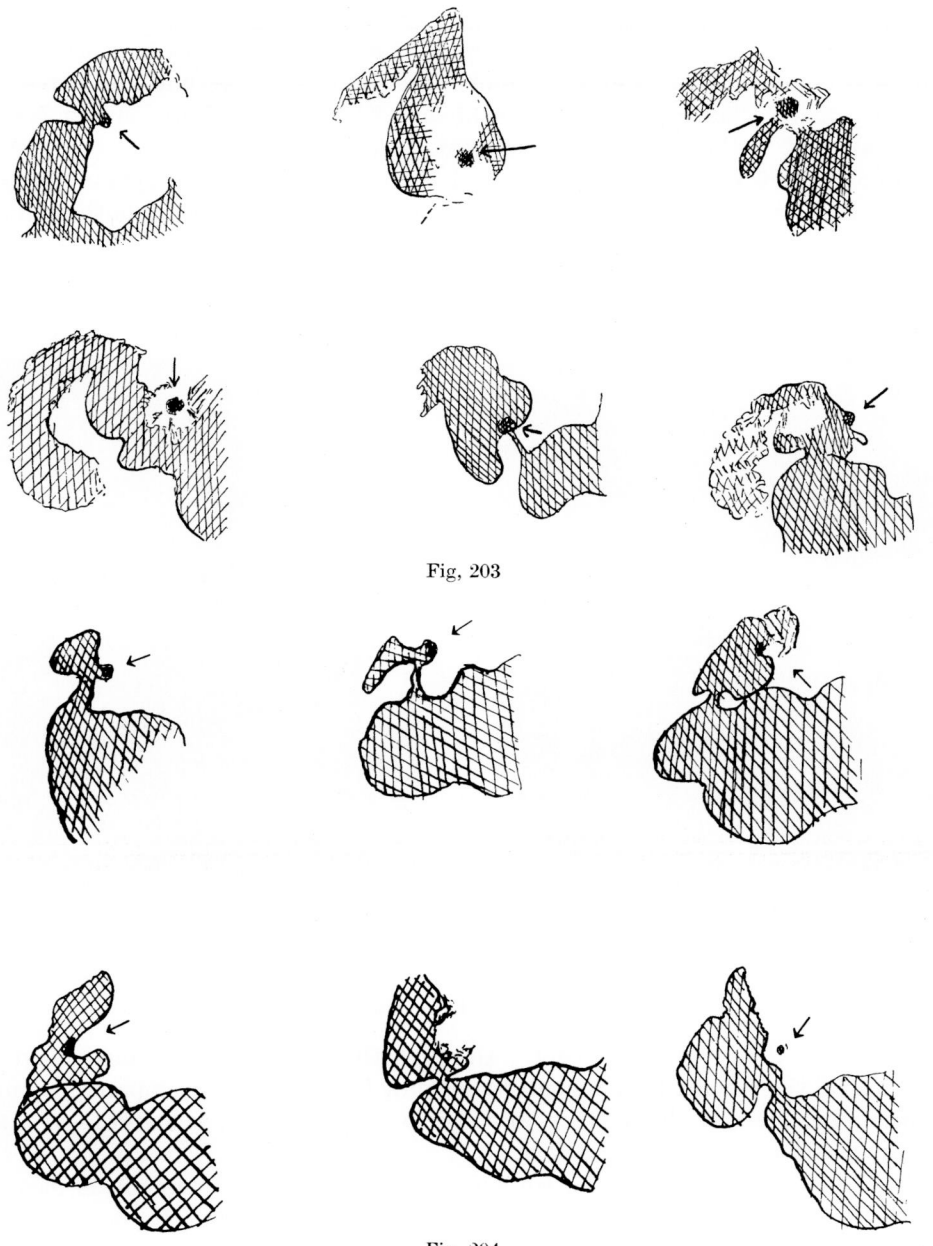

Fig. 203

Fig. 204

Figs. 203, 204. Diagrams from tracings of duodenal ulcer cases. The resulting deformities are legion and often it is extremely difficult, if not impossible, actually to detect the ulcer crater. In many of these cases the crater was not shown in the radiograph and was only with difficulty made out on the screen by palpation.

Different clinics give very varying figures for the percentage of cases in which the niche is demonstrable. Burch (71) quotes the following: Åkerlund, 60 per cent. in 1923 and 75 per cent. in 1931; Albrecht, 90 per cent.; Berg, 50 per cent.; Carman and Sutherland, 13·27 per cent.; Clark and Geyman, 54 per cent.; Diamond, 66·6 per cent.; Ettinger and Davis, 50 per cent.; Geyman, 64 per cent.; Kirklin, 15·24 per cent. The Mayo Clinic figure for fifteen months ending

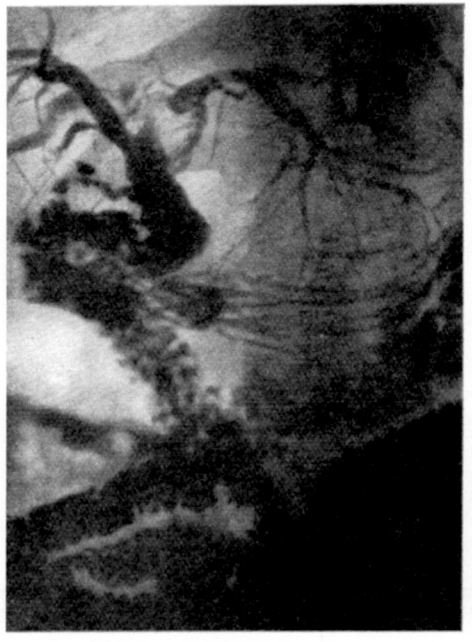 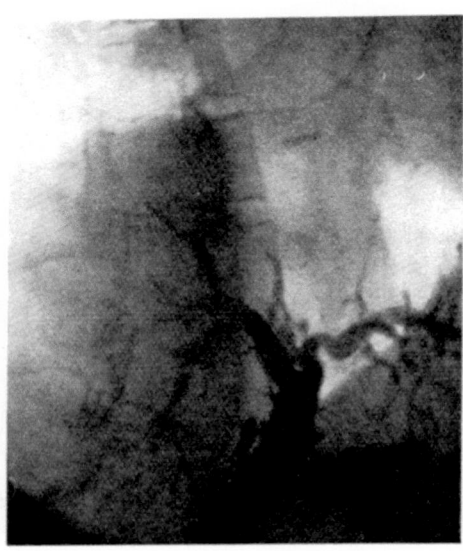

Fig. 205   Fig. 206

Fig. 205. A duodenal ulcer in a woman aged 47 has apparently perforated into the cystic duct; the opaque meal has flowed into the hepatic duct and right through, almost into the capillary hepatic ducts.
Fig. 206. Lateral view of same case. (Contributed by H. Graham Hodgson).

March 31st, 1935 is 17·7 per cent. Although the technique used must have a bearing on the results, it is difficult to account for this wide discrepancy. Some workers believe that the niche is only visible when the ulcer is active, and that its disappearance indicates healing.

Duodenal ulcer seems to be from four to six times as common as gastric ulcer (p. 230). It is more common in men than in women. Many cases are "silent", others give symptoms that last over many years, a few dating sympto-matically from childhood. Cases have been operated on as early as ten years of age (Brice Smith, Crymble and Allen (300)). In fact, Berglund (61) gives figures from post-mortem examinations that indicate an incidence of one per cent. in children under thirteen, while Dietrich (109) found six cases in 8534 post-mortem examinations in children under ten. The majority of cases, however, are found about middle age.

Some cases of duodenal ulcer seem to be associated with a long stomach, such as used to be called "gastroptosis" (cf. p. 282), and in these cases the right kidney is said to be mobile and dropped. There may be some connection between the "ptosis" of the kidney and the duodenal ulcer, for the symptoms have been known to disappear completely after nephropexy.

Perforation into biliary passages

A few cases have been recorded in which a duodenal ulcer has perforated into the biliary passages (Figs. 205 and 206). In the case illustrated, from Dr Graham Hodgson's department, the opaque food had travelled in a most extraordinary manner, passing right into the hepatic passages and giving well-defined outlines of the ducts far out into the liver substance. How such a thing could be possible with the ordinary opaque food is difficult to imagine. On the face of it the suggestion is that some negative pressure must have been responsible, for the pressure in the duodenum could not conceivably have forced this far-flung distribution. Clinically there was no suggestion of interference with the function of the liver. There was slight indigestion, with occasional stabbing pain below the ribs, brought on by such things as pickles. There had been no serious illness, and operation did not seem to be justified on clinical grounds. This was a most extraordinary case and, by a curious coincidence, two other friends sent me similar examples, but in neither of them had the opaque food passed much beyond the junction of the hepatic ducts. Some of the food had, however, passed into the gall-bladder in one of the cases.

Lönnerblad (221) reviews 40 published cases and describes two of his own.

(5) POST-OPERATIVE ULCER: JEJUNAL ULCER

The incidence of ulcers after operation seems to vary widely in different clinics. Carman (81) records the presence of gastro-jejunal ulcer in 200 (5·3 per cent.) of a series of 4146 cases operated on at the Mayo Clinic. In a certain proportion of these the primary operation was performed elsewhere. The sex incidence was 93 per cent. male and 7 per cent. female. The primary lesion was duodenal ulcer in 89 per cent. and gastric ulcer in 4·5 per cent.; about the remainder there was no definite information. 96 per cent. had had a posterior and 4 per cent. an anterior gastro-enterostomy. The time interval between the operation and the onset of symptoms varied from 6 weeks to 21 years, the period between the first and fourth years showing the highest percentage. Some of the ulcers were at the site of the anastomosis and involved both stomach and jejunum, but more frequently they involved the jejunum only and were, perhaps, several inches from the anastomosis. The diagnosis at that time depended entirely on indirect signs and was not satisfactory.

Goodall[137] states that gastro-jejunal ulcer follows over 2·8 per cent. of duodenal and 0·8 per cent. of gastric cases. D. P. D. Wilkie, in a personal communication, says that he has come to the conclusion that gastro-jejunal ulcer hardly ever develops after gastro-enterostomy for old-standing duodenal ulcer with stenosis, but that it is especially apt to occur in cases of irritable ulcer with high gastric acidity and hypertonic stomach, and that these patients complain of acidity and water-brash almost from the day of operation. For this reason he has of late years always preferred to do a gastro-duodenostomy in cases without stenosis. He has never had a gastro-jejunal ulcer after an anterior

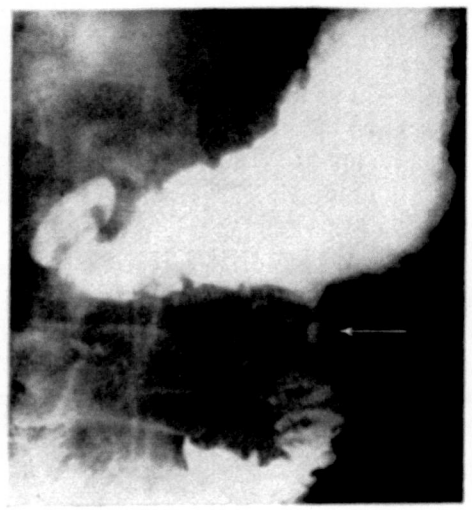 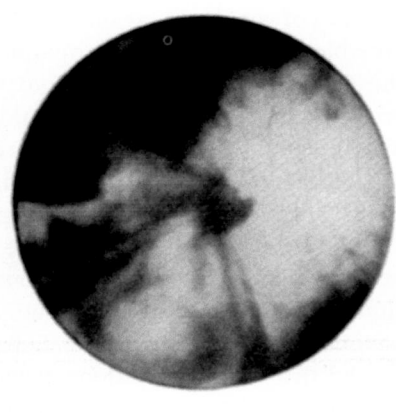

Fig. 207. Post-operative jejunal ulcer crater. (Contributed by J. D. Camp.)

Fig. 208. Post-operative jejunal ulcer crater. Note the converging folds of the mucous membrane. (Contributed by H. Berg.)

gastro-enterostomy, but gives the incidence of gastro-jejunal ulcer after the posterior operation as about 5 per cent.

Unfortunately I have no recent experience of the detection of jejunal ulcer, but in the past it has been unsatisfactory. The indirect signs on which an ulcer used to be suspected were gastric enlargement, six-hour retention, hyper-peristalsis and duodenal dilatation. These were, however, entirely unreliable, and the only satisfactory diagnostic point is the demonstration of the ulcer crater. Carman[81] discovered the crater in only one case, but in more recent years numerous observers have recorded success. Ström[305], for instance, examined 300 cases after operation and was able to demonstrate niche formation in a small number. Scott (295) has also recorded three cases in which he demonstrated the crater by "whitewashing" (i.e. obtaining mucous membrane relief pictures). Buckstein (69) summarises the literature on the subject up to 1932 and, from his own cases, demonstrates that the direct diagnosis is possible. Kirklin (201) now holds that a niche can be demonstrated in two-thirds of the cases.

The essential radiographic technique is one of intensive manipulation and judicious application of pressure in varied directions over the suspected area. Converging folds centring on the ulcer crater can be detected (Figs. 207 and 208). Berg was, I believe, the first to describe these, in jejunal as well as in duodenal ulcers. It is very unlikely that jejunal ulcers could be demonstrated by ordinary radiography, but with a technique such as Berg employs the diagnosis, in skilful hands, may become as accurate as that of duodenal ulcer. It will, however, always require expert procedure to make certain of the crater in the mottled shadow of the food passing over and lodged between the folds of mucous membrane. The patient should always be re-examined and the observations confirmed before diagnosis.

CHAPTER XVI

NEW GROWTHS OF THE STOMACH AND DUODENUM

Radiographically, new growths involving the stomach are of three distinct types:
 (1) Ulcerative.
 (2) Fungoid.
 (3) Linitis plastica.

They are practically all carcinomata; sarcoma of the stomach is very rare, but an interesting case has recently been described by Gage and Hunt (126). Wilbur (337), in reporting three cases of cancer under the age of forty, says, "Approximately 95 per cent. of gastric carcinomas afflict persons who are between the ages of forty and sixty-nine years, according to Eusterman, who found that the average age of men with carcinoma is fifty-four years, and that of women is fifty-three years. The records of the [Mayo] Clinic show that before 1930, there were 250 verified cases of gastric carcinoma involving patients less than forty years of age. Osler and McCrae reported that in 2 per cent. of cases the condition afflicts patients less than thirty years of age".

Carcinoma in the body of the stomach is frequently quite symptomless until far advanced. A case was recently reported in which it seemed that the carcinoma had been latent for 37 years before the patient came to operation (see p. 275). Spasm is not a prominent feature, except sometimes at the pylorus. In order to determine what degree of deformity of the shadow is due to spasm, belladonna has been exhibited, but has not, in my hands, been of assistance. In the pyloric region, however, symptoms are apt to occur early and lead to pyloric obstruction (cf. p. 265). Klason (206) analysed 201 cases of cancer in various regions of the stomach and found marked retention of food in 31 per cent. of cancers in the pyloric region. Retention was only marked in 11 per cent. of 258 cases of duodenal ulcer. Delay in emptying is discussed on p. 263.

The examination for new growths proceeds on the same lines as the routine for the detection of ulcers. A large growth presents no difficulty in diagnosis: it invades the cavity of the stomach, displacing the opaque food and causing a large filling defect (Fig. 215). But an early growth is often almost, if not quite, impossible to diagnose. A curious and unexplained feature of cases of gastric neoplasm of all types is the fact that, in contrast with the delay so frequently noted in gastric ulcer, the stomach tends to empty very rapidly.

(1) THE ULCERATIVE TYPE

A malignant ulcer appears as a definite niche which, in its early stages, is indistinguishable from that of peptic ulcer. The larger the crater the greater the probability that the ulcer is malignant (cf. Fig. 173). Differential diagnosis can only be made on the mucous membrane pattern. In a peptic ulcer, particularly if fairly large and indurated, the rugae tend to be drawn in to the affected area and to converge on the ulcer (Fig. 209). In a malignant ulcer they are not so displaced: sometimes they can be seen to be, as it were, cut off, but more often they fade away in their normal courses as they approach the indurated area, the mucous membrane being destroyed by the underlying growth (Fig. 210). When, however, the ulceration progresses the growth tends to be heaped up around the ulcer, and although there is still a definite niche, it is wider, flatter and usually

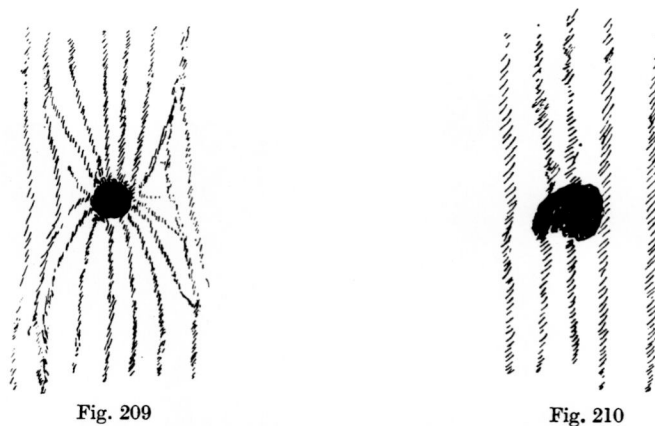

Fig. 209   Fig. 210

Fig. 209. Diagram to indicate the way in which the mucous membrane is distorted in peptic ulceration.

Fig. 210. Diagram to suggest the way in which a malignant ulcer invades the mucous membrane but does not necessarily distort the rugae.

not so deep as a chronic peptic ulcer. The appearance distinctly suggests the morbid anatomy: surrounding infiltration and heaping-up of the wall around the niche. The outline may exactly resemble the indentation of a peristaltic wave; but it is stationary and there is no corresponding wave on the greater curvature.

On palpation, even if nothing is definitely felt or seen, there is an impression of thickening which is not likely to be present even in a very chronic callous ulcer surrounded by adhesions. Moreover, the mucous membrane will probably show an irregular mottling round the ulcer as the opaque food is displaced by pressure. The patient should be turned so that the effect of palpation can also be studied as far as possible in profile. As most ulcers occur near the lesser curvature it is usually possible to see both projections of the shadow.

A plaque of growth in the wall, even if it does not show itself by a filling defect, may cause an interruption of the peristaltic wave, as described by some of the earliest workers. This is not easily detected on the screen, and is best observed by making a series of films with the patient rotated in such a way that the suspected portion is on the profile. A simple method is to make two exposures on one film at an interval of, say, ten seconds, while the patient holds his breath. The double outline will show the progress of the peristaltic wave, and an unaltered shadow at the suspected point will show that the wave is interrupted in its course. The appearance, although very suggestive, is not diagnostic of a growth, for a chronic indurated ulcer may give the same sign.

Later on, as the growth develops—slowly as a rule in these cases—it obliterates the niche, and the appearances become those of the fungoid type.

The differential diagnosis of early malignant from simple ulceration is often

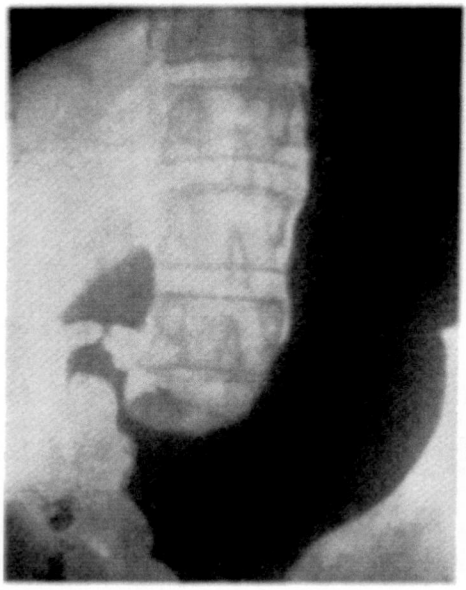 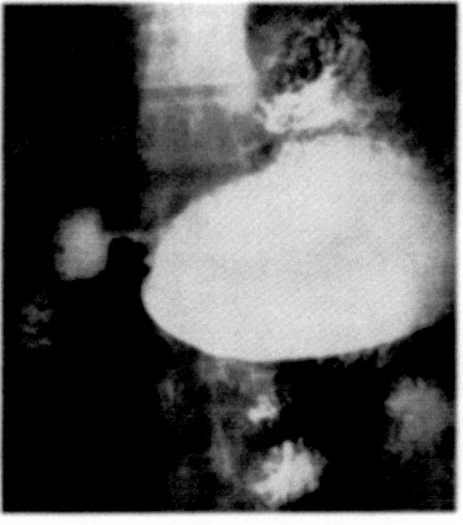

Fig. 211. New growth involving the pyloric portion of the greater curvature. Patient symptom-free and quite well in 1932. (Contributed by G. E. Richards.)

Fig. 212. Early growth involving the pylorus, but apparently not yet causing marked obstruction. (Contributed by Arial W. George.)

quite impossible, and if there is any doubt the radiologist should express it quite definitely for the guidance of the surgeon. In most cases, however, the clinical history will make the radiological differentiation quite unnecessary.

(2) THE FUNGOID TYPE

Here the growth, starting in the walls of the stomach, invades the cavity. It is usually of an active type, spreads rapidly, and frequently gives no clinical indica-

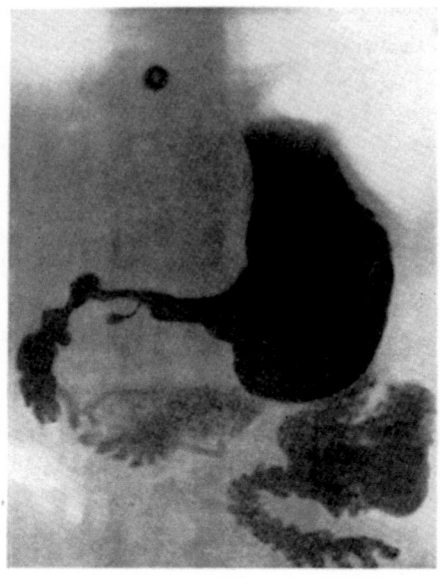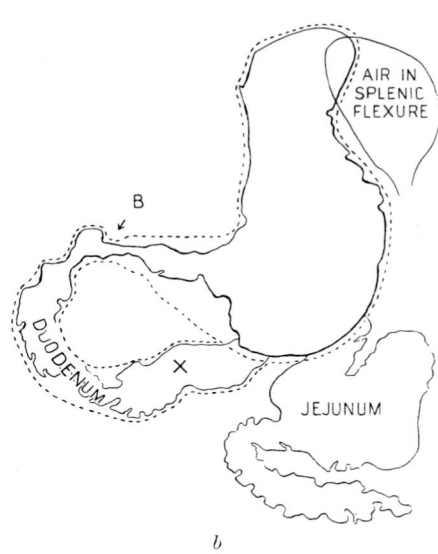

a   *b*

Fig. 213. *a, b.* Radiograph (touched up) and tracing of extensive carcinoma involving the pyloric end of the stomach. The dotted line in the tracing suggests the probable outline of the external wall. *B,* Pylorus. The small tag below the pylorus is probably a perforation.

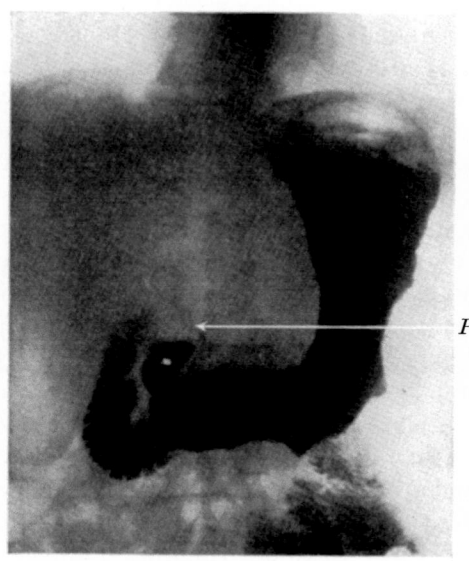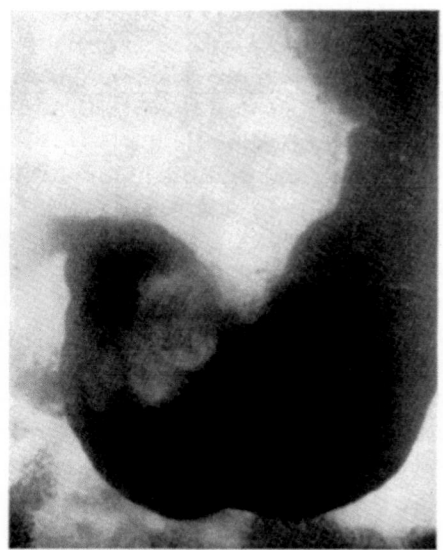

Fig. 214. Infiltrating growth of the leather-bottle type involving the greater part of the stomach wall but not extending to the pylorus. The food has rushed through to the jejunum, and the duodenum is distended. *P* = Pylorus.

Fig. 215. Growth involving the anterior or posterior wall of the pyloric antrum, causing a filling defect that appears as a more trans-radiant area in the opaque food. It gave rise to no localising symptoms. (Contributed by G. E. Richards.)

tion of its presence until it is quite advanced, almost obliterating the lumen. I once found the cavity almost completely obliterated in a girl in her early twenties.

The radioscopic picture is the reverse of that of the ulcerative type in its early stages, for the growth displaces the opaque food and, instead of a niche, there is a notch, a filling defect where the opaque food is displaced (Figs. 212–214). Such a growth may originate in any part of the stomach; there is no site of election. The cardiac end is frequently invaded and, if the patient is not examined in the recumbent position, even a large tumour may easily be missed. As the growth pursues its irregular, polypoid invasion, it occupies more and more of the cavity, leaving irregular channels and spaces that are filled by the opaque food. When the tumour is on the profile the shadow looks as if a portion had been torn out of it, leaving an irregular outline like that of a piece of coral.

If, however, the growth is not very extensive and only involves the anterior or posterior walls, it will not be seen until palpation is used. Pressure over the stomach at once reveals the unequal thickness of the cavity by producing relatively transradiant areas, which tend to appear and disappear as peristaltic waves sweep past over the opposing wall (Fig. 215).

Success in the detection of early growth depends on the radiologist's skill in palpation and manipulation of the first mouthful as it canalises the empty stomach. He will probably note deformity of the ordered channels of the rugae, which run in the length of the stomach, and perhaps some displacement of the opaque food. He may be able to detect resistance due to the growth, and he will attempt to discover whether or not there is undue fixation caused by infiltration into the surrounding tissues. Palpation is of great service in these cases in gauging the extent of the growth and the equally important question of involvement of surrounding tissues. Growths of this type vary greatly in consistency and, while some quite small ones are definitely and easily sensed under the palpating fingers, others, even large ones, give no sense of resistance at all. Soft tumours, however, are relatively rare.

By co-ordination of the senses of sight and touch the limits of the growth can be defined with a considerable degree of accuracy, especially in the upright posture. Palpation is greatly assisted by respiratory movements. If the radiologist exerts just insufficient pressure to prevent the mass coming down on deep inspiration, he can feel it slip under his fingers. In this way he can not only estimate the size of the growth, but form a shrewd idea of the direction and degree of its extension beyond the stomach wall. With this object, he should be sure to manipulate from each side in turn. If palpation is carefully carried out, even a small fungoid growth should be recognised without difficulty, provided, of course, that the stomach is empty and that the opaque meal is unmixed with retained food and gives a heavy clean-cut shadow. Palpation seldom gives much definite information about secondary deposits, but it does tell whether the growth is fixed and whether other organs are invaded by it, and thus gives guidance on the possibility of excision. Naturally, the radiologist will examine the lungs for secondary deposits, and will also note whether the liver shows any signs of enlargement.

Differential Diagnosis of Fungoid Cancer

An undigested bolus of food, curdled milk, a phytobezoar or a hair ball might be mistaken for this type of cancer, but there is seldom any doubt. If the observer cannot make certain by palpation, he can always expose the fallacy by comparing radiograms made on two successive days. I have seen polypi that gave the appearances of cancer, but they are very rare. One polypus was pedunculated, and could be moved about over the wall of the stomach. Syphilis should also be borne in mind (cf. p. 272).

The observer should not forget that the outline of the normal greater curvature is not always regular; it is quite often crenated, giving the appearance of the jagged inroads of an extensive growth. Palpation, however, reveals the absence of any tumour, and it may be possible actually to palpate out the cause of the crenation, which is an oblique, or perhaps a crinkled, disposition of the rugae over the profile instead of the more usual parallel arrangement. It has been suggested that this marked crenation is due to gastritis. Whether this is so or not, I do not know, but I well remember one case in which the crenations concealed an ulcer that I had failed to detect.

The examination should, of course, include the whole alimentary tract, even though a diagnosis of gastric cancer has been made. The complete examination quite often shows that not only the stomach but also the large intestine is involved. On several occasions this discovery has contra-indicated operation. The reverse is equally true, for a gastric invasion is sometimes found in patients sent for investigation of the colon. In a current journal I find the following:

X-ray examination revealed a filling defect involving the middle of the transverse colon. It was not thought necessary to make an examination of the stomach because of the lack of gastric symptoms.... Exploration showed a carcinoma involving the transverse colon, which was tightly adherent to the greater curvature of the stomach as well as to a loop of the small bowel.

(3) LINITIS PLASTICA: SCIRRHOUS OR FIBROID CARCINOMA

This is a relatively rare type of growth that, infiltrating the stomach wall, gives rise to what is known as the "leather-bottle stomach". There has been much controversy about its nature, some maintaining that it is syphilitic, others that it is merely a diffuse fibrosis. In many cases the sections have shown a scirrhous condition, in others there was no indication of malignancy, the structure being apparently entirely fibroid; but, whatever the microscopic report may have been, one thing is certain: the patient invariably dies. That is the acid test of malignancy. From the radiologist's point of view, therefore, I think these conditions can be classed together; in any case they cannot be differentiated radiologically.

The condition progresses slowly, and the obvious fact is that some part, or perhaps the whole length, of the stomach cavity is narrowed down to a tube with a smooth lining. It is thick-walled and nothing of the mucous membrane pattern could be made out in the cases I have seen (Figs. 216 and 217). The food tends to run straight through and the pylorus appears to exercise no restraining influence. There is no peristalsis in the affected part of the wall. The appearances are quite typical and there is no condition with which it is likely to be confused.

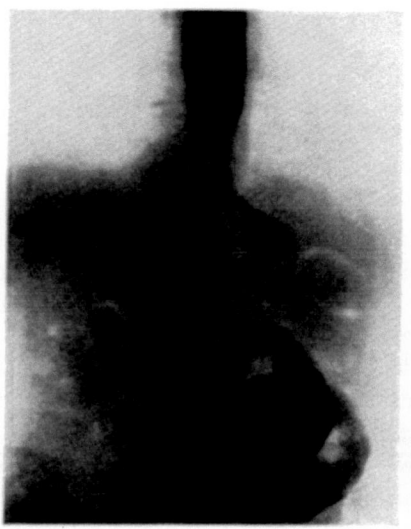 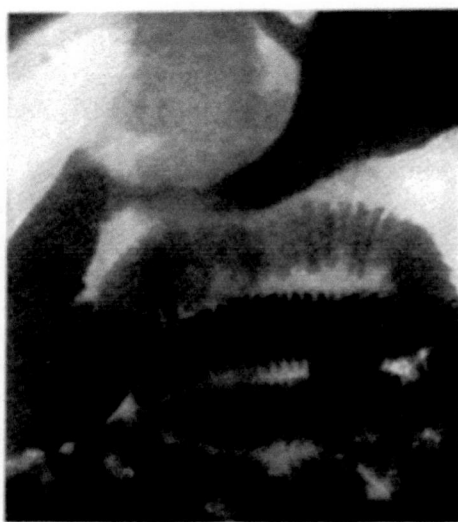

Fig. 216   Fig. 217

Fig. 216. Leather-bottle type of stomach. The food runs straight through, but there is, nevertheless, some back-pressure to the oesophagus.

Fig. 217. Leather-bottle type of scirrhous carcinoma of the stomach. Clinically there were no symptoms except loss of weight and lethargy. (Contributed by H. M. Tovell.)

THE RELATION OF CANCER TO ULCER

The possibility of cancer arising in a pre-existing ulcer has been much debated in recent years. At one time it was seriously contended that carcinomatous change inevitably took place in chronic ulcers, and that all gastric ulcers were potentially, if not actually, malignant. The early writers regarded the association of the conditions as rare, but Zenker (343) in 1882 propounded the extreme view that nearly all cancers of the stomach originated in ulcer. Wilson and

PLATE XII

A.

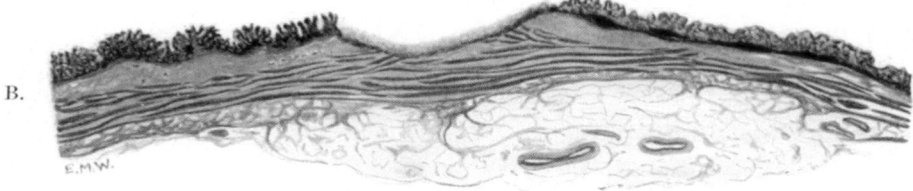

B.

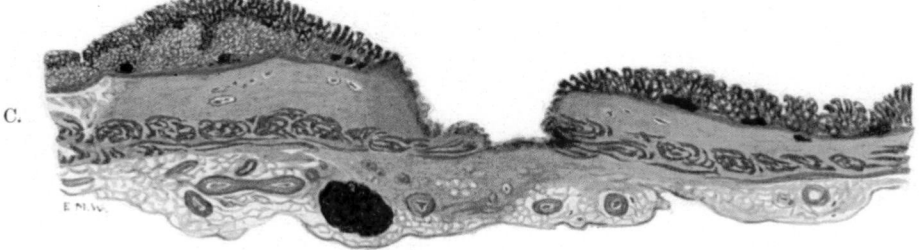

C.

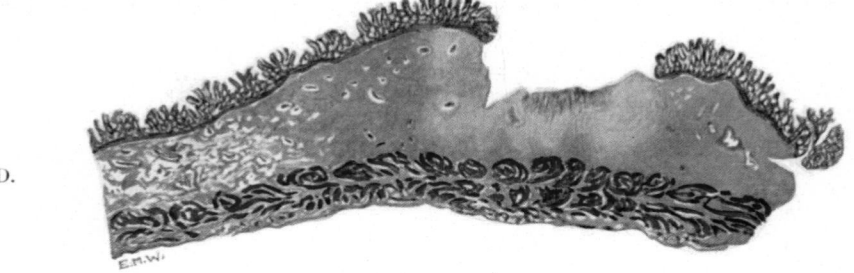

D.

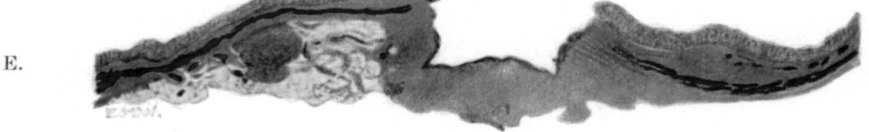

E.

Plate XII.

Fig. A. Section of an acute ulcer. There is a shallow ulcer-crater lined by necrotic material. The mucous membrane here is completely destroyed, together with the muscularis mucosae, while the sub-mucosa is congested and oedematous.

Fig. B. Section of a medium-sized sub-acute ulcer. The characters are those of a recent ulcer, but invasion of the muscular coat is beginning. × 3.

Fig. C. Section through an early chronic ulcer of the stomach. The muscular coat has been breached over quite a small area, but considerable subserous fibrosis is already present. The dark purple mass in the subserous tissue is a slightly enlarged lymphatic gland. The patient, a man of 61, had had pain in the epigastrium for five months only. Partial gastrectomy. The ulcer, of small size, was on the lesser curvature $3\frac{1}{2}$ inches from the pylorus. × 3.

Fig. D. Section of an ulcer which, although it has not yet invaded the muscular coat, shows well-marked fibrosis of the sub-mucosa and other evidences of chronicity, including the presence of numerous eosinophil cells. (Mallory's connective-tissue stain.) From a woman of 26, who had had upper abdominal pain for two years. Excision of ulcer from the middle of the lesser curvature. This is probably to be regarded as a chronic ulcer in which the lesion has not passed beyond the sub-mucous coat, a very unusual state of affairs. × 3.

Fig. E. Section of a chronic gastric ulcer stained by Mallory's connective-tissue stain. There is an extensive breach in the muscular coat, the severed ends of which terminate in the lateral walls of the ulcer. The floor is formed of a dense mass of fibrous tissue derived from the subserosa. Two years' history. Partial gastrectomy. The ulcer, which was fully half an inch in long diameter, was on the lesser curvature 3 inches from the pylorus. × 2.

(Contributed by A. F. Hurst and Matthew J. Stewart. By the courtesy of Oxford Medical Publications.)

Fig. A. Very chronic, densely sclerosed, but nevertheless healing ulcer. The crater has flattened out and marginal epithelialisation has made considerable progress, as shown by the comparative width in the mucosal and muscular gaps. From a man of 40 who had had intermittent attacks of dyspepsia for five years. Partial gastrectomy. (Mallory's connective-tissue stain.) × 3.

Fig. B. Section of a large chronic duodenal ulcer from the posterior wall. There is a densely sclerotic floor, buttressed by pancreas (*purple*) and lymph glands (*blue*). From a man of 62, who had had indigestion for years and who died three weeks after profuse haemorrhage. The ulcer was an inch beyond the pylorus, and had given rise to a severe grade of duodenal stenosis. × 3.

Fig. C. Section from a scar. It is of longer standing, and shows more complete healing, with fusion of the muscularis and muscularis mucosae at the margins, and a well-restored mucosa. (Masson's trichromic stain.) × 3.

Fig. D. Section across a well-healed linear scar from a case of very advanced hour-glass contraction of the stomach, showing well-restored mucous membrane and fusion of muscularis and muscularis mucosae. (Masson's trichromic stain.) The patient, a woman of 59, gave a twenty years' history of pain in the stomach. Each attack lasted from one to three months and was accompanied by vomiting. Partial gastrectomy. There was extreme hour-glass contraction $4\frac{1}{2}$ inches from the pylorus. × 3.

(Contributed by A. F. Hurst and Matthew J. Stewart. By the courtesy of Oxford Medical Publications.)

Note: These sections probably do not represent the appearances during life, when, owing to the action of the muscularis mucosae, the membrane is heaped up round the ulcer. (See p. 236.)

PLATE XIII

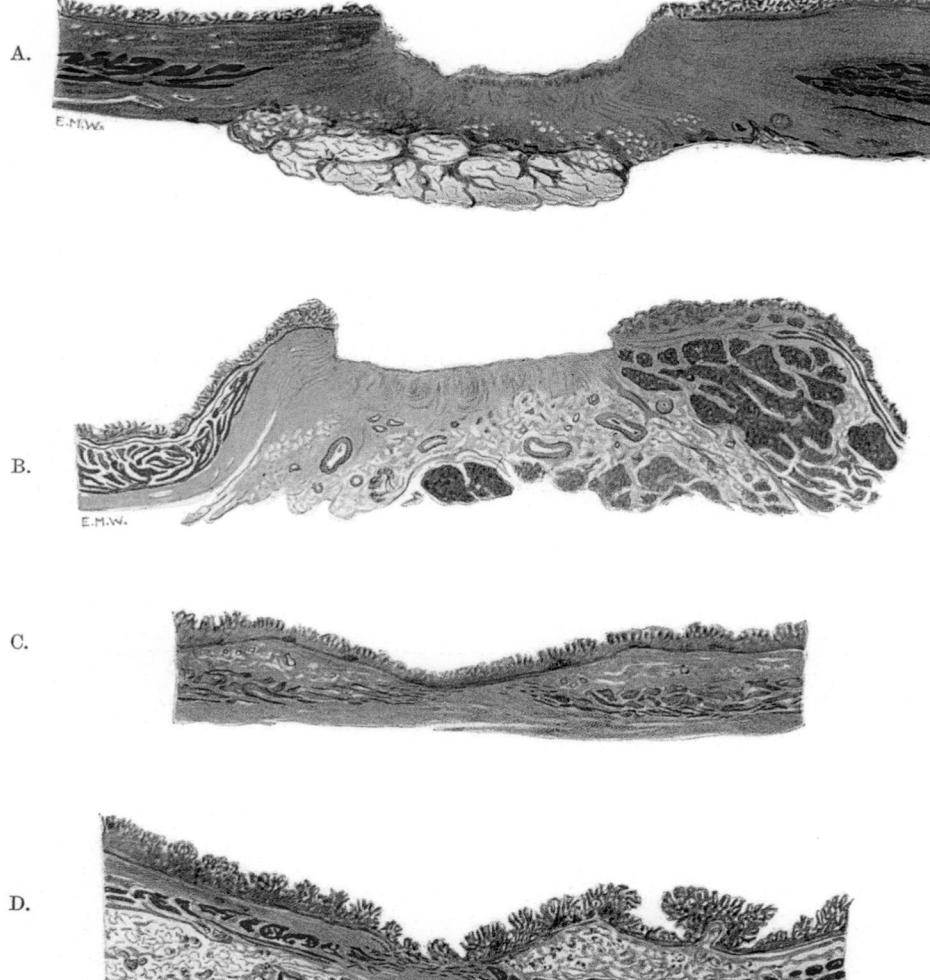

A.

B.

C.

D.

MacCarty (340) of the Mayo Clinic gave this view much publicity and support in 1909–10; in their series of 153 "undoubtedly malignant" cases 71 per cent. "presented sufficient gross and microscopic evidence of previous ulcer to warrant placing them in a group labelled 'carcinoma developing in a preceding ulcer'".

Stewart (181) states that 15·7 per cent. of his 70 cancer cases arose in ulcers and that 6·1 per cent. of his 180 cases of chronic ulcer showed cancerous changes in the margins; he figures some very convincing instances and believes that the active process of chronic ulceration is the factor responsible for the formation of cancer. Kirklin (202) points out that benign intragastric tumours commonly ulcerate, and that three-quarters of all gastric lesions are carcinomatous.

Thurstan Holland (156), on radiological and clinical grounds, emphatically rebutted Zenker's theory. He does not agree that malignancy commonly arises in chronic ulceration or that ulcer is a predisposing cause of cancer. Later writers, particularly J. Ewing (115), have concluded that cancer grafted on ulcer is an unusual condition—"probably not exceeding 5 per cent."

The pathological side of the subject is well summarised and illustrated by Stewart (181). Cabot and Adie (73) have analysed the figures of no less than 82 observers:

39 per cent. of observers say that cancer arises in ulcer in less than 5 per cent.
50·6 per cent.   ,,   ,,   ,,   ,,   ,,   ,,   ,,   10 per cent.
18 per cent.   ,,   ,,   ,,   ,,   ,,   ,, over   50 per cent.
Cabot and Adie's own figures of 56 cases gave a figure of 9 per cent.

Surveying the end-results of 454 cases of pyloric ulcer, Luff (222) states that "no case of carcinoma developing at the site of an ulcer has been reported in the whole series of cases". Most authorities now hold that not more than 5 or 10 per cent. of ulcers become malignant. Hurst (177) points out that there is no evidence that carcinoma ever develops in the scar of a healed ulcer. There is, however, a tendency to regard ulceration occurring elsewhere than on the lesser curvature as more likely to be potentially malignant, and to submit such cases to operation with a view to excision. In fact, I am informed that this is now an accepted principle of operative procedure in some centres.

Experience in radiological departments entirely confirms the views of Thurstan Holland, expressed twenty years ago. My own impression is that carcinoma rarely develops on ulcer. The original diagnosis may have been wrong, so that a case diagnosed as ulcer may subsequently prove to be cancerous, but in my experience as a radiologist I have found that an ulcer is either peptic or malignant and remains so throughout its whole course. I cannot recall a single case of gastric ulcer, diagnosed by X rays, which has come back to the radiological department after operation with any suggestion that malignancy has supervened, despite the very large number of cases that have been examined again for recurrence of symptoms.

It is for others to decide whether this opinion, which is common to most radiological departments, can be set against the evidence afforded by microscopic sections of ulcer-cancer. There may be fallacies in the histological method. Certainly Stewart's sections (Colour-plates XII and XIII) seem to indicate that the growth is starting in the crater of the ulcer, but it is possible that cells which are histologically malignant may not be malignant in life. Moreover, a cancer may arise independently near an ulcer and invade it, and a section through the place where the growth impinges on the ulcer wall might well give the impression that this was the site of origin. Newcomb (258), in discussing the criteria on which a diagnosis of ulcer-cancer can be based, analyses the findings in 100 cases of carcinoma of the intestines and says: "The only certain criterion for the diagnosis of ulcer-cancer is fusion of the muscularis mucosae with the muscularis at the edge of the ulcer, each of the other suggested criteria being present in at least 6 per cent. of the control cases."

NEW GROWTH OF THE DUODENUM

Primary new growth of the duodenum is extremely rare, as the following quotations from personal communications show:

Lord Moynihan says: "I have only come across two cases of primary new growth of the duodenum. One I am not quite sure about, as there was no post-mortem."

Prof. A. H. Burgess says: "I have always regarded primary malignant growth of the duodenum as excessively rare—at any rate in our part of the world. I can recall only two cases in my own experience, and I have looked through the statistics of the Manchester Royal Infirmary for the last five years without finding a case. It seems strange that it should be so rare considering the frequency of gastric carcinoma—which will stop dead at the duodeno-pyloric junction."

Mr A. J. Walton says: "I have been more and more coming to the conclusion that there is practically no such thing as a primary carcinoma of the duodenum. I have been quite convinced that the carcinomata that I have seen in this situation, and almost as certainly convinced that those which are described in the literature really commence, either in the stomach and spread downwards, in the ampulla of the common bile duct and spread inwards, or in the jejunum and spread backwards. This being the case, I cannot really say that I have seen a single example of a primary carcinoma of the duodenum. It is of interest, however, that one does see localised papillomata which apparently commence definitely on the duodenal side of the pylorus. I have made a precisely similar statement in my book *The Surgical Dyspepsias* (p. 156)."

Dr H. Courtney Gage informs me that there are two cases on record at St Mary's Hospital during the last thirty-three years, but none has been found in the last 3,000 autopsies.

The published literature on the subject gives the following figures:

Perry and Shaw (268) found ten cases of primary carcinoma of the duodenum in 18,000 necropsies.

Jefferson (186) found forty-three cases in 109,201 autopsies (0·04 per cent.) from eight European hospitals. Of all the cases of cancer of the intestines that he could collect, only 3·1 per cent. occurred between the pylorus and ileo-caecal valve. Of the 71 cases in the small intestine 48 per cent. were in the duodenum and 52 per cent. in the jejunum or ileum.

H. D. Rolleston (284) collected 41 cases of primary carcinoma of the duodenum; 8 of these were in the first part only, 24 in the second, 4 in the third, and 5 involved both the first and second parts.

The combined figures of Mayo, Rolleston, Geiser and Fenwick, quoted in Osler,* show 22·15 per cent. in the first part of the duodenum, 65·82 per cent. in the second and 12 per cent. in the third.

A very small number of primary sarcomata of the duodenum are also recorded.

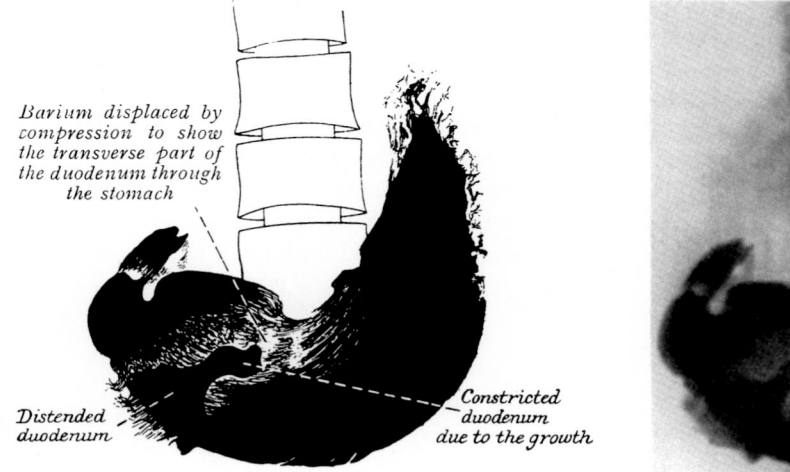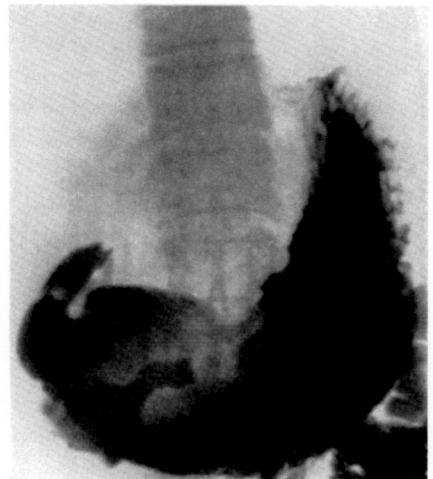

Fig. 218. Carcinoma of transverse part of duodenum (tracing and radiograph).
(Contributed by H. Courtney Gage.)

New growths are less rare in the region of the duodeno-jejunal flexure, but I do not know whether these are in fact primary or have spread from the jejunum as Walton suggests. One of my own cases was a ring carcinoma localised to the flexure as in the case illustrated (Fig. 218), the growth in which involves the same region but extends further back into the third part of the duodenum. I also know of another case in which the growth was just distal to the duodeno-jejunal flexure (Dr G. W. Mitchell). The papilla of Vater is not an uncommon site for malignancy which subsequently spreads into the duodenum. There are numerous islets of pancreatic tissue beneath the mucous membrane of the suprapapillary portion of the duodenum and some authorities hold that primary carcinoma only develops in these. Bland-Sutton (64), however, scoffed at this idea.

Since malignancy is so rare, neoplasm arising in a duodenal ulcer must be almost a curiosity. Rolleston (284) collected 10 cases and to these Jefferson (186)

* *Modern Medicine*, 1926, vol. III, p. 634.

added 20 more, but is doubtful of the reliability of some of them. Arisz [23] has recently reported two cases of men in whom X-ray diagnosis of duodenal ulcer had been made. In one case the origin of the cancer in the ulcer seems to be quite definite, for the ulcer had been observed three years previously, and a section showed the origin of the malignant changes in its base.

Diagnosis

As the region is too high for palpation, neoplasm of the duodeno-jejunal flexure cannot be diagnosed except as a probability when there is definite obstruction. In a case which I saw recently, the symptoms were at first intermittent. There were attacks of copious and quite painless vomiting that became more frequent. When I saw the patient the first time, I noted nothing abnormal in the duodenum, but a few days later I found it distended and exhibiting an intermittent writhing peristalsis. The growth was annular and the surgeon removed it extremely delicately, but the patient did not recover consciousness, although he did not appear to suffer unduly from shock. To the onlooker it certainly seemed as if, even though the growth came away so easily, the sympathetic nervous system, which is complex and abundant in this region, had been fatally injured.

CHAPTER XVII

OTHER CONDITIONS OF THE STOMACH AND DUODENUM

DELAY IN EMPTYING

In the early days the radiologist used to consider that delay in emptying had definite pathological significance, but he was then dealing with a large proportion of old-standing cases in which this feature was very conspicuous: often practically the whole of the food remained in the stomach after twenty-four hours. This was with a bread-and-milk meal. Nowadays these extreme cases are rare; moreover, with the emulsion type of food there is much less liability to retention. For this reason, when testing for delay, I rely on the second opaque meal, which is made up as a real food. Small residues are not uncommon and are neglected, but a fairly large residue is of some importance.

Whenever definite delay is confirmed, the radiologist should review the case and make the most searching investigation of the whole stomach, because, for some unknown reason, delay is often associated with ulceration elsewhere, even at some distance from the pylorus. In carcinoma, on the other hand, rapidity of emptying is usual. In only a comparatively small number of cases will the cause be traced to the pylorus, and other causes must be sought. If an unusually large collection of food is found behind the ileo-caecal valve, the delay may be referred from irritation in the appendix region. The possibility of gall-bladder inflammation must also be investigated, and the teeth should be scrutinised and probably radiographed. If the patient is suffering from head-ache, extreme nervousness or similar troubles, the delay is likely, to some extent at least, to be attributable to psychic causes. Worry of any kind may cause delay, and if the patient is examined after a holiday, disordered or even pathological appearances may have disappeared. Professor Pembrey and his colleagues (3) found that severe muscular exercise delayed the passage of food through the stomach of man, rats and mice. Similar work before food had no effect, but anaesthesia produced marked delay. Gentle exercise and congenial company appeared to increase the rate of passage. Gianturco (131) observes that after fundusectomy the emptying time (in cats) is shortened.

In a Stomach of Good Tone

The presence of retained food or secretion is at once indicated by the shape of the air space, the segment of a circle bounded above by the diaphragm and below by a fluid line that can be shaken and splashed. This is, of course, the picture that is seen after an ordinary meal. The succussion sign of olden days can be obtained in any normal stomach containing the requisite proportions of fluid and air. If, however, instructions have been carried out, this fluid level should not be noted when a patient first comes for examination. One patient, I recollect, upset my routine by fortifying himself for the examination with two large whiskeys and soda on his way to my rooms.

The retention of opaque food beyond six hours in a J-shaped stomach is not usual, and should always be confirmed, especially if the peristalsis is of the intermittently powerful type. More often, however, such delay is associated with an inert condition in which peristalsis is not seen for long periods and in which when it does occur the waves are not at all powerful. The cause is then more likely to be found elsewhere than in the stomach.

In a Stomach of Poor Tone

In the atonic type of stomach, in which delay in emptying is common, the air space is typical: it is pear-shaped, and its thinned-out lower end narrows and becomes ill-defined, or perhaps ends in a half-inch-wide fluid level. It is usual to find a residue of food or secretion in such stomachs. As the opaque food is given, it slides downwards and forwards from the cardiac orifice to the narrowed neck—the lower end of the pear-shaped air space—and then drops off in blobs or in a thick stream through the retained food. The outline of the wide sac of the lowest part of these atonic stomachs is typical (cf. p. 86). It forms the arc of a circle, usually low down in the pelvis, and is very often almost unbroken by peristaltic waves. The character of the peristalsis should be carefully watched, for it may be a very important clue (cf. p. 267).

In these cases it is often exceedingly difficult, if not impossible, to fill the pars pylorica satisfactorily, as it lies so high up in relation to the food, and only well-calculated posturing on the couch will make the opaque food flow into it. Moreover, the manipulation tends to mix the opaque with the retained food, so that the shadow is poor and ill-defined.

It is a remarkable fact that, in spite of quite considerable delay in emptying, the patient may suffer only slight indigestion and may go on year after year in the same condition, a sub-standard dyspeptic who is seldom free of the feeling that he has a stomach and must always be on his guard about the food he eats. In most, if not all, of these cases I am quite confident that the atony is merely the response to a sedentary life or to some psychic or similar cause that leads to deficient muscular tone and disordered balance of gastric secretion. The sense of a weight and the "food hanging heavy on the stomach" has a very definite foundation in fact.

The mere retention of food is not necessarily an indication for a short-circuiting operation, which is, in fact, an admission that the cause has not been found.

The search for the cause may reasonably include, I conceive, all possible sources of debility and of reflex spasm, not only in the alimentary tract, but also in the other systems. Dental sepsis and other sources of toxic absorption are the most likely causes, and on a number of occasions investigation has revealed unsuspected advanced pulmonary disease that has been masked by the gastro-intestinal symptoms.

In some of the early cases of hour-glass stomach due to ulcer I found such marked delay in the lower sac that I reported pyloric obstruction in addition. In some of these, definite evidence of ulceration in both situations was found, while in a few the surgeon could find nothing to account for the delay. Several of these were examined subsequently on account of persistence of symptoms, and it was found that the delay in the lower sac was still present. In at least two, a further operation revealed that the pylorus was by then definitely thickened. Whether the ulceration which had led to this cicatrisation had actually been present at the time of the first operation and had shown no indication on the peritoneal surface, was not determined, but well-marked delay is evidently a sufficient indication for a gastro-enterostomy even if the surgeon does not find sufficient justification in the external appearance of the pylorus. If he does not follow out this procedure, a number of these patients will probably come back to him. This indication, however, does not apply to the long, atonic stomach in which the delay is suspected to be due to the mechanical difficulty of raising the food to the pylorus. With present-day technique it ought to be possible, by persistent posturing and manipulation, to make almost, if not quite certain of the presence or absence of pyloric and duodenal ulceration, even in atonic stomachs.

PYLORIC OBSTRUCTION

The part that defective tone plays in delayed emptying is so difficult to assess that I do not feel able to analyse with certainty the various stages of pyloric obstruction. The radiological pictures seen can, however, be grouped into acute and chronic, and the latter can be divided into three types.

Acute Cases

The onset of an acute obstruction is seldom observed, but I shall never forget one of my very early cases, in which the activity of the peristalsis was dramatic in the extreme. The stomach, in addition to being segmented by the extremely violent and rapid waves, writhed and twisted as if in an agony of struggle to overcome the obstruction. The distortion was far greater than that in Plate fig. 192. The stomach was successful in its efforts when I first examined the patient, but at a later examination there was marked delay in emptying and, doubtless, had an operation not been performed, the tone would eventually have given way and left the usual type of atonic stomach that is seen in chronic obstruction. In this, as in another similar case, the cause of the trouble was a carcinoma of the pylorus. So far as my information goes, this stage of acute obstruction lasts only a short time. The stomach fails to evacuate the contents and the X-ray picture soon becomes that of a chronic obstruction.

Chronic Cases

There seem to be three types of chronic obstruction; the first two are very rare and perhaps are merely stages in the failure of the gastric muscle to cope with the obstruction.

(*a*) In the first type the stomach is apparently normal, with unusually powerful and sometimes intermittent peristalsis. When the patient is feeling well, this is generally effective, and the stomach is emptied in a reasonably short time. When the patient has symptoms, the stomach is still normal and the peristalsis powerful, but it is not effective and there is a considerable residue after the five-hour interval. It is therefore very advisable in such cases to compare observations made when symptoms are present and absent.

(*b*) Occasionally a stomach with good tone contains large quantities of retained food; the opaque food lies in the lowest part for long periods, unmoved by peristalsis. It is impossible to evoke any peristaltic movement, and I have seen fully a half of the opaque meal still present after twenty-four hours. I do not know the explanation of this curious appearance. Such cases as have been operated on have shown definite pyloric lesions. Whether they form a group on their own or are, as one would expect, a transitional type before tone relaxes, I do not know.

(*c*) Practically all the cases of chronic obstruction that we see fall into this group: the "dilated stomach" of former days, which sags down far into the pelvis and gives the typical appearance of the grossly atonic stomach (cf. p. 86).

ABNORMAL PERISTALSIS

The force and rhythm of peristalsis may vary considerably within the limits of normality and are subject to various influences apart from the local factor of gastric contents (p. 149). Hence, too much stress should not be laid on this phenomenon unless the appearances are very definite. Slight variations should be disregarded.

In any obstructive lesion there are two local factors at work, namely, the propelling force and the size of the passage relative to that of the bolus that is held up. One of the strongest points of evidence is the character of the peristalsis. In ordinary circumstances, peristalsis does not seem to be a propulsive force, but when powerful and obviously propulsive waves are persistently ineffective, in association with definite delay in emptying, the suspicion of an organic lesion must necessarily be strengthened. If a succession of these powerful waves gradually dies away, giving place to a period of rest that is followed by another succession of waves, the presence of an organic obstruction is strongly suggested. This intermittent and powerful peristalsis is almost characteristic of long-standing obstruction.

Even in the thinned-out atonic stomach which results from the persistent retention of food, the waves are still unexpectedly powerful at times. The periods of rest may be prolonged, and the food lies stagnant in the lowest part of the stomach, appearing as an unbroken semi-circular shadow low in the abdomen. If, after prolonged observation coupled with manipulation of the stomach, these powerful waves do not show themselves, the cause will probably be found in the pylorus, but it is possible that inertia due to reflex or psychic factors may play an unsuspectedly large part in producing the delay. It is advisable to re-examine such patients, and quite often the second observation will not reveal such marked delay, especially if the patient is encouraged and relieved from apprehension. I have very occasionally seen the powerful type of peristalsis, which almost segments the stomach, in definite association with purely reflex causes, but it seems to be rare.

Reverse Peristalsis

In reverse peristalsis the waves are first noted as indentations perhaps an inch or more from the pylorus and then progress backwards towards the fundus. This used to be fairly common in long-standing cases, and it was always associated with an extensive lesion in the neighbourhood of the pylorus. The rhythm did not appear to be very stable, and any interference, such as rubbing the abdomen, might check it. In fact, on several occasions, by tickling the abdomen over the greater curvature, I have not only stopped the reverse peristalsis but started the rhythm in the normal direction. I have never seen really powerful reverse peristaltic waves. Nowadays, reverse peristalsis is seldom seen, probably because cases are submitted to radiological examination at an earlier stage.

VOMITING

In the early days the radiologist saw far more patients who were in the habit of vomiting than he does now. Perhaps the habit has gone out of fashion or possibly the experimental types of food then used may have had something to do with this; some of them were extraordinarily distasteful.

Observations of vomiting in patients during the course of routine examinations are naturally unsatisfactory, as the occasion is fraught with urgency not only to the patient but to the observer! It seems, however, reasonably clear that there are two types of vomiting, distinct both in causation and in mechanism.

(1) The first is that produced by voluntary stimulation of the pharynx. Everyone knows that vomiting can be accomplished as a mechanical reflex by tickling the back of the throat: a necessary routine in the Gargantuan feasts of Roman days when a vomitorium was provided in adequately equipped houses. Vomiting of this kind is not necessarily associated with nausea and is purely mechanical. The stimulation causes retching, with very powerful jerky movements of the diaphragm and abdominal wall which, if the stomach were full, could reasonably be expected to expel the contents. I have watched this mechanism on many occasions, although not to the extent of actual vomiting. The stomach appears to be passive; it is simply squeezed and shaken by the abdominal wall and diaphragm. The chief feature is retching; nausea, the nausea of sea-sickness, is absent.

(2) The other type of vomiting is characterised by preliminary nausea. The most striking example I have met was a man who said that he could vomit at will and who actually made an appointment with me for a demonstration under the X rays. Unfortunately, however, he suddenly lost his ability. This was particularly disappointing, as his vomiting was not of the mechanical type, but depended on a nausea produced entirely by auto-suggestion. In this type there is absence of peristalsis and an extremely rapid secretion of gastric juice, to which swallowed saliva is added before vomiting occurs. The tone of the stomach can be seen to relax so that the lowest part of the greater curvature drops several inches (cf. p. 85). The patient is conscious of this and feels the weight of the food in the stomach. The air space becomes elongated and pyriform, so that the superimposed fluid does not show up on the screen. After this, powerful peristaltic waves—or perhaps spasmodic contractions—appear and alter the contour of the shadow; they are associated with the violent and jerky retching movements of the diaphragm and abdominal wall, but the conditions of an examination do not usually admit of further observation. The stomach is jerked up mainly by a contraction of the gastric muscle itself, and this may be assisted by the action of the abdominal muscles. On a few occasions, however, I have seen vomiting occur as a result of this gastric contraction alone, without any aid from the abdominal muscles. The stomach visibly contracted up and expelled its contents, while very marked contractions, resembling peristalsis, indented its outline. I have myself seen and two observers have told me that they have noted a spasm of the stomach starting at the pyloric end and pushing the contents upwards, the patients stating that they felt they were about to vomit. Once I thought that the stomach was going to be completely segmented in the middle by one of these contractions and that food would be ejected from the upper part only; this was, however, in a case of suspected ulcer, and the appearance may

have been merely an accentuation of the spasmodic hour-glass contraction due to ulceration. In cicatricial hour-glass stomachs vomiting occurs, I believe, only from the upper sac but, surprisingly enough, some patients with spasmodic hour-glass stomach also vomit from the upper sac only (even when subsequent operation has shown absolutely nothing to account for the contraction), the discomfort and desire to vomit passing off as soon as the upper sac is emptied.

An interesting personal experience was related by the late Dr Deane Butcher (28):

Some years ago he accidentally swallowed an irritant poison. He rushed into the surgery and hastily swallowed several tumblers of hot water containing permanganate of potash. The first vomit was clear, pink, and unmixed with food. Only after three or four repetitions did food appear in the vomit, although a copious dinner had been taken three-quarters of an hour before. This unintentional experiment seemed to prove the occurrence of an hour-glass contraction of the stomach as a consequence of irritation.

In vomiting, the upper part of the food is expelled first. If there has been little retching, the first mouthfuls brought up will consist of the over-lying secretion and fluid that has settled out from the food-stuffs, but if there has been much retching the whole contents are churned together and the mixed mass is expelled at once. Even the most violent and persistent vomiting may fail to empty a large atonic stomach in which the food lies well down in the pelvis; I have seen quite a large residue of opaque food remain in such a stomach for nearly a week despite persistent vomiting.

On one occasion I observed the action of vomiting in a patient who had malignant disease of the pylorus. Whenever he retched, a spasmodic contraction divided the stomach, and extremely powerful peristaltic waves appeared. This seemed to originate at the biloculation, and sometimes it passed in a reverse direction upwards and at other times downwards, while occasionally waves would start from the contracted zone in both directions at the same moment.

I have several times seen food return from the duodenum to the stomach, sometimes in the process of vomiting and sometimes independently of it. In one case, in which the duodenum was overloaded on account of a growth at the duodeno-jejunal flexure, the distended duodenum was emptied back into the stomach, but the reflux was only sometimes followed by vomiting. In another case the food had a much longer journey, for the obstruction was an annular growth in the jejunum 12 inches beyond the duodeno-jejunal flexure. The coil of jejunum behind the obstruction became more and more distended, until at last sudden contractions forced the food out of it back into the duodenum and then into the stomach. These contractions were not associated with much pain, but when the patient felt that he was going to be sick, the X ray revealed a more violent type of contraction that cleared the coils almost entirely and swept the contents into the stomach, whence they were voided in the usual manner by the combined effort of voluntary and involuntary muscles. The X-ray appearances well bore out the patient's own description: "When I vomit I feel as if I have to bring it up from the very bottom of my stomach." There was no nausea in this case.

Merycism (Rumination: Cud-chewing)

This curious habit, normal in the ruminants, is very rare in man. It may date from infancy and is said to be sometimes hereditary. No case has been studied radiologically, but Magee (231), working under considerable difficulties, has observed it in the goat. The habit in man—a habit about which he is usually reticent—is partly voluntary and partly involuntary, and may be practised for a few minutes only or for more than an hour after meals, especially after meat.

GASTRITIS

At one time gastritis was the usual diagnosis for all gastric conditions that were not sufficiently severe to be labelled gastric ulcer. The diagnosis has fallen out of fashion this century but recently there has been a revival owing to the detailed investigation of the mucous membrane pattern by the radiologist. To-day, the diagnosis of gastritis is made not on hypothesis but on the observation of definite facts: widening of the rugae and disorders of the mucous membrane pattern. In one instance, perhaps twenty years ago, long before demonstration of the mucous membrane pattern was routine, I noted extremely marked crenation of a large section of the outline of the greater curvature. It was far more definite and persistent than I have ever seen, either before or since: its pattern remained approximately unaltered for several days. I reported that the appearance probably represented a pathological condition of the mucous membrane. To-day it would have been diagnosed as a case of marked gastritis. At the operation an ulcer was found on the greater curvature and the surgeon told me that he had found marked inflammatory changes of the mucous membrane.

The intensive study of the mucous membrane is leading to great advances in our knowledge but, although it is easy to diagnose a fully developed disease involving the mucous membrane, it is difficult to recognise its earliest stages. Köhler took for his book the title of "Grenzen des Normalen und Anfänge des Pathologischen im Röntgenbilde", and no title was ever better selected, for the borderland between the normal and the pathological is no wider than a hair, even in such gross conditions as cancer. The muscularis mucosae that is responsible for the changes in the form of the mucous membrane pattern is probably infinitely more sensitive and responsive to local and remote stimuli than the comparatively gross musculature of the stomach wall. Its capacity for producing changes that are within the limits of normality is probably infinite.

Moreover, who shall say where gastritis and other relatively slight and possibly transitory changes in the mucous membrane begin? What opportunity have most radiologists for confirming the interpretation they place on the mucous membrane pattern? As yet there is a gap, a gap that will need a great deal of filling, between the variations of the normal mucous membrane pattern and the diagnosis of those conditions which do not produce definite and well-recognised changes in the morbid anatomy. Clinically, the diagnosis of gastritis rests on very slender foundations; a background of intensive study of non-hospital subjects is, to my mind, essential before such pathological conditions are diagnosed with any degree of precision. I trust that I am not too conservative in suggesting that radiologists exercise restraint in this new method of investigation, at any rate until they have adequate proof that the changes they see and believe to be pathological do in fact consistently represent the conditions to which they are ascribed. My own studies of the mucous membrane in students are not extensive, but they are quite adequate to assure me that a very wide range of changes in the mucous membrane pattern of the stomach is met with in normal healthy subjects.

In the last few years, however, Henning (152) has had the opportunity of correlating the radiographic appearances of the gastric mucosa with photographs made by the gastroscopic camera. His opinions and descriptions are therefore based on his own experience and his results are convincing. For him, at any rate, chronic gastritis is a definite morphological change in the mucous membrane. Radiographically he describes the rugae as larger, broader and more irregular than normal. They are not easily altered in shape by palpation and distension. In atrophic gastritis they are abnormally tenuous.

Westphal (335), also combining histological, radiological and gastroscopic examination, distinguishes two grades of excessive function in what he describes as a hyperergic irritable stomach. In Grade I, patients are young, the gastric juice is moderately hyperacid, and mucosal folds are steep, tortuous and somewhat broadened. In Grade II, the folds may be a finger-breadth across. The hyperergic stomach may develop gastritis as a result of intensive alkali therapy, but the broad, high folds are not due to gastritis, but to purely functional alterations of the muscularis mucosae, blood supply and interstitial cell content.

Holmes and Schatzki (159) describe three definite types of gastritis: (a) a hypertrophic form in which there is thickening of the rugae, which are also increased in height, and are somewhat rigid. Such changes may be localised but are more often general. These authors point out that "the differential diagnosis may be extremely difficult. Lymphoblastoma and congenital giant rugae have to be considered—it must be emphasised that the appearance of large rugae alone is not sufficient to make a positive diagnosis of gastritis". (b) An atrophic form, which cannot be diagnosed radiologically because "normal cases may shew thin rugae similar to those which we sometimes find in atrophy, and there may be normal rugae in cases with complete atrophy of the mucosa". (c) An ulcerative erosive form in which, with much difficulty, the authors have been able to detect numerous ill-defined craters that are masked by the marked secretions.

The X-ray diagnosis of gastritis is therefore possible but should be made with reserve, for it is not yet on a sound footing. Moreover, the condition is not a common one, as is shown by the fact that Holmes and Schatzki, looking for it in a large hospital service, only diagnosed it 13 times in a year (1934).

SYPHILIS

The differential diagnosis of gastric carcinoma from gastric syphilis is, I believe, not possible from X-ray observation, but any invasion of the shadow picture which does not cause some degree of resistance or palpable thickening should suggest the possibility of syphilis, and a Wassermann test should be made.

There is a considerable literature on gastric syphilis in France, Germany and America, but in this country the condition must be extremely rare. Carman[80], Le Wald[323, 325] and other workers in America and Germany have recorded a number of cases, in some of which the history suggests that there can have been no mistake. The X-ray appearances are those of neoplasm, but these authorities state that even large gummatous masses in the stomach are not easily palpated (Figs. 219 and 220).

On the strength of the entire absence of any resistance on palpation I once made a tentative diagnosis of syphilis in a man of 41 who had such extensive filling defects of the whole stomach that the opaque food, although not markedly obstructed in its passage, gave only a mottled or widely reticulated outline of the stomach. The patient grudgingly admitted that he had had anti-syphilitic treatment and had been discharged "cured" a year previously. Anti-syphilitic treatment was renewed, the patient made a remarkable rally and was soon back at business. Three months later, however, he had relapsed and, when I again examined the stomach, the picture was not markedly changed but the whole mass had become hard, nodular and quite unmistakable. Operation was not indicated and the patient died shortly afterwards; no post-mortem was obtained. My impression of this case is that it may possibly have been a primary syphilis with superadded malignancy. It is, however, the only instance in which I have even suspected syphilis.

Carman quotes a number of cases seen in the Mayo Clinic in which the evidence of a positive Wassermann is taken as presumptive evidence that the gastric tumours were syphilitic. Le Wald has also recorded cases and summarises the diagnostic points:

(1) Diminished size, accompanied by the almost immediate evacuation of most of the stomach contents. There is often *compensatory dilatation of the oesophagus* in this type of case.

(2) Fairly symmetrical deformity of a large portion of the middle of the body of the stomach, producing a *dumbbell-like appearance*. When this is found in the young person, or in an older individual without the characteristic appearance of cachexia commensurate with a malignant involvement of the stomach to the extent indicated by the X-ray findings, syphilis should always be suspected. If a positive Wassermann reaction is obtained, the diagnosis is established with reasonable certainty.

(3) In cases showing a remarkably small *tubular* stomach (linitis plastica, cf. p. 257) the problem is more difficult, as this condition even in the young may denote carcinoma. In other instances it may be fibromatosis or syphilis.

(4) In another class of case the X-ray appearances are very similar to those of carcinoma and consist of localised areas of infiltration of the stomach wall, but the lesion may be as extensive in syphilis as in carcinoma.

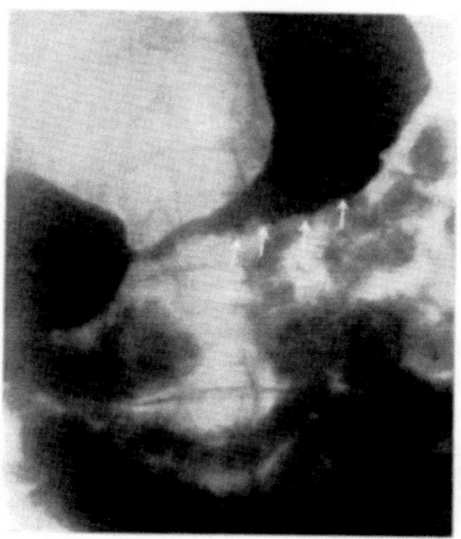 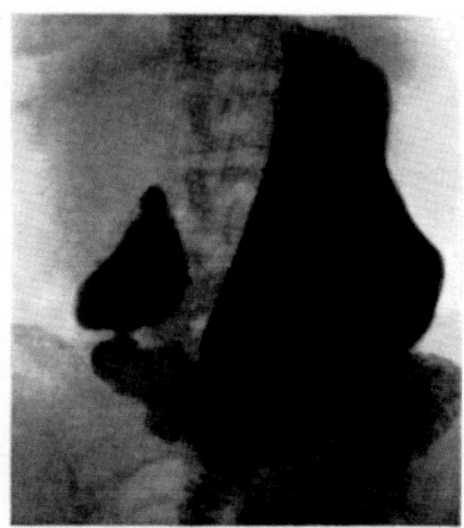

Fig. 219   Fig. 220

Fig. 219. Extensive syphilis involving the greater curvature. In November 1925, when the radiograph was taken, the stomach wall was markedly fixed. Later films, up to March 1932, showed that the stomach became nearly normal in appearance under anti-syphilitic treatment, and the fixation was not nearly so marked. The patient is now (1932) quite well and the diagnosis of syphilis seems to be proved. (Contributed by G. E. Pfahler.)

Fig. 220. Syphilis of the stomach. Deformity of the pyloric end of the stomach involving both curvatures. A complete disappearance of the deformity followed anti-syphilitic treatment, and five years later the stomach appeared to be quite normal. (Contributed by L. T. Le Wald.)

(5) The lesion may be situated at the pylorus and produce marked stenosis and gastric retention, resembling ulcer or carcinoma, but always more extensive than simple ulcer.

Speaking of gastric syphilis in general, Redding says (280): "The skiagrams reproduced are identical with those due to scirrhous carcinoma—an opinion which does not seem to be disproved by the subsequent history of the recorded cases."

Whatever may be the case in other countries where disease forms may be different, I am convinced that in this country syphilis of the stomach is extremely rare, if it occurs at all.

TUBERCULOSIS

Tuberculosis of the stomach is rarely seen in the X-ray department; so far as I know I have never examined a case. It is only likely to be found in patients with advanced and well-recognised tuberculous lesions elsewhere.

ADHESIONS

Adhesions occasionally distort the outline, but in such cases the clinical history, together with palpation, will make the diagnosis clear. Doubt may be caused by the crenated appearance of the greater curvature due to distortion of the rugae, but again careful palpation will reveal the nature of the irregularity.

The diagnosis of adhesions depends upon the fact that, under normal conditions, it is possible to manipulate the stomach through the abdominal wall and to determine more or less accurately its fixity or mobility. Like all other observations on the stomach, the presence of adhesions must be confirmed at a subsequent examination. More than once my second examination has revealed a perfectly normal stomach where I had been quite confident that adhesions were present.

Extensive adhesions occasionally cause inroads into the gastric cavity that are almost impossible to distinguish from those of carcinoma. Palpation in the upright position is the most valuable means of determining whether irregularities in outline are due to adhesions or to new growths, for in this position it is nearly always possible to detect the size and extent of a growth. Where adhesions are present, no definite tumour can be felt but only an indefinite sense of resistance; if, however, the transverse colon is also full of opaque mixture, the observer can usually obtain fairly accurate and helpful knowledge of the possible relative movements. A history of peritonitis in childhood may throw light on very puzzling appearances. The presence of adhesions fixing the transverse colon into the pelvis is best demonstrated on the couch with the hips raised. With forcible respiratory and abdominal movements the transverse colon should come up out of the pelvis. If it does not, it is anchored by adhesions. A careful inquiry into the history is as necessary in this as in any other gastric case, in order to avoid fallacies in the interpretation of the radiographic findings.

POLYPI

Multiple polyps are rare and I have only seen one case. The relief picture of the mucous membrane shows a dappled appearance, the usual longitudinal arrangement of the channels and folds of the mucosa being lost. This appearance of

Plate XIV

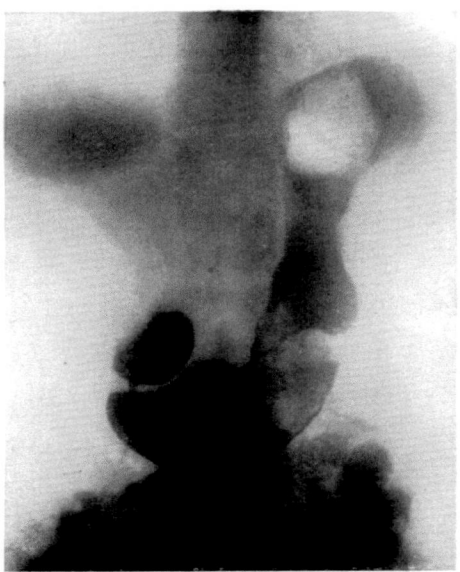

Fig. 221. Pedunculated adenoma of the stomach. On palpation the tumour was movable above the opaque food and the site of the attachment to the pedicle on the greater curvature was localised by screen examination.

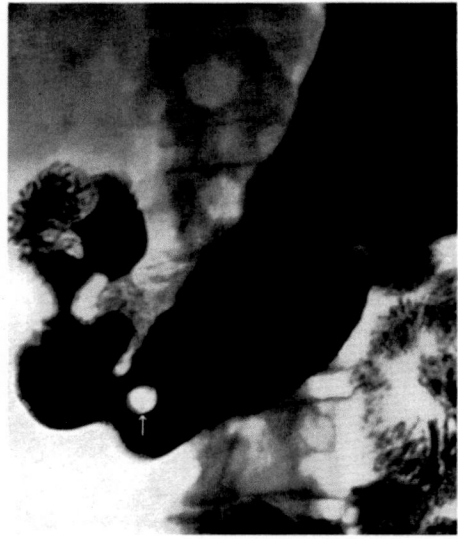

Fig. 222. Papilloma of the pyloric end of the stomach. Clinically, there was marked loss of weight and anorexia (three months), but no localising signs. Operation showed a mass the size of a walnut attached to the anterior wall of the stomach. Microscopical sections showed that it was a papilloma undergoing mucoid degeneration. (Contributed by J. Currie McMillan.)

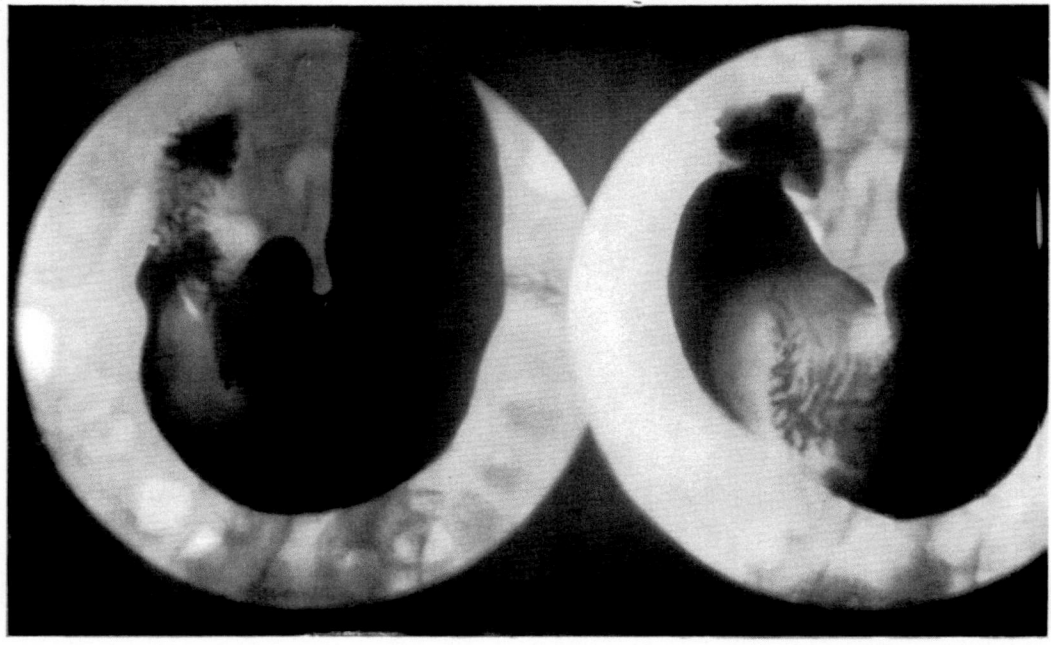

Fig. 223. Large simple fibroma of the stomach. There was no suggestion of infiltration. See Fig. 142. (Contributed by H. Graham Hodgson.)

multiple filling defects is quite distinctive from that of carcinoma, which is almost invariably a single mass. The condition may affect the whole of the stomach or be limited to one part.

Single polypi of the stomach, both sessile and pedunculated, are also seen very occasionally (Plate figs. 221–223). The sessile variety causes a filling defect which cannot be distinguished from that caused by some carcinomata. The pedunculated polyp is distinguished by the way in which it can be moved about in the opaque food. In the only case that I have seen the diagnosis was not difficult, for the point of attachment of the polyp formed an indentation on the greater curvature, and the filling defect caused by the mass could be moved about this point and was obviously adherent to it.

Some figures from the Mayo Clinic state that 20 per cent. of fifty-eight benign tumours investigated were polyps (Priestley and Heck (275)). In another series an incidence of 4·5 per cent. of all benign tumours was recorded. McRoberts (230) regards adenomas as a low-grade malignancy, to be treated as merely a stage in the development of malignant disease. Alvarez and Judd (16) state: "No matter how certain we may be that the tumour is benign, experience shows that such tumours are very liable to be of a low grade of malignancy or to become malignant. The rate of growth is not by any means a certain criterion, as carcinoma of low malignancy may develop very slowly and cause no symptoms for years." A striking instance was reported by these authors, together with Wilbur and Baker (17): they removed an ulcerated polypoid carcinoma which had a 37 years' history. The case had been under X-ray observation for 34 years.

FOREIGN BODIES

A great variety of swallowed objects are found in the stomach—such as coins, toys, false teeth, pins, marbles and buttons—and the only point in diagnosis is to determine that they are actually in the stomach. This is very readily done by giving a few mouthfuls of opaque food and noting whether it does or does not reach the foreign body. They very seldom give rise to any trouble and in due course they find their way out. Even complete upper sets of false teeth may pass through the whole length of the alimentary tract and be voided normally. Only a very small proportion of swallowed needles and pins cause symptoms. I have, however, come across two cases in which pins gave trouble.

In one, a girl of 18, the pin, swallowed a week before, was located in the stomach. On the following day some gastric trouble was present and opaque food showed a very marked hour-glass contraction of the stomach at the site where the pin had been seen (Plate fig. 224). Next day the patient was feeling rather better and the hour-glass contraction was not nearly so persistent; it relaxed almost completely with massage. Four days later I again saw the girl and again located the pin, but this time in the region of the caecum. The gastric symptoms persisted. On re-examining the stomach I again found the hour-glass condition. The case is of academic interest and importance as illustrating the relation of spasm to trauma and of symptoms to spasm.

In the other instance, one of my colleagues discovered a pin in a case where the symptoms were those of duodenal ulcer. This pin was located as having perforated the lesser curvature, the head being still embedded in the wall of the stomach, the point in the lesser sac of the peritoneum. The localisation was accurate and the removal of the pin relieved the symptoms (Plate fig. 225).

A *bezoar* is a concretion of any kind in the stomach.

The *phytobezoar*, or food-ball, is rare, and is a concretion of skin, seeds, fibres, etc. from fruit and vegetables, matted together. Potter (273), who recorded a case recently, could only find references to ten others.

Hair-ball

The *trichobezoar* or hair-ball is also very rare and seldom diagnosed, even tentatively. It simulates inoperable growth but its surgical removal is perfectly straightforward. The following case, described (32) in 1913, is the only one I have ever seen and is, I believe, the first to have been definitely diagnosed radiologically.

A woman aged 28 was referred for examination on account of a swelling in the abdomen. The history was that for a few weeks she had complained of weakness, loss of appetite, and attacks of abdominal pain which were indefinite, not severe but usually accompanied by vomiting. In the left hypochondrium there was a very distinct hard mass extending to the epigastric, left lumbar and umbilical regions. Its upper limit could not be defined. It was not tender and was freely mobile.

On X-ray examination the opaque food was diverted from its course and found its way down the greater curvature (see Plate fig. 226), showing very clearly that the tumour was not the spleen. At this stage the appearances suggested advanced carcinoma. Presently, however, the food also found its way down the lesser curvature, surrounding the mass, which was therefore evidently in the stomach. Moreover, the mass was freely movable within the stomach; Plate fig. 227 shows how it could be displaced by pressure from below, the top of it rising above the level of the bismuth food and showing as a rounded shadow in the clear air-space in the fundus of the stomach. In order to demonstrate the nature of the tumour still more clearly the fundus of the stomach was distended with carbon dioxide, and the tumour was pushed up into the large air-space thus obtained (Plate fig. 228). It gave a heavy shadow, because of the coating of bismuth it carried up with it.

The diagnosis was therefore so complete that even the size of the hair-ball could be predicted: 9 inches long by 3 inches wide, while the predicted shape corresponded closely with the actual shape. The process of the hair-ball that occupied the pyloric canal formed an acute angle with the rest, and in the physical examination this angle felt like a notch in the border of the tumour, more or less in the position of the notch in enlargements of the spleen.

An interesting point at the time was that the shape of the hair-ball corresponded almost exactly with that which radiologists consider to be the shape of the normal

PLATE XV

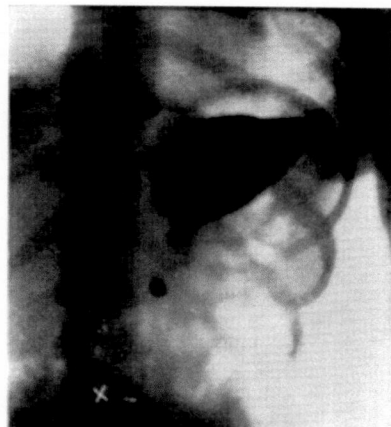

Fig. 224. Spasmodic contraction of the stomach due to trauma. The swallowed pin was located at the site of the contraction. Although the pin passed on, the spasm persisted for three weeks.

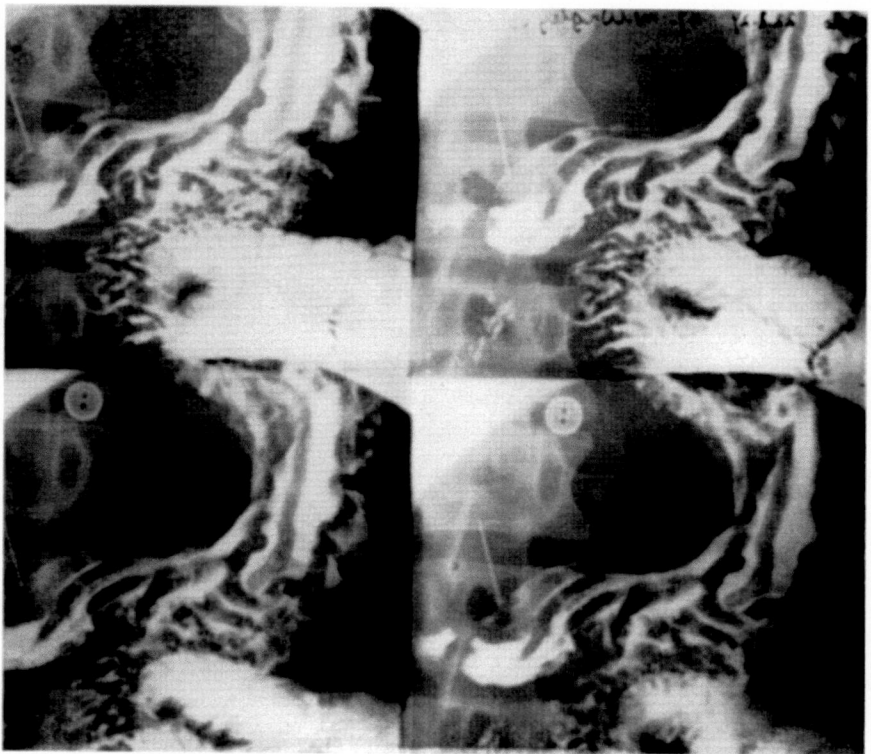

Fig. 225. Serial views showing a pin that has perforated through the lower end of the lesser curvature, the head remaining embedded in the mucosa. The symptoms were suggestive of duodenal ulcer.

PLATE XVI

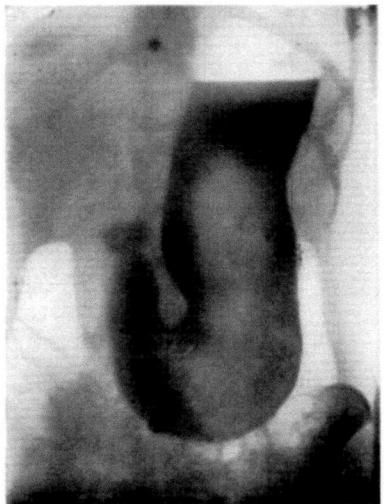

Fig. 226. Hair-ball in stomach surrounded by opaque food.

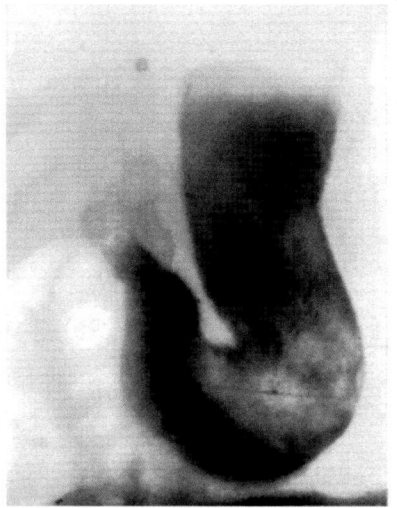

Fig. 227. Hair-ball pressed up from below.

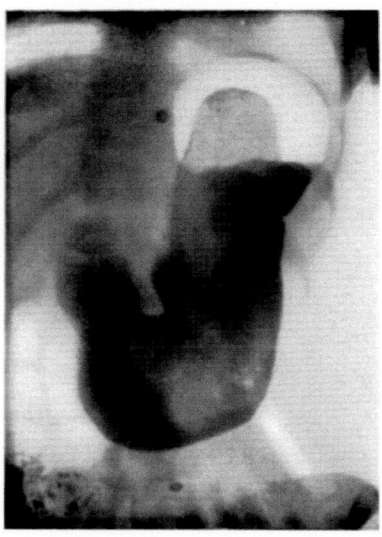

Fig. 228. Hair-ball after distending the stomach with carbon dioxide. The top of the tumour is pressed up into the air space and the actual shape of the mass can be mapped out.

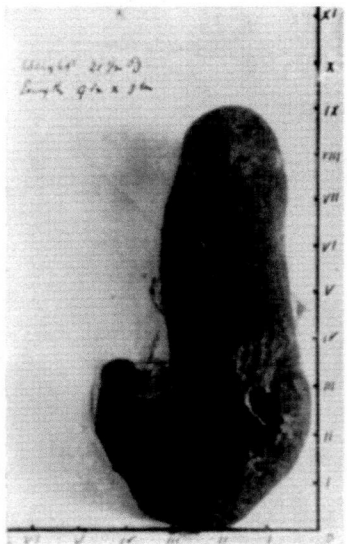

Fig. 229. The hair-ball after removal.

stomach, and there was no suggestion in its markings that the stomach was other than one undivided cavity. At that time there was a very heated controversy in the medical press, some anatomists and surgeons holding very strongly that the stomach was normally a bilocular organ.

I gave a definite report that the tumour was a hair-ball in the stomach. The patient denied that she had been in the habit of eating her hair. After the operation, however, we learned that when she was eight years old she had had scarlet fever. In this illness she had lost practically all her hair. Prof. A. H. Burgess enucleated the mass without difficulty and the convalescence was quite uneventful.

This hair-ball is now a dried and shrunken mass of felt and, as a museum specimen, is a mere caricature of the giant hair-ball that was removed twenty years ago (Plate fig. 229).

Rare conditions notoriously appear in "runs". A little time before I saw this case I had visited Dr Thurstan Holland (157, 158) in Liverpool and he had shown me beautiful radiographs of what was supposed to be inoperable carcinoma. The possibility of hair-ball was suggested, and in fact operation subsequently confirmed this diagnosis. Within a few days, the case I recorded came to my department, and not very long afterwards Dr Holland saw yet another case.

EXCESS OF AIR IN THE STOMACH

The collection of air that is practically always seen as a clear area just below the dome of the diaphragm is still called the "air shadow", although in fact it is photographically a high light, because of its transradiancy. The Germans call it the "Magenblase", or stomach sac. In the supine position it disappears, the air being spread out below the anterior wall. Presumably this air that is trapped above the cardiac orifice has some function; possibly it forms a buffer, an air cushion, associated with the balancing and "springing" of the stomach, that saves it from undue shaking, particularly when it is full of food. Abnormal quantities of air are found in the stomach as a result of air-eating, air-swallowing and air-sucking.

Air-Eating

It is usual to take in a certain amount of air with food and drink, particularly when the meal is hurried. When watching the opaque food pass down the oesophagus, the radiologist frequently sees a bolus of air in the midst of the opaque shadow. Quite apart from any pathological condition or disorder of function, the quantity of air swallowed may be considerable and may distend the cardiac end of the stomach. This distension causes slight discomfort and the patient eructates, noisily or otherwise. I have often seen superfluous air escape from the stomach noiselessly without any conscious effort and without the patient's knowledge; this, however, is unusual, for the patient is made aware of the air passing up between the collapsed and moist walls of the oesophagus by a bubbling sound and sensation, and generally voids it audibly, by belching.

Aerophagy—Air-Swallowing

The swallowing of excessive quantities of air is a habit which is sometimes carried to extreme limits. The patient is usually a neurotic woman. She believes that all the gas is being produced in the stomach and is quite unaware of the mechanism by which she swallows it. Often she is secretly rather pleased about the condition; it excites sympathy, for the "indigestion" must indeed be severe when all this gas is being produced by fermentation in her stomach! She complains of attacks of flatulence with abdominal distension and discomfort, and her eructations may be so noisy and violent as seriously to distress not only herself but those around her. I have heard of cases where mill-workers refused to work alongside sufferers from this condition. A few air-swallowers, however, do not bring up the accumulated air noisily, but let it escape without muscular effort.

The condition may easily be missed at an X-ray examination for, unless the patient is "performing", the quantity of air in the stomach may be quite small. When there is a history of severe flatulence, the observer should tell the patient that some air is present in the stomach and that it would assist his observations if she could bring it up. This suggestion is nearly always effective, and he can watch the whole procedure. Subconsciously the patient shuts her mouth and swallows air, which may be drawn in through the nose, and he sees this air rapidly distend the stomach, often to a surprising extent. Then, with a violent explosive eructation, most of it is noisily expelled and the process recommences, the stomach filling again at once. I have sometimes seen patients fill the stomach with air until it extends far down the abdomen, well below the umbilicus, in efforts which they think are designed to expel air (Figs. 230 and 231). It would seem impossible to produce this appearance unless the lower part of the stomach is anchored down by adhesions, but I have not been able to satisfy myself on this point, although adhesions were certainly present in one of the cases in which the air filled the stomach almost completely. Sometimes the whole of this air is belched up in an objectionable and unnecessarily noisy manner, but more often only a part is expelled and, having started, the patient goes on eructating air that she seems to swallow almost in the act of bringing it up. In severe cases this noisy procedure may go on for hours at a time. Some device such as a cork between the back teeth, or, better, a pencil held between the molars, to keep the mouth from shutting and thus prevent swallowing, is usually effective. I have not succeeded in making any of these patients "perform" when lying down; they will empty wind out of the stomach, but only severe cases seem to be able to take it in.

Sometimes the stomach is so distended that the air passes through into the intestine, but not so frequently as in air-suckers, who seem to create a negative pressure in the abdomen. I have often noted slight aerophagy in connection with appendicitis which appeared to be causing gastric symptoms.

Leven (216), in an extensive treatise on air-swallowing, described analyses of the gases brought up, showing that the eructations produce only air and that gastric fermentation could not possibly evolve the enormous quantities.

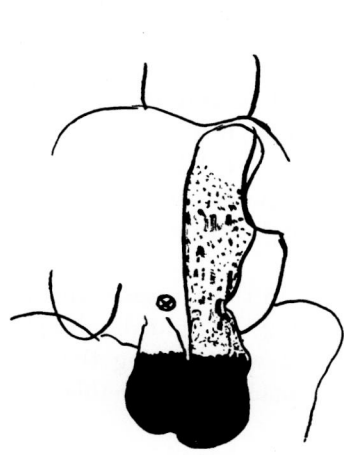 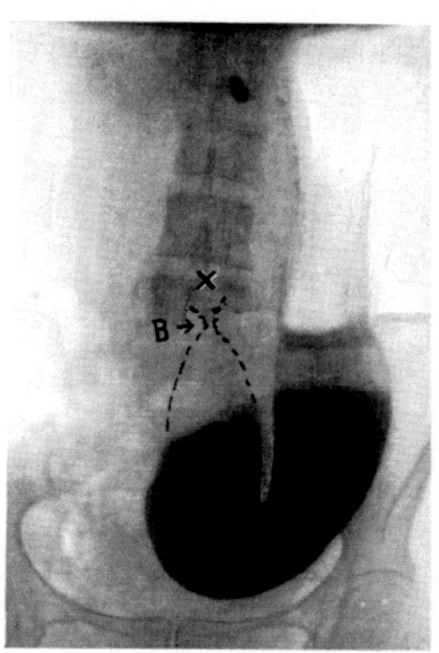

Fig. 230   Fig. 231

Fig. 230. Tracing of a long type of stomach; the upper two-thirds are filled with air. Flecks of opaque food are adhering to the mucous membrane—the subject was an air-swallower. Note the indentations caused by the spleen and kidney, which were well outlined on the film. The pylorus appears to be low in this case.

Fig. 231. Air-swallowing. The subject swallowed all the air shown in the radiograph in her efforts to bring up flatus. *B*, Pylorus.

Oesophageal Aerophagy

Some patients suffer from persistent eructations and yet show no increase or decrease in the air space of the stomach. When examining these subjects in the semi-lateral position, however, the radiologist can usually make out that the swallowed air is taken down as far as the cardiac orifice and distends the oesophageal ampulla to a considerable extent. This may produce precordial discomfort.

Air-Sucking

Air-sucking is frequently encountered in horses and is, I believe, so serious that the animal has to be destroyed. In man it is rare. The clinical picture is much the same as in air-swallowing, but the mechanism, and consequently the treatment, are entirely different. It does not depend on the act of swallowing at all, for the air is drawn down the oesophagus into the stomach. The mechanism is complicated and, so far as I can make out, is as follows. The patient draws the abdomen in and fixes it. Correspondingly, the diaphragm rises on both sides, but particularly on the right, and is fixed in this position. The patient then expands the chest, sucking the left diaphragm high up into it, the upper level reaching two or three inches above the right side and possibly four or even five inches above the normal level. This causes a negative pressure in the abdomen, and air rushes in through the oesophagus and distends the stomach, which follows the left side of the diaphragm as it is sucked up into the chest. The patient is quite unconscious of the inrush of air, and the stomach is filled up in a few seconds. The air is then expelled or, in severe cases, to judge from the clinical picture, it may be passed on into the intestine to cause extreme abdominal distension and be voided as flatus.

The mechanism of expulsion of air from the stomach in these cases seems to be as follows. Without relaxing the abdomen, and keeping the right diaphragm fixed, the patient bears down by contracting the chest wall, forcing the left diaphragm down and squeezing the air out of the stomach with forcible and exceedingly noisy eructations.

The movements of the diaphragm in air-sucking can be explained in two ways: (1) that there is separate voluntary control for the two sides (as we now know may be the case), or (2) that the diaphragm is largely passive, its movements being dictated by the pressure exerted by the abdominal and chest walls. The liver seems to be stabilised by its attachment and held in position by the fixation of the abdominal wall, while the stomach, having free access to the atmospheric pressure, carries up the left side of the diaphragm with it when the chest is expanded. Probably the latter explanation is the correct one.

The act of air-sucking, therefore, seems to depend on the chest expansion, and a tight belt round the chest should make it impossible for the patient to perform this distressing feat. It is a most unsatisfactory and trying condition to deal with.

Gastric Borborygmi

The annoying and persistent "rumbles" in the abdomen from which some people suffer, and which are very audible to bystanders, are generally supposed to be due to collections of air in the intestine. Sometimes they are, but the "repetitive" type is more often due to air in the stomach. They are usually located by the patient—generally a tall, thin woman—on the left side, at about the level of the umbilicus. Sometimes, when she can repeat them at will indefinitely—for ten minutes or more—the bubbling can actually be felt through the abdominal wall, but only when she is in the upright position. In the normal stomach the movements of the diaphragm are automatically compensated by a concertina-like contraction of the gastric walls, with the result that there is very little alteration in the appearance; the organ becomes a little wider as its length diminishes but the lower border hardly moves at all, even with forced respiration (cf. p. 92). When, however, the stomach is atonic, its walls come into contact a few inches below the level of the cardiac orifice, leaving a pyriform air space above. The walls of the collapsed portion, as it comes downwards and forwards over the kidney, are in contact and kept moist by the secretions. They separate the air in the fundus from the food-stuffs that lie in the lowest part, which rests on the contents of the pelvis and therefore does not move as much as the rest.

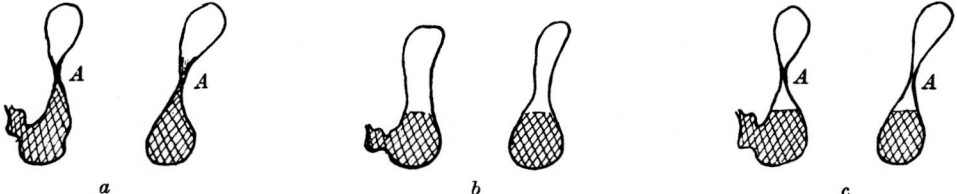

Fig. 232. Diagram to illustrate the mechanism of gastric borborygmi. *a*. Standing. Just below the air the walls are in contact at *A*, i.e. the air is separated from the gastric contents. *b*. Inspiration, leaning forward. The air is pressed down and the whole cavity of the stomach is opened up. *c*. Standing again. The walls are again in contact at *A*, but some of the air is shut off below this point. The borborygmi are caused by this air bubbling up between the collapsed walls at *A*.

When the mechanism is watched on the screen, inspiration is seen to produce a very marked change in the shape of the air space: the air is pressed downwards, and opens out the collapsed walls. Its lower border is then seen to be bounded by the fluid which lies beneath it and which could not be seen before (Fig. 232*b*). On expiration the stomach again elongates and the middle portion is once more stretched over the kidney and collapsed. When a portion of air is nipped off below the collapsed region borborygmi occur, for this air, in escaping, bubbles up between the moist collapsed walls, with the typical noises and sensations.

The mechanism was at one time particularly common in waitresses who, taking a breath as they leaned forward to serve a guest, naturally opened out the collapsed wall and brought the fluid and air into contact. Then, when they stood up straight, the walls collapsed again over the left kidney and the bubbling occurred. In these days one has no opportunity of observing this mechanism, for the pale-faced waitress of the old days—with an atonic stomach and tight corsets—is no longer to be found.

The sounds can be stopped at once by a little pressure on the lower abdomen, i.e. by supporting the lower part of the stomach. This was, in fact, the clue that led to the detection of the mechanism. No sooner was the patient placed in position in front of the apparatus and, as usual in those days, directed to press the abdomen against the screen, than the sounds ceased and nothing was observed but elongation of the air space with each inspiration. The "rumbling" only took place when there was no pressure on the lower abdominal wall. Even slight pressure of the hand on the lower abdomen was sufficient to prevent the air from coming low enough to be nipped off.

The text-books that I have consulted state that gastric borborygmi are the result of over-active peristalsis. This is manifestly not true, for in the patients I have observed peristalsis was comparatively feeble, owing to the thinning-out of the gastric muscle that is part of the atonic condition with which these sounds are associated.

The same kind of sound and sensation is made by gas bubbling from one coil of intestine to the next, but it is not usually repetitive.

GASTROPTOSIS

A considerable number of authorities, accepting the work of Goldthwait (135), Coffey (100) and others, so admirably summarised by Bedingfield (56), believe that gastroptosis is a definite clinical entity. To most radiologists, however, the question is whether or not there is such a condition as gastroptosis. In many normal subjects, particularly women, the lower border of the stomach extends far below the umbilicus, even to the level of the symphysis pubis. The pylorus in these cases may occupy a correspondingly low position or it may be found about the usual level, i.e. much above the most dependent part of the stomach (Figs. 70, 76). When this form of stomach was first seen, the conception of visceroptosis and particularly of gastroptosis was very prominent, and naturally these long stomachs were accepted as the radiographic evidence of a condition that was very frequently diagnosed. The appearances confirmed the hypothetical conception of gastroptosis that there must be difficulty in emptying because the pylorus was so high in relation to the food. Many cases were treated on the prevailing theory of the supposed mechanical disability which appeared to be obvious. Some were even subjected to operation, a section being excised to make the stomach shorter. Later, it was recognised that delay in emptying was not necessarily associated with this type of stomach and that it was, in fact, a variation of the normal. Yet, looking back to the early days, one remembers many cases in which the effects of massage and exercises not only had a beneficial effect on the patient but the stomach was found to be an inch or two higher. In these it certainly looked as if the "gastroptosis" had been the cause of the symptoms. But in others who were equally benefited, no such change was noted in the stomach as the result of treatment. It had to be realised that, although the patient had benefited, the "gastroptosis" had not been the cause of the symptoms.

Then there was the other supposed effect of gastroptosis: drag on the pyloric and duodenal attachments. Here again it was easy to accept such a plausible mechanical explanation of symptoms and, in fact, in some of the cases it looked as if there was a definite drag distorting the duodenum. In some of these I was quite convinced of the facts: I could only get the duodenum to fill satisfactorily either by pressing on the abdominal wall and thus relieving the drag, or by laying the patient down. Individual cases stick in my mind: a tall thin woman in whom this drag seemed to be definite and the operation showed adhesions about the duodenum and evidence of a long-standing ulcer. Was the ulceration due to the drag or was the long stomach merely incidental? At the time and for many years afterwards I was on the look-out for cases of duodenal ulcer associated with the appearances suggestive of drag from a long stomach. The suspicion of a causal relationship between the two conditions has not, however, been confirmed. It is with regret that one abandons the delightfully simple explanations offered by the mechanical disabilities of the long stomach, but they cannot be substantiated.

As the transverse colon hangs from the greater curvature of the long stomach, it is naturally very low in the abdomen or even in the pelvis. The low transverse colon was spoken of as "coloptosis" and it was assumed that this must be a cause of constipation. Moreover, as the ascending and descending colon have little or no mesentery, it was argued that there must be a tendency to kinking. It must be categorically contradicted that a low position of the colon, coloptosis, is in any way responsible for constipation or that kinking of the colon ever occurs as a result of the supposed dropping of the abdominal contents. The sooner these and similar plausible explanations of symptoms are eliminated the better.

DIVERTICULA OF THE STOMACH

These are rare. For the most part they are found high up on the lesser curvature, just below the cardiac orifice. The appearances are those of a deep "penetrating" type of ulcer, but a diverticulum is likely to be much more freely movable both by respiration and, if it is accessible, by palpation, than an ulcer, for ulcers of the size of such diverticula as I have seen in illustrations would surely be adherent to underlying structures (Fig. 233). In some recorded cases, radiologists have demonstrated a neck or pedicle (Fig. 234) by which the diverticulum could move both in relation to the stomach and to surrounding parts (Hurst and Stewart (181)). In one case that I saw demonstrated, the pocket was quite

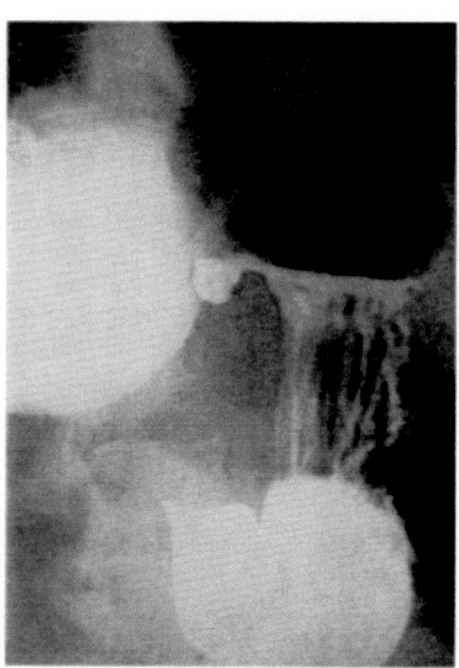

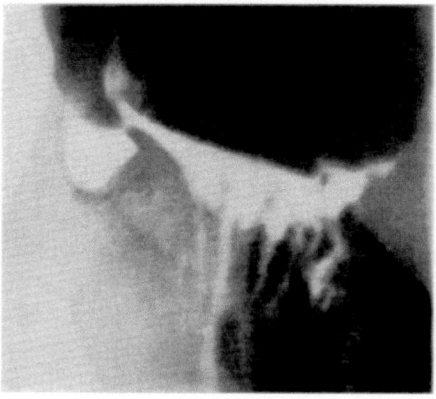

Fig. 234. Radiograph of a diverticulum close to the cardiac orifice, showing the neck.

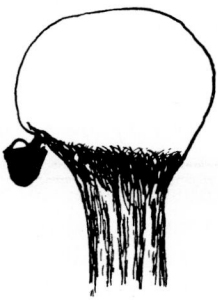

Fig. 233. Diverticulum of the stomach. The diverticulum lay behind the lesser curvature and the neck did not show.

Fig. 235. Tracing of a radiograph of a diverticulum.

separate from the stomach. It contained an air-bubble as well as the opaque food (Figs. 234 and 235). I understood that it was not producing any symptoms.

HYPERTROPHIC STENOSIS OF THE PYLORUS

E. W. Twining (316) has recently published a study of this condition in adults. The symptoms are those of vague indigestion, which may simulate pyloric or duodenal ulcer, or carcinoma of the stomach. X rays reveal a long, narrow prepyloric segment, sometimes with fluid in the fasting stomach and moderate hyper-peristalsis. A tumour cannot usually be felt, but if there is palpable thickening it is much less marked than it would be with a carcinomatous filling defect of equal size. The prepyloric defect should cause suspicion of chronic hypertrophic stenosis whenever it is found. Frequent findings are (*a*) a constantly narrowed but contractile prepyloric segment, (*b*) crescentic indentations of the base of the duodenal cap (Kirklin (204), Fig. 237 *a*), (*c*) a smoothly rounded intragastric projection of the proximal end of the mass, (*d*) a projection of barium from the stenosed lumen, usually on the greater curvature side.

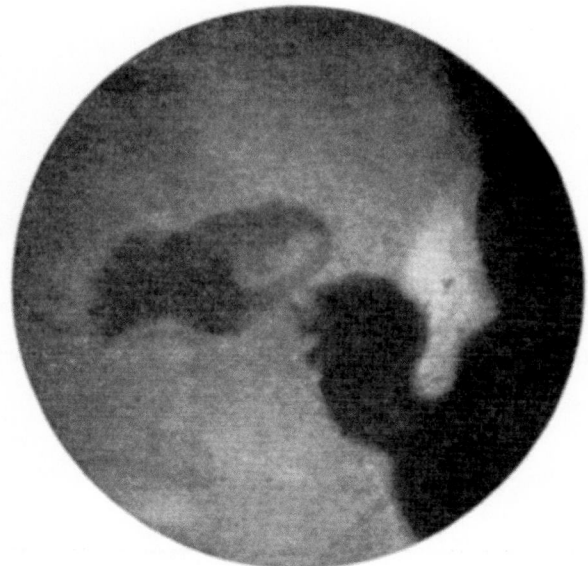

Fig. 236. Filling defect in the duodenum of a man aged 62, due to hypertrophied basal mucosa (cf. Fig. 238). The appearance might be mistaken for polypus. (Contributed by E. W. Twining.)

A crescentic indentation of the base of the duodenal cap may occasionally be found in other conditions than pyloric hypertrophy. The diagrams (Fig. 238) relate to a case observed by Twining, in which the bulbar indentation was apparently due to thickened mucosal folds (cf. Fig. 236).

Congenital Pyloric Stenosis

In these cases it is not usually possible to make out detail of the pylorus, and in fact it is not necessary, as the clinical picture is so typical. It is interesting that, in one case of congenital pyloric stenosis which I saw, operation was declined, and I noticed a persistent collection of air behind the ileo-caecal valve. Treatment was directed towards overcoming this trouble, and the results were quite satisfactory; the child is now healthy.

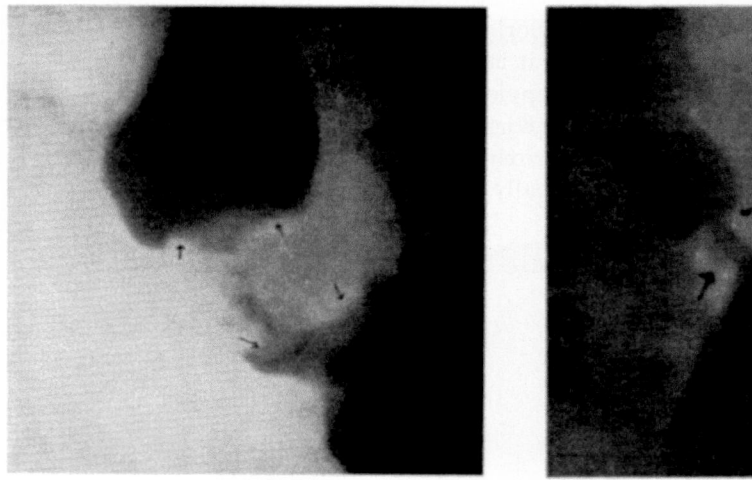
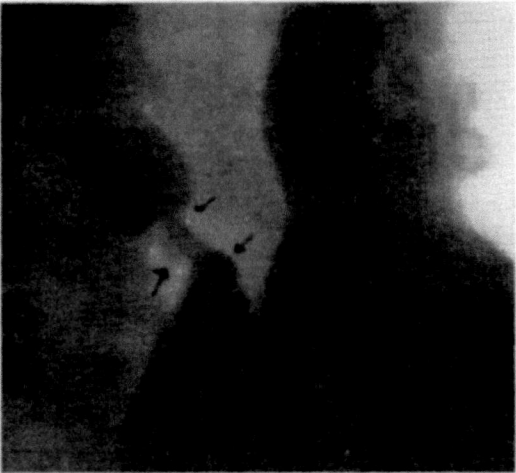

Fig. 237 a   Fig. 237 b

Fig. 237 a. Chronic hypertrophic stenosis of the pylorus in a man aged 55. The arrows point to basal indentations of the bulb (Kirklin's sign). (Contributed by E. W. Twining.)

Fig. 237 b. Chronic hypertrophic stenosis of the pylorus in a woman aged 43. (Contributed by E. W. Twining.)

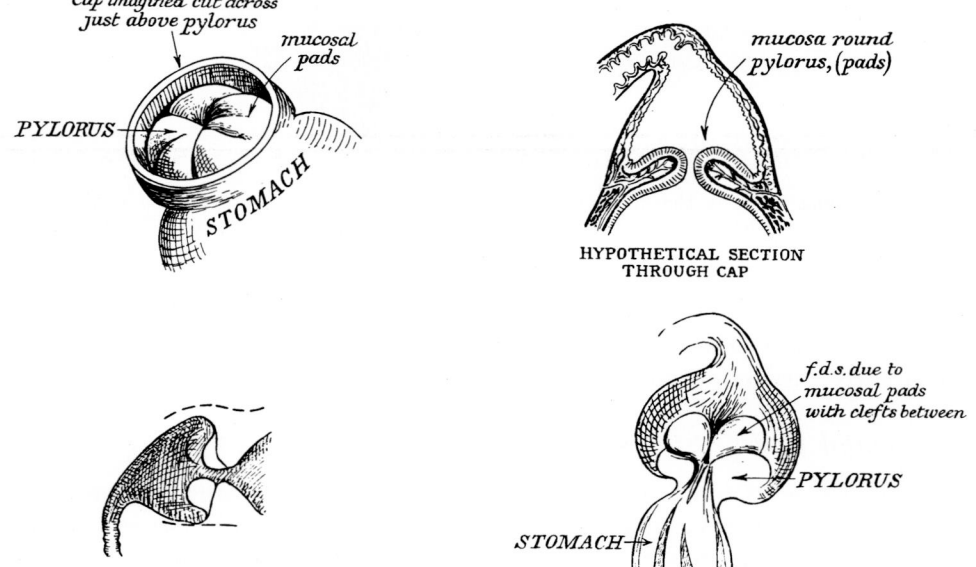

Fig. 238. Bulbar indentation due to thickened and prominent mucosal folds. There is no hypertrophy of the muscle (cf. Fig. 236). (Contributed by E. W. Twining.)

THE POST-OPERATIVE STOMACH

Before the advent of X-ray examinations, any failure of a gastro-enterostomy, which was at that time performed on all and sundry patients presenting gastric symptoms, was attributed to the formation of a vicious circle through the duodenum; though of this there was never any proof. Then came the suggestion that the cause was the formation of jejunal ulcers at or near the stoma (cf. p. 249). About 1914 such ulcers were common in Leeds and unknown in Manchester, and even at the present day, although operative technique is so standardised, I believe

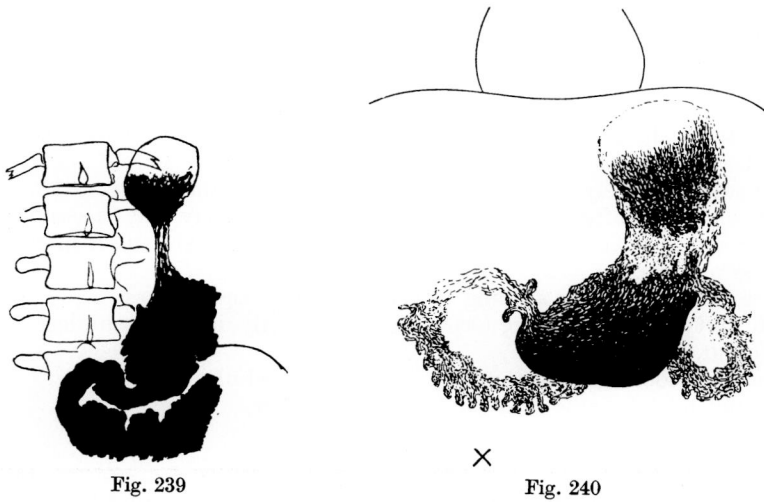

Fig. 239   Fig. 240

Fig. 239. Tracing of a radiograph from a medical student in whom the pylorus had been resected at the age of 8 days. He presented himself as a normal subject, having forgotten this early incident in his life.

Fig. 240. Tracing from a case of gastro-jejunostomy. The position of the stoma is not usually as low as in Fig. 239, and is sometimes found high up on the greater curvature, as in this case; its position may vary from day to day. The food was passing out by both the pylorus and the stoma.

that the incidence of this condition, like that of duodenal ulcer, has a geographical variation (cf. p. 231). The two points that were noted in the unsatisfactory cases were: (1) That the food poured straight through into the small intestine and overloaded it; the stoma failed to develop any sphincteric action. (2) The stoma was wrongly placed, so high that, if there was pyloric or duodenal obstruction or if the surgeon occluded the pylorus, perhaps by excision, a large residue was held in the stomach below the stoma, from which peristalsis tended to carry it away. The surgeon always maintained that he had placed his stoma in the most dependent part of the stomach, yet, on examination, I often found it well up on the greater curvature. I have, indeed, found a stoma in one patient high up on one occasion and quite well placed on another. Presumably this displacement is due to local thickening and rotation of the stomach wall (cf. p. 63). Whatever the cause, the distal end of the stomach was a cul-de-sac. Nowadays, thanks to selection, improved technique and after-care, operative failures are not so common. The food still pours through into the small intestine and overloads it but, after a time at any rate, it does not appear to distress the patient (Figs. 239 and 240). In most cases, however, the stoma appears to develop a certain degree of sphincteric action.

Kirklin[201] in a recent paper describes the technique of investigating the alimentary canal after operation. His recommendations may be summarised as follows:

(1) The history of the type of operation should be known.

(2) The first mouthful should be watched with infinite care; especially the lines of suture should be searched.

(3) The stoma should not be regarded as non-functioning till it has been observed after a rest.

(4) The stoma is likely to be irregular for some time after the operation.

(5) For some time after the operation there is often atony and excess of secretion.

(6) After a time evacuation takes about the usual six hours and is intermittent, as through the pylorus.

(7) In carcinoma there is a filling defect, stiffening, and a mass.

(8) Deformity about a healing ulcer is not necessarily due to fresh ulcer. The crater must be found.

(9) A niche is found in two-thirds of cases of jejunal ulcer.

(10) Do not mistake a fleck in the folds for an ulcer.

(11) Intussusception into the stoma may occur.

Cochrane Shanks[297] has also published recently a valuable study of the radiology of the post-operative stomach and duodenum and of the varied conditions that are found.

Strange causes for operative failure are sometimes found. I have seen two cases in which the stoma has been made directly into the large intestine (both war relics) and, if I recollect aright, there was another in my department in which the reputed gastro-enterostomy had not been done on the stomach but on a distended colon! The failure is sometimes attributed to the persistence of duodenal or pyloric ulceration. Certainly the deformity of the duodenum often persists after operation, and I have occasionally noted this persistence in patients who were quite well and had lost all the symptoms for which the operation had been performed.

The formation of adhesions to the coil just beyond the stoma is sometimes a source of trouble. The coil is found distended and shows occasional forceful movements suggesting obstruction.

This table, for which I am indebted to Dr S. C. Shanks, and which was published in the *British Journal of Radiology* (Vol. IX, No. 105, Sept. 1936, p. 559), represents the normal and abnormal results in 150 consecutive barium meal examinations of posterior gastro-jejunostomy in two London general hospitals and private practice, operated on by many different surgeons. They represent an average sample from most of the surgical centres of London and some of the provincial schools. The number of abnormal results found by examination considerably exceeds the total number of cases. In many cases more than one abnormality was found, e.g. recurrent duodenal ulcer and jejunitis.

Results of posterior gastro-jejunostomy: 150 cases.

Normal		23
Dumping stoma		12
Inflammatory sequelae:		
gastritis	4	
gastro-jejunitis	19	
jejunitis	17——40	
Ulcerative sequelae:		
recurrent duodenal	25	
lesser curvature	16	
jejunal	11	
posterior wall	6	
pyloric	2	
stomal	3——63	
Gastro-entero-colic fistula		3
Stenotic sequelae:		
Stenosis of stoma	22	
Obstruction of stoma	9	
Stenosis of efferent limb	5	
Stenosis of afferent limb	3	
Duodenal ileus	6	
Jejunal ileus	2	
Contracture of pyloric antrum	5	
Pyloric stenosis	1——53	
High mal-placed stoma		2
Carcinoma supervening		2
Retrograde jejuno-gastric intussusception		1
	Total	199

OTHER DUODENAL CONDITIONS

Duodenitis

In certain cases, clinically diagnosed as duodenal ulcer, the duodenum was apparently in an irritable condition. No deformity of the cap could be detected and yet the appearances gave the definite impression that some pathological condition was present. A small stomach showing unusually active peristalsis was usually found. It emptied rapidly, and yet the opaque food would not fill the duodenal cap properly and was persistently ejected from it. I laid considerable stress on this condition in my book *The Alimentary Tract*, and considered

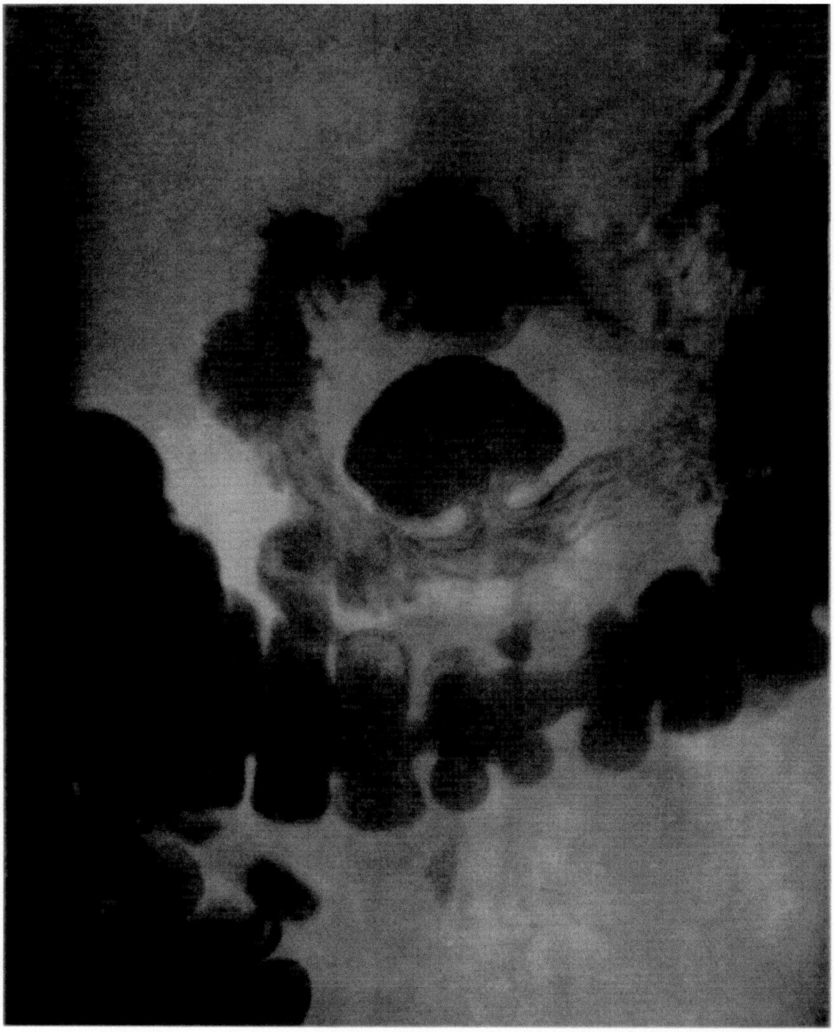

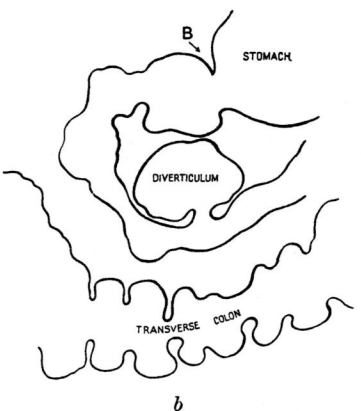

a

b

Fig. 241. *a*. Large diverticulum of the third part of the duodenum.
b. Tracing from *a*. *B*, Pylorus.

it as a possible precursor of duodenal ulcer. In several of these cases, reported as duodenal irritation, the surgeon was so convinced that ulceration was present that he opened the viscus, to dicover only some ill-defined signs of inflammation with swelling of the mucous membrane but no indication of ulceration. I was inclined to regard these cases as a pre-ulcerative stage.

With the extensive material at the disposal of the Mayo Clinic, Kirklin (200) has now defined the condition as duodenitis. Its chief characteristic is irritability of the duodenum manifested in intense spasticity and hypermotility. The barium races through so rapidly that there is scant opportunity to inspect the shadow. The bulb is frequently small and grossly deformed, both on its mesial and lateral borders, and the configuration of the deformity may vary from

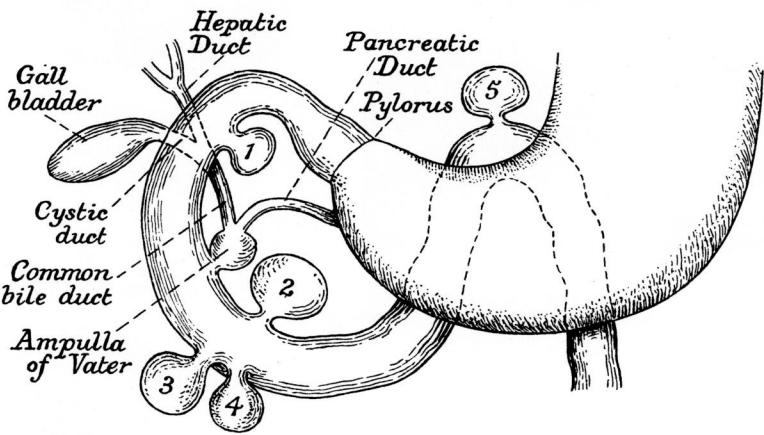

Fig. 242. Diagram of the common sites for diverticula: 1, 2, 3, 4, 5.
(After Schinz, Baensch and Friedl.)

moment to moment. Further, the bulbar shadow lacks the density commonly seen in cases of frank ulcer; it is thin and indistinct, and its margins are hazy. A second characteristic is the mucosal pattern, which is coarsely and irregularly reticular, and is depicted as translucent islets lying in a denser network. This appearance is perhaps attributable to puckering of the mucosa by spastic contractions of its muscularis. A third characteristic of simple duodenitis is the absence of an ulcer-crater. Neither marginal niche nor persistent central fleck can be seen. Finally, uncomplicated duodenitis is marked almost invariably by absence of gastric retention or other evidence of obstruction, whereas such obstruction occurs in more than 25 per cent. of cases of true ulcer. The stomach in these cases was small and hypertonic, with active, sometimes disordered peristalsis. Gastritis was found in none of the thirty-two cases which Kirklin describes in his paper. Eight patients were operated on for severe symptoms which had lasted on an average seven years. During the period covered by this series, radiological diagnoses of duodenitis had been made in ninety-two cases. Medical treatment is ordinarily preferable to surgery.

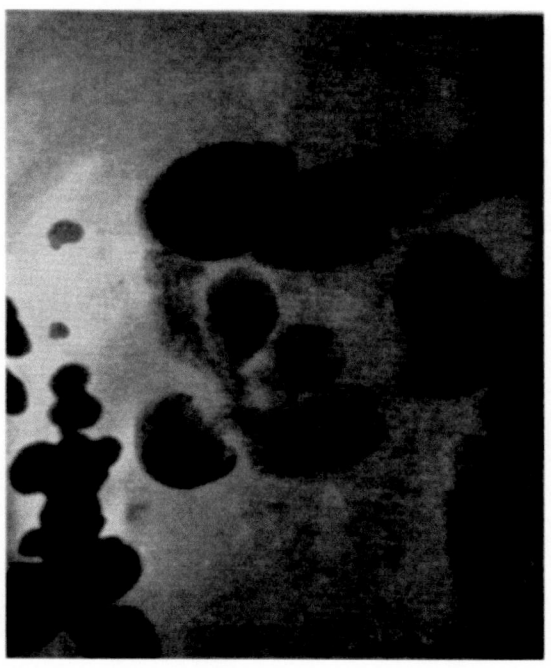

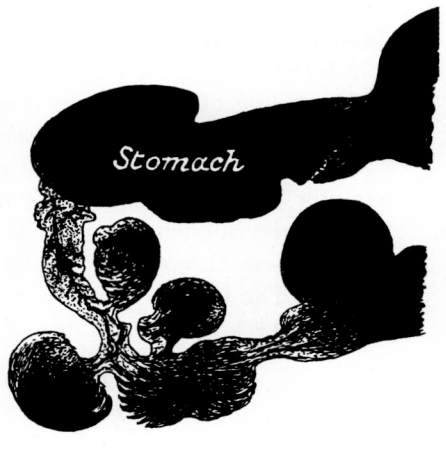

Fig. 243 a. Multiple diverticulum of the duodenum. Note the way in which the mucous membrane appears to be infolded into the diverticula.

Fig. 243 b. Tracing of Fig. 243 a.

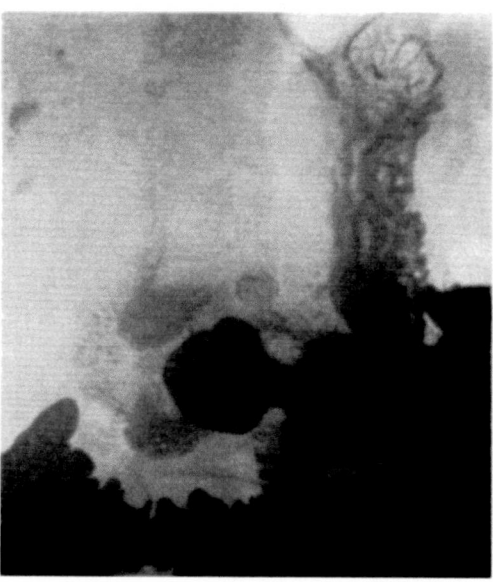

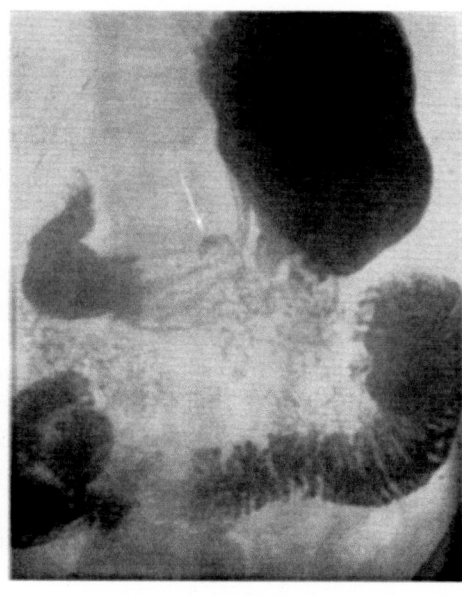

Fig. 244. Duodenal pouch close to the duodeno-jejunal flexure, patient standing.

Fig. 245. The same case as Fig. 244. Patient lying down.

Adhesions

Adhesions about the gall-bladder are common, and many of them give rise to deformities of the duodenum which are almost, if not quite, indistinguishable from those caused by ulcer. Palpation of the food in the duodenum and the detection of undue fixation are the only way in which the radiologist can attempt to arrive at a reasonably accurate diagnosis (cf. p. 335).

Duodenal Diverticula

Diverticula may occur in any part of the duodenum (Figs. 241–245) and also in the small intestine, but they are relatively rare there and are probably less often associated with symptoms. In the duodenum they are comparatively common; some are symptomless while others have symptoms like those of duodenal ulcer. At the Mayo Clinic [163] in 1930 duodenal diverticula were found at 2·8 per cent. of all autopsies. In about 10 per cent. the diverticula were multiple, 58 per cent. occurred near the ampulla of Vater, 26 per cent. at the minor papilla (the duct of Santorini) and 16 per cent. at varying distances distal to the major papilla. All lay on the inner side of the duodenum in close association with and often penetrating into the head of the pancreas. The smaller sacs invaginate the pancreas head and in many instances are entirely surrounded by pancreas.

The entry of the bile duct into the duodenum is usually about two-thirds of the way down, but may be higher; sometimes the opening gets filled with opaque food and looks like a small diverticulum.

Up till 1911 only about a hundred cases had appeared in the literature. Since then a number have been reported, most of which had been accidentally discovered. Several were recorded by Case [92] and Spriggs [303]. Spriggs attributed the symptoms to eighteen out of thirty-eight cases and Gibbon [133] to 70 per cent. of the twenty cases he records. The most common symptoms were distension, heaviness or dull pain in the epigastrium, and vomiting. Friedenwald and Feldman [124] remark that dyspeptic symptoms were present in all their cases and many showed signs of subhepatic and duodenal adhesions.

The pocket of the diverticulum is usually about the size of the end of a finger and is most frequently found about the junction of the first and second parts. It is more readily identified on the screen than on the X-ray film. Anatomically the walls usually consist only of mucosa, muscularis mucosae and connective tissue, but in early diverticula there are a few muscular fibres near the fundus of the sac. Horton and Mueller [163] conclude that "although duodenal diverticula are not congenital, they are, nevertheless, probably due to a congenital muscular defect caused by dystopia of the pancreatic tissue". From the clinical standpoint duodenal diverticula probably seldom cause symptoms or serious complications.

Pseudo-diverticulum of the Duodenum.

Sear has drawn attention to a transient condition that may simulate diverticulum of the duodenum. In the radiographs that I have seen the condition resembles Fig. 246 but, I understand, Sear (295a) has seen these pseudo-diverticula in other places. He attributes them to irregular peristalsis but they appear to be more probably due to two contractions holding the duodenal contents between

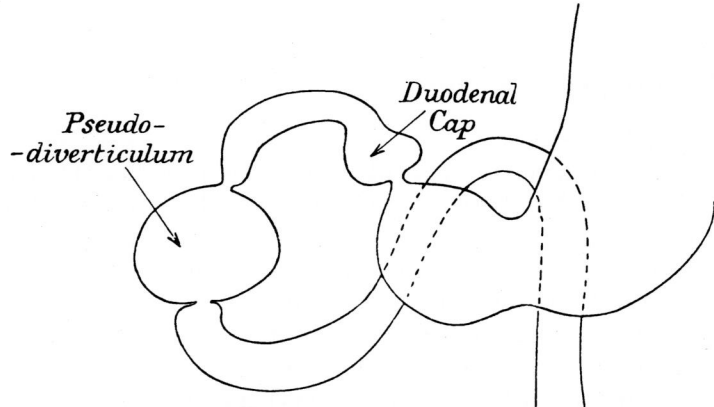

Fig. 246.   Diagram illustrating pseudo-diverticulum.

them. The appearance is constant for a time so that spasm seems the more likely explanation. In some of Sear's cases the appearance so closely simulated a diverticulum that, had he not re-examined, a mistake would have been made. He suggests that this condition is the explanation of those cases in which the

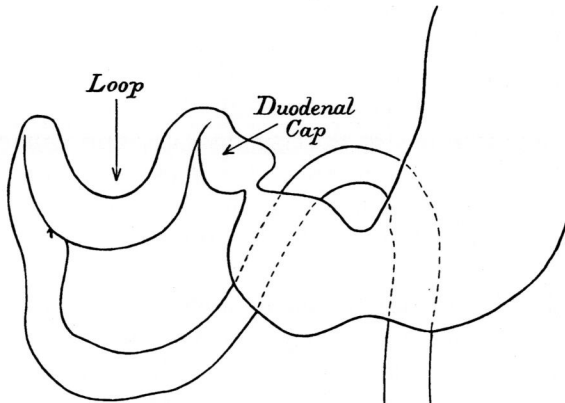

Fig. 247.   Diagram to indicate looping of the duodenum.

surgeon does not find duodenal diverticula that have been observed and radiographed.

The Looped Duodenum

Dropping over and twisting of the junction of the first and second parts may give rise to symptoms of duodenal ulcer and to appearances rather similar to those of a diverticulum (Fig. 247). This anomaly is not readily appreciated on the screen and is not always recognised as a possibility on the operating table. Gastro-enterostomy has been entirely satisfactory in two cases I have followed.

The duodenum is one of the very few parts of the alimentary tract in which I believe I can recognise "kinking" as a definite phenomenon, and even here this mechanical obstruction is rare. The two points where it may occur are (1) just beyond the cap; (2) at the junction of the duodenum and jejunum, giving rise to duodenal ileus. Kinking at the first point may be the result of a drop of the stomach when the pyloric and duodenal attachments have not come down correspondingly, or the result of the abnormal development of mesentery, which allows the top of the loop to drop over, thus giving the appearance of a pouch resembling looped duodenum. It is not easy to recognise with certainty, because the pressure or posture used to fill the cap is almost certain to relieve the obstruction.

Duodenal Ileus, Chronic Intermittent Obstruction and Duodenal Stasis

Kinking at the duodeno-jejunal flexure may be caused by adhesions and results in a blocking of the duodenum; the whole loop may sometimes be filled up. This condition is not very rare but is sometimes not recognised; it may give rise to definite duodenal symptoms. The duodenal loop is distended and its contents are churned and segmented. Writhing movements are often seen, and the food is sometimes even forced back into the stomach, but there is a residue in the lower part of the loop. Gilbert Scott observes that in duodenal ileus proper the second part of the duodenum is unduly long.

Unless duodenal ileus is well marked, the radiologist will be wise to regard it as of no pathological significance; a slight degree should certainly not be regarded as significant. As often as not it will be absent when he re-examines, particularly if the circumstances are more nearly normal than at the first examination. Rapid emptying of the stomach due to hunger or purgatives often causes such appearances, especially if the opaque food is particularly fluid.

Miller and Gage [236] have published a careful study of chronic duodenal ileus in children suffering from enlargement of the stomach, and regard it as a definite source of symptoms. The condition has not received much attention in this country but in France both clinicians and radiologists are inclined to lay considerable stress on duodenal ileus as a definite pathological entity. I always used to regard the appearances of duodenal ileus as of definite significance, possibly indicating a spasmodic or organic lesion in the duodeno-jejunal region. It appears, however, that this view is open to doubt and that ileus may be of no pathological significance whatever. In the course of anatomical demonstrations, I have come across several students in whom all the typical appearances were persistently present. The subjects did not suffer from any gastro-intestinal disturbance. Moreover, it was not just a temporary overloading of the duodenum due to too rapid emptying of the stomach, for it persisted even when the stomach was nearly empty. It is clear, therefore, that too much stress should not be laid upon the radiological appearances of this condition unless the clinical picture points definitely to the duodenum as the source of the symptoms. It is quite likely that symptoms have been ascribed to what is, in reality, a normal but unusual variation of the duodenal mechanism.

Chronic duodenal stasis was reviewed in a recent editorial in *The Lancet* (346). Anatomical abnormalities, congenital or acquired, ileus and disordered balance of the autonomic nerves are given as aetiological factors. The main symptoms in children are lack of appetite and vomiting, with malnutrition and failure of growth. The typical symptoms of the adult are cyclical crises of abdominal pain, bilious vomiting, a sensation of weight and distension in the epigastrium and general toxic symptoms such as headache after meals, loss of weight and loss of energy. Cholelithiasis, appendicitis and chronic duodenal ulcer may be simulated. The final diagnosis, which is radiographic, is based on delay in passage through the duodenum, dilatation of the duodenum, and abnormal peristaltic and anti-peristaltic waves. The leader-writer suggests that many patients labelled as "nervous indigestion" or "visceroptosis" may be suffering from mild duodenal stasis, but admits that the true incidence of the condition is the most doubtful thing about it.

N. Ratkóczi (278), of Budapest, describes a condition of intermittent stenosis of the duodenum which may arise from various causes yet gives a constant radiological picture: the opaque meal flows to the duodeno-jejunal flexure and is there obstructed, the lower part of the duodenum becoming almost distended. A strong anti-peristaltic wave then sweeps the food back into the bulb of the duodenum and even into the stomach. The process is repeated, the duodenum being again filled and emptied in the same manner, for from two to twenty minutes, the appearance being that of complete organic obstruction at the duodeno-jejunal flexure. Then, without any warning, the obstruction gives way and the food in the duodenum flows into the jejunum. There may be no repetition of the obstruction, but if, as frequently happens, it is repeated, there will be delay in emptying of the stomach which may extend to several hours beyond the normal limits. Ratkóczi says that this condition may be associated with gastroptosis and elongation of the mesentery, accentuated by lordosis, in which case the obstruction disappears if the patient lies on one side or in the knee-elbow position. It may also be caused by a tumour near the flexure. I have, however, seen this intermittent obstruction in association with ulcer of the first part of the duodenum and chronic appendicitis. In the course of these operations, nothing abnormal could be detected in the region of the duodeno-jejunal flexure.

TUMOURS OUTSIDE THE GASTRO-INTESTINAL TRACT

Many tumours arising within the abdomen but outside the alimentary canal may be elucidated by the opaque meal and enema, e.g. hydatid cysts and other rare conditions. By determining the displacement of the alimentary canal it is usually possible to form a fairly correct idea of the anatomical position of the growth, and this alone may give the clue to the diagnosis. For instance, neoplasms of the head of the pancreas are apt to extend forwards and displace the duodenum, and in a number of cases the loop of the duodenum has been

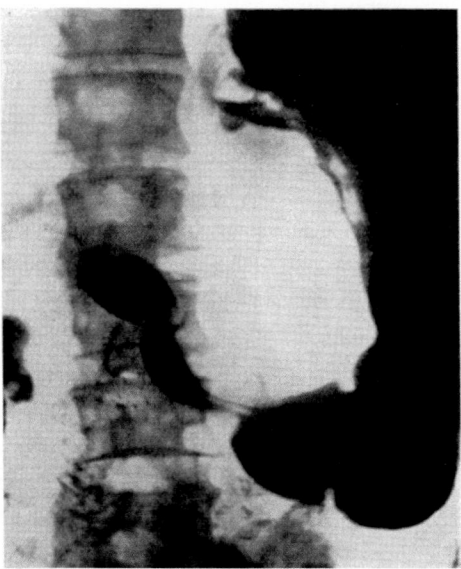

Fig. 248. Displacement of the stomach by a large renal tumour. Note the pressure on the pyloric end of the lesser curvature displacing the opaque food in the stomach. (Contributed by H. Courtney Gage.)

seen encircling the mass. Tumours arising from the lower surface of the liver and sub-hepatic abscesses displace the lesser curvature and the duodenum, and the radiologist can say that there is something abnormal between the liver and the stomach (Fig. 248). There may even be some clue to indicate whether it is intra- or retro-peritoneal. Mesenteric growths and cysts are occasionally seen, and the surgeon always wants to know the anatomical displacement and also whether the mass is movable in relation to the viscera. In fact, in every case of abdominal tumour both an opaque meal and an opaque enema are needed to throw as much light as possible on its nature and extent. A friend told me of an abdominal tumour thought to be either in the spleen or in the colon; only an enema was given, and the operation revealed a hair-ball in the stomach!

CHAPTER XVIII

THE SMALL AND LARGE INTESTINE

SMALL INTESTINE

Colic

Colicky sensations mostly appear to be associated with the small intestine. A wave of peristalsis sweeps the food along to some spasmodic or other obstruction and the pain comes when the tension is at its height. In the large gut the same thing happens, but is seldom seen radiographically unless conditions are very far from normal. The contractions of the large intestine that can be seen through the abdominal wall in cases of obstruction are a very late result and close precursors of disaster. I have occasionally seen them, and they have given me the impression of a series of mass movements throwing the churned contents against an obstruction from which they rebounded. The contents were very fluid and there was abundant gas. Perhaps three of these active movements would be seen and then once more there was a still-life picture: the opaque food and the air lying in pockets in the distended colon. Doubtless similar activity in lesser degree is the cause of the colicky pain that precedes an attack of diarrhoea and is often associated with some forms of colitis.

Organic lesions of the small intestine

These are rare. Symptoms are vague or absent and there are seldom any localising signs. The food is so divided when it passes through the small intestine that it is not liable to serious delay or obstruction until a comparatively late stage. The lesions that have been found at operation have always shown marked organic narrowing. In some cases colicky pains are associated with distended coils in which the food is tossed backward and forward, but the distension passes off and nothing abnormal is found on re-examination. Probably it is due to some temporary spasm.

The symptoms are very vague; the only one that may suggest organic disease is vomiting which "seems to come from the pit of the stomach" (cf. p. 269). The diagnosis depends entirely on the detection of a definite coil that is persistently distended and from which peristaltic movements fail to pass the opaque food onwards. The radiologist attempts to isolate this coil by manipulation and palpation and to note if the distal end of it is fixed and if there is any tumour. If a coil is found fixed, the diagnosis lies between adhesions, cicatrisation or ulceration, and growth. Apart from the resistance of a tumour there are no differentiating signs.

PLATE XVII

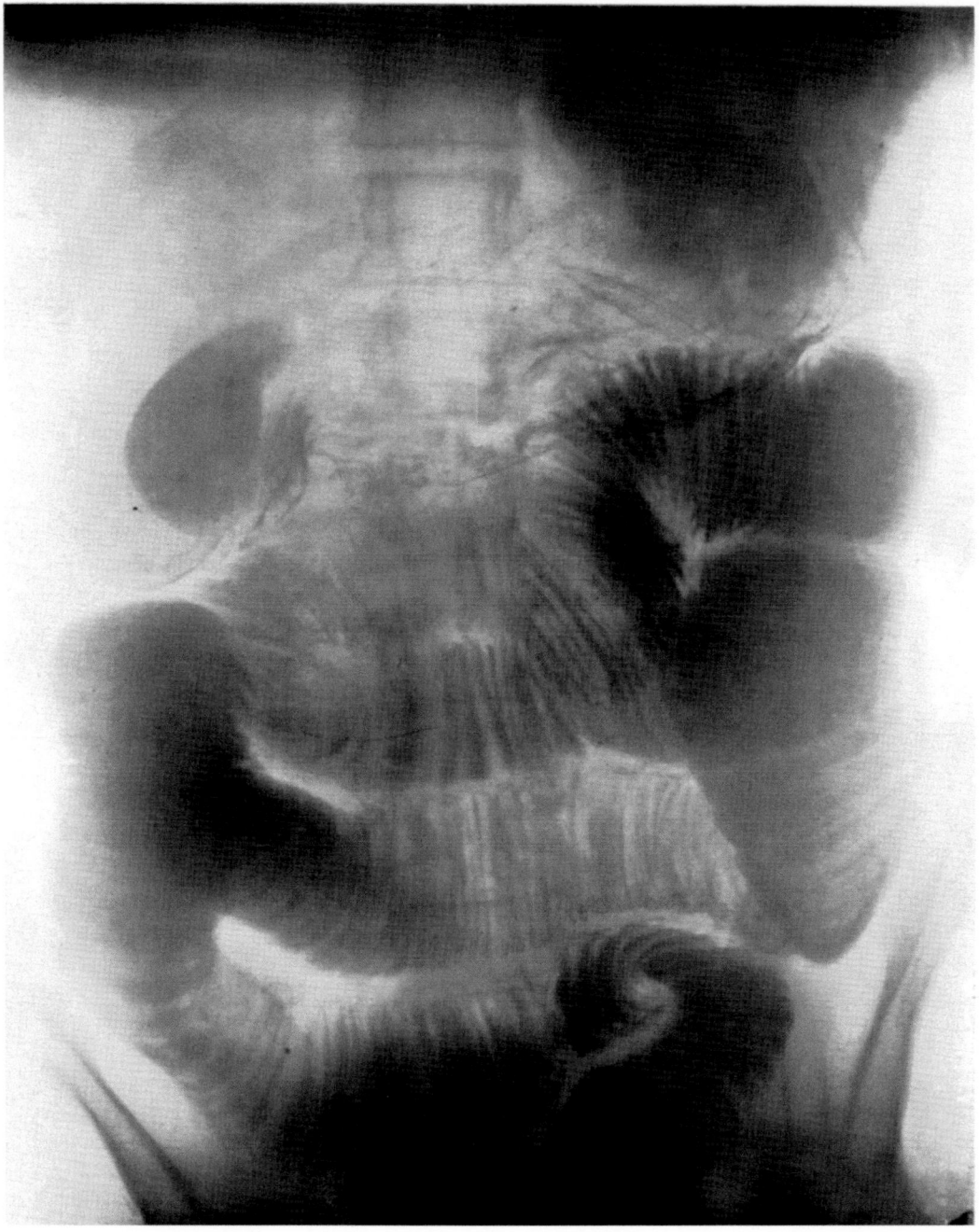

Fig. 249. Laddering effect in a case of obstruction due to a mass of inflammatory glands near the ileo-caecal valve. The intestine is distended and the opaque food lies between the folds of the mucous membrane, which are disposed transversely to the lumen of the gut. Supine position.

An advanced obstruction is, however, always indicated by a number of irregularly scattered air spaces in the abdomen, each with a horizontal fluid lower margin like the air space in the stomach (Fig. 250); these are seen at the preliminary examination in the upright position. In the horizontal position a curious laddering effect is produced (Plate fig. 249). Unless a purgative is

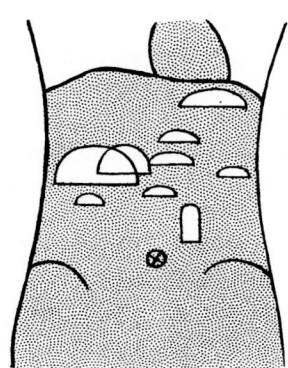

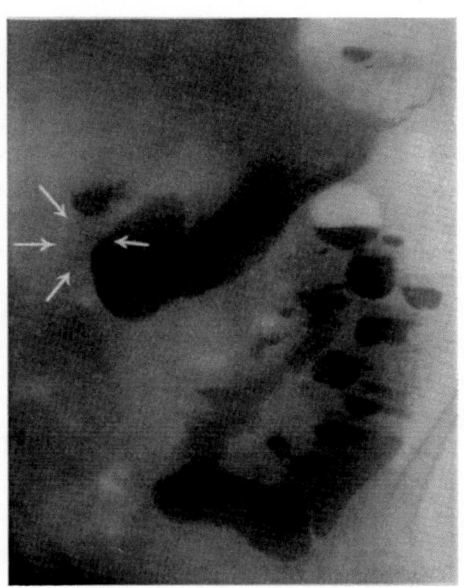

Fig. 250. Diagram to indicate the types of air-pocket noted in the abdomen in cases of obstruction. The lesion in this case was low down in the large intestine.

Fig. 251. Case of multiple diverticula of the jejunum. There is also a diverticulum near the cardiac orifice. Multiple gall-stones are also shown, indicated by arrows. Diverticula verified at gall-bladder operation. (Contributed by J. T. Case.)

still acting, such a picture indicates an obstructive lesion, not necessarily organic, in some part of the intestinal tract, perhaps even as low down as the rectum. The situation may be urgent even though the clinical picture is still vague and does not apparently call for urgent measures. Whether the radiologist should attempt to locate the lesion is doubtful; the responsibility for pursuing the examination, which would necessarily entail delay, should be placed on the surgeon.

In tuberculous and other forms of adhesive peritonitis, there is an initial hurrying of the food into the intestine and an appearance suggesting that the fragmentation mechanism is defective and that the coils are distended. This appearance may be physiological, but in disease it tends to persist and some coils may show writhing movements as the result of definite obstruction. When the appearance is merely due to hunger, for instance, the aggregations of food are dissipated fairly rapidly and in half an hour the doubtful appearance has disappeared.

I have notes of numerous interesting cases in which the small intestine was suspected but in which confirmatory observations gave contradictory results. The cases included well-marked mucous colitis, dental sepsis and lead poisoning. The colic of plumbism may be very difficult to distinguish from that of organic obstruction. In one woman of 45 who very nearly came to operation, the appearances seemed to be precursors of mental derangement, for the intestinal symptoms entirely disappeared when the delusions became definite. In another case of similar type, I was convinced that there was some definite small intestine lesion but, fortunately, operation was deferred, and symptoms of general paralysis of the insane developed. The gastric crises of tabes dorsalis may closely resemble acute intestinal obstruction, both clinically and radiologically.

Intussusception of the small intestine can be recognised radiographically. Knoepp (208) reports a case due to submucous lipoma of the ileum. X rays after a barium enema showed a somewhat varying but persistent filling defect in the terminal part of the ileum, and a correct diagnosis was made on these appearances.

The diagnosis of lesions of the small intestine calls for great discretion and the confirmation of all observations.

Jejunal Diverticula

Diverticula of the jejunum are not common, and may be single or multiple. The first case diagnosed radiographically, and confirmed at operation, was reported by Case (88), who later (91) published other cases and summarised the literature and his experience of ten cases. L. A. Rowden reported a case of multiple diverticula in 1917 but it was not operated upon until 1922, when it was published by Braithwaite (68) together with the radiographs and diagram that had been made five years previously. About a quarter of Case's patients complained of symptoms: mild, prolonged dyspepsia, bilious attacks, loss of appetite, nausea and vomiting. Two of them underwent operation. The diagnosis depends on the detection of the pockets, which are unmistakable (Fig. 251).

Meckel's Diverticulum

In about 2 per cent. of all individuals the intra-abdominal portion of the yolk sac fails to disappear completely. The persistent remnant is known as Meckel's diverticulum and forms an intestinal tubular appendage of variable length. The proximal end opens in the ileum about two or three inches above the ileo-caecal valve. The distal end may still be attached to the umbilicus. It is very seldom that this congenital diverticulum is recognised in the routine examination of the alimentary canal. I have not myself seen one.

THE TERMINAL ILEUM

Some delay at the ileo-caecal valve is normal (cf. p. 166) and there is no precise definition of ileal stasis. With the technique I employ, provided that the stomach is empty, any shadow composed of a number of coils that cannot be readily separated at the five-hour examination suggests delay. If the residue is again seen after seven or eight hours, ileal stasis is fairly definite, especially if, in the interval, the patient has had some food. If not, it is a good plan to send him out to get tea. Too much stress should not, however, be laid on the appearance of ileal stasis, for there are so many possible contributory factors, not only in the tract above but also in the caecum and large intestine.

Obstructions in this region are not very rare; most of them are due to adhesions following operation or old appendicular trouble. Typhoid ulceration is not a likely cause, as the lesions are longitudinally distributed. The indication of an obstruction in this region is the accumulation of food in the terminal coils. This may also be associated with gastric delay. In the later stages the appearances are those of obstruction (cf. p. 299).

A curious condition of the terminal ileum was described by T. I. Candy [75]. It was strongly reminiscent of the leather-bottle stomach. The symptoms were very indefinite, and the screen showed a persistently narrowed terminal ileum with some delay in the coils behind it. Microscopically, there was an abundance of fatty deposits between the muscle fibres. The patient recovered satisfactorily, and had no recurrence for at least nine years. Possibly this was a case of Crohn's disease [342a].

APPENDIX

The value of an opinion in appendicular trouble depends entirely on the technique and experience of the radiologist. Given a standard technique, the radiologist can determine whether or not there is delay behind the ileo-caecal valve. Its presence is of some importance. He should palpate the filled caecum and terminal ileum; if he finds it to be abnormally fixed, this point also is of some importance. To determine it, he may have to employ posture in addition to palpation, in order to bring the caecum out of the pelvis. A definitely tender spot located to the site of the appendix provides evidence of the utmost value.

In the detection of the site of origin of pain, the radiologist has a very great advantage over the ordinary clinical observer, for there is often some superficial rigidity and even tenderness, which are aggravated by palpation, and the patient cannot relax. The result is that, more often than not, the exact localisation of the site of the pain is unsatisfactory. Under X-ray observation no preliminary blind palpation is necessary. The radiologist sees where the base of the appendix lies and goes straight to it, before the patient has warning or has time to resist.

Those for whom I worked for many years were quite satisfied and placed reliance on the findings. There is, however, a school which entirely discredits the X-ray diagnosis of appendix lesions. Their view is that not only is the X-ray evidence of chronic appendicitis fallacious and untrustworthy, but that the pathology of the condition is unreliable. What is needed is a very careful follow-up of all cases diagnosed as appendicitis. The immediate results of operations are apt to be misleading and a follow-up a year later may throw unexpected light on the ultimate results. Whether it will confirm or disprove the radiological diagnosis of chronic appendicitis I cannot say, but in those occasional cases which I have been able to follow up, the ultimate results seem to indicate that, with the technique I have adopted, the radiological diagnosis is quite reliable. I have not come across one case that has made me question the matter, although others, particularly in the Mayo Clinic, are entirely sceptical and have abandoned the attempt to make an X-ray diagnosis of appendicitis. The pendulum of fashion swings backwards and forwards and the present phase suggests that many normal appendices have been removed, the immediate benefit being in many instances merely psychological. Scoffers say that no surgeon will ever admit that an appendix or a gall bladder that he has removed shows no signs of abnormality.

Chronic Lesions

Three points—ileo-caecal delay, abnormal fixation, and localised tenderness—taken together, if they are all positive, justify a definite diagnosis of a chronic appendicular lesion. Tenderness localised to the exact site of the appendix is the one conclusive sign. The filling and visualisation of the appendix itself are not of great moment. If the radiologist sees it (Figs. 252–256), he can palpate and note whether it contains concretions, whether it is fixed in the pelvis or retro-caecal or in any abnormal position, but none of these findings has necessarily any immediate pathological significance. The appendix is usually of more or less uniform diameter but in the foetal form it is relatively wide and tapers down to the usual diameter towards its distal end.

If, however, the radiologist has the opportunity of observing the patient for some days, and finds that the opaque food is retained for a prolonged period, he is probably justified in saying that the appendix is not functioning normally. The longest period during which I have seen opaque food remain in the appendix is three weeks. During the game season it is not uncommon to find shot, perhaps quite a number of them, lodged in the appendix for long periods; they will probably pass out in time without any untoward result.

Acute Conditions

The acute appendix is seldom seen in the X-ray department. It gives rise to so much localised irritation that the caecum and terminal ileum are found

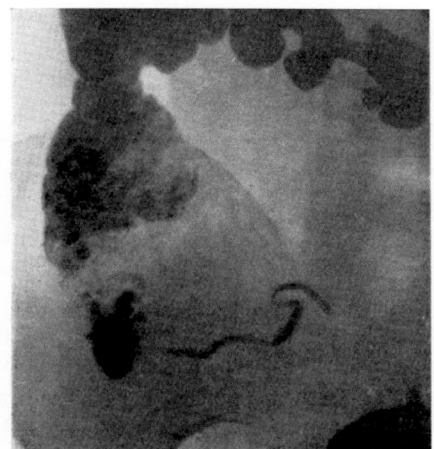

Fig. 252. Long appendix lying free. Lower end of the caecum contains non-opaque food.

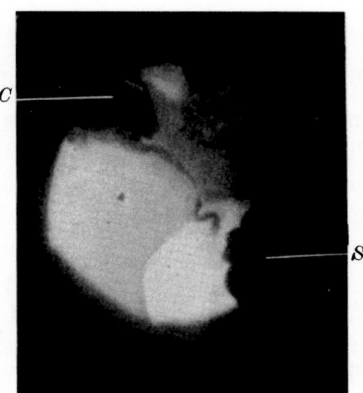

Fig. 253. Long appendix with tip fixed to sigmoid. *C*, Caecum. *S*, Sigmoid.

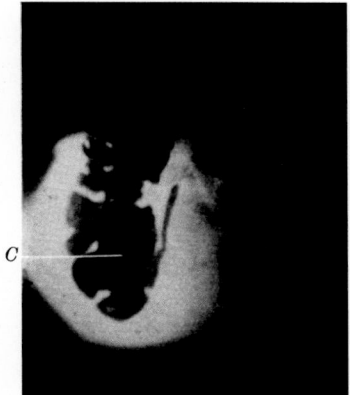

Fig. 254. Adhesions about appendix. The tip was fixed to coils of intestine. *C*, Caecum.

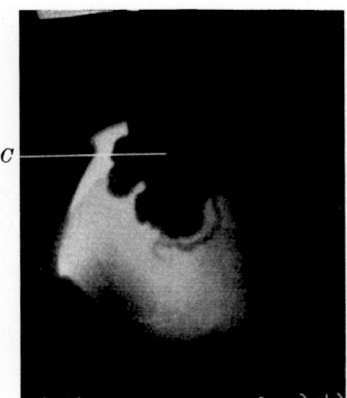

Fig. 255. The appendix bound down to the lower end of the caecum, *C*.

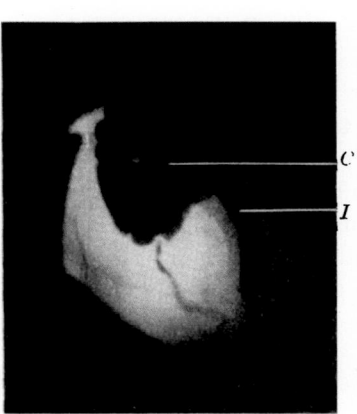

Fig. 256. Tip of appendix adherent in the pelvis. *C*, Caecum. *I*, Ileum.

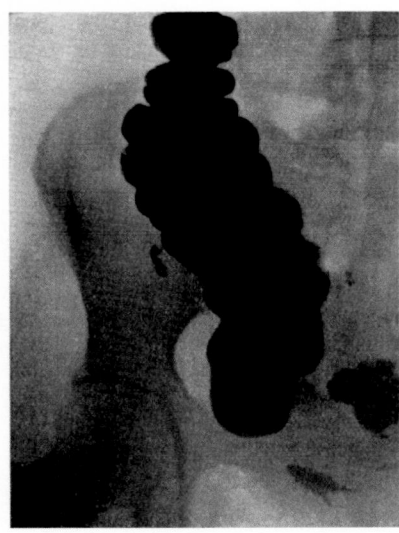

Fig. 257. Adherent appendix, lying external to the caecum. (Contributed by C. G. Sutherland.)

empty at a time when they should be filled, as would be expected if the "gradient" theory (p. 157) of Alvarez is accepted. This appearance suggests at least some irritative condition in the caecum or thereabouts, if not a comparatively acute appendicular lesion, but it is also seen in tuberculous disease of the caecum, an infection that is rare apart from obvious tuberculous disease elsewhere.

For some unknown reason spasm of the pelvic portion of the descending colon is very frequently associated with appendicular trouble. It can readily be detected by palpation, the gut feeling like a sausage as it slips under the fingers. The enema shows that the lumen is either narrowed or that this section is persistently empty. The spasm is very easily mistaken for a neoplasm, but the tumour is not constant and sometimes it can be felt to come and go.

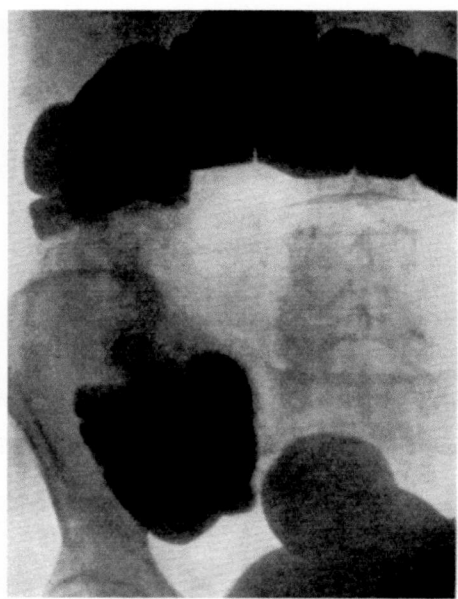

Fig. 258. Growth of the caecum. (Contributed by F. Haenisch.)

CAECUM

Neoplasm is rare and is detected in its later stages by the definite filling defect and the tumour, which is usually evident on palpation (Fig. 258). In the early stages filling defects are extremely difficult to be sure of, for the normal outline of the caecum is so very irregular. The only suggestive point in the early stages would be sharply angular margins to the filling defect, but this appearance might be produced by adhesions.

Chronic Hyperplastic Tuberculosis

This condition is most frequently found in the ileo-caecal region, and is characterised by extensive proliferation of tuberculous granulation tissue in the intestinal wall. The resulting tumour is dense and usually felt with ease through the abdominal wall. It cannot be distinguished from neoplasm either by the naked eye or radiologically and the condition is, in fact, usually diagnosed as new growth. Stenosis of the lumen is the first indication, but there is generally tuberculosis elsewhere. Some observers hold that there is something in the nature of a physiological sphincter of the caecum near the ileo-caecal valve (see p. 168) and that it is at this point that carcinoma develops, whereas tuberculosis tends to develop at the lower pole. Hence in carcinoma there is apt to be a division of the caecum by the ingrowing mass, whereas in tuberculosis the lower pole becomes more or less obliterated by the growth of hyperplastic tubercle.

Migratory caecum

Buckstein (70a) has described a condition in which he says that the caecum is abnormally mobile and may cause attacks of colicky pain on the right. The free movement is due to an abnormally long mesentery, which is the result of failure of absorption during development. There may also be chronic constipation, sometimes alternating with attacks of diarrhoea, and a tumour in the caecal region. X-ray examination reveals the abnormal mobility with dilatation and stasis. I have no personal experience of the condition and, knowing the extra-ordinary ranges of mobility that are possible in the normal healthy subject, I should be very sceptical of mobility as a source of symptoms.

CONSTIPATION

Whether to regard constipation as a pathological condition or as a physiological variation is a point that has been debated. Eventually I considered that it should fall rather under physiology than pathology and accordingly it has been dealt with in Part II (p. 176).

COLON

COLITIS

"It soon became evident that appendicitis was on its last legs, and that a new complaint had to be discovered to meet the general demand. The Faculty was up to the mark, a new disease was dumped on the market, a new word was coined, a gold coin indeed: COLITIS! It was a neat complaint, safe from the surgeon's knife, always at hand when wanted, suitable to everybody's taste. Nobody knew when it came, nobody knew when it went away.

Many sins have been committed both by doctors and patients in the name of colitis during the early stages of its brilliant career. Even to-day there is not seldom something vague and unsatisfactory about this diagnosis."

AXEL MUNTHE, *The Story of San Michele.**

"This disorder (mucous colitis) is given the least space in the standard works and the most synonyms of any important disease; to wit, mucous colitis, mucous colic, tubular diarrhoea, chronic exudative enteritis, chronic muco-colitis, fibrinous diarrhoea, pellicular enteritis, pseudo-membranous enteritis, membranous enteritis, membranous colitis, membranous enterocolitis, muco-membranous colitis, enteritis membranacea, myxomembranous colitis, myxorrhea coli, myxoneurosis intestinalis. What other disease is so well buried under the verbal débris of several centuries? But this is not all. A prominent authority in a three-volume work on *Diseases of the Rectum, Anus and Colon*, 1923, states: 'To eliminate confusion relative to the nomenclature of so-called membranous entero-colitis and mucous colic, the author designates these conditions as myxorrhea membranacea and myxorrhea colica.' We would suggest that after each of these names the author's name be appended in recognition of an outstanding feat in etymology. This distinguished writer, at a time when verbal ingenuity seemed to have been exhausted, invented not simply one combination, but two perfectly new word-complexes to apply to one rather obscure disease. What there is about mucous colitis to stimulate activity in its etymology instead of its pathology is a question for the psychologist. Perhaps the disease will yet have a chance if this verbiage can be swept into the innocuous desuetude originally provided for political rubbish. It would be practically impossible to follow this disease through the literature were it not for the saving fact that, whatever name an author has invented or prefers, he, almost without exception, uses also the term mucous colitis."

A. W. CRANE (105).

Yet in the same journal Kantor (192) states: "Colitis is a common disorder of digestion: and is susceptible of precise röntgen demonstration." But this observer holds much more definite views than I do (cf. p. 178) as to just how the colon should act, and any deviation from his standard is abnormal:

"When the upper alimentary tract transport is normal the caecum begins to fill four hours after the standard opaque barium meal. At six hours, the head of the barium column reaches the region of the hepatic flexure; the tail is still in the ileum. At nine hours, the head reaches the splenic flexure, and the tail has cleared the terminal small intestine. At twenty-four hours, the bowels have moved once, and the left-sided shift has occurred—that is, the barium has cleared the proximal colon in whole or in part, and has become distributed throughout the distal colon. By forty-eight hours, the bowels have moved twice, and the colon is clear except for traces of the barium.

Any departure from the above schedule is abnormal. If the change is in the direction of stasis, a diagnosis of some variety of constipation is in order. If, on the other hand, the colonic transit is hastened, there exists a state of colonic irritability which is the essential motor expression of colitis. Colitis may therefore be diagnosed, or at least suspected, from the röntgen findings."

He details the findings from which he deduces colitis purely from the rate of progress of the opaque food. He states that in three-quarters of the cases

---

* London, John Murray, 1929, p. 33.

there is also ileal stasis. He then summarises the points in the appearance of the colonic form on which the diagnosis can be made: alterations in the size, shape and distribution of the haustra leading to irregularity in the distribution and, in severe cases, to a ragged, twisted or distorted appearance of the faecal column. When the faeces are watery there is often a trail left in the otherwise empty lumen. He also calls attention to the gas in the colon in these cases and to the "streaks of barium which may occasionally assume a characteristic stringy or ropy appearance", which Case has shown to be due to barium in strings of mucus and which Crane calls the "string sign" (Plate fig. 259). Later on he says:

"Colitis, in the sense in which the term is here employed, implies simply an abnormal irritability of the colon. This irritability, though fixed in the organic form of infection and ulceration, is more often a purely transient, functional phenomenon as observed in many patients suffering from obscure or patent digestive disorders."

Both Kantor and Crane are clinicians of wide experience in the diagnosis of colonic conditions and they balance the clinical with the radiological findings. But the average radiologist sees only one side of the picture and I am fully convinced that he should err on the side of omission rather than of commission in the diagnosis of conditions that are not very definitely pathological. I hold therefore that he should turn a blind eye to appearances that suggest colitis unless

(1) The symptoms are fairly definite.

(2) There is rigidity or tenderness over the suspected colon.

(3) The observations are definitely confirmed.

In many cases the confirmatory examination will make him thankful that he has not committed himself to a diagnosis and perhaps given the patient the foundation for an introspective state that might almost be termed mental colitis. More or less mucus is normal in the large intestine and, one would suppose, the variations in amount would be comparable with those in the secretion of saliva with which we are all familiar, dictated not only by the type of food but also by a variety of reflex and psychical influences.

One of the greatest difficulties in the large intestine is its close connection with and subjection to the central nervous system. One person suffers from constipation if he takes a railway journey, another dreads travelling because of the diarrhoea that is certain to develop even before the train starts. Many people suffer from loose stools or even severe diarrhoea in response to suspense or emotion. On the other hand, diarrhoea—or in fact any condition affecting the large intestine—is extraordinarily apt to produce remote symptoms of lassitude, depression and headache. Some of these may be definitely toxic, but the symptoms which develop if a man is a quarter of an hour late in the time he goes to stool are assuredly not. In no sphere of symptomatology is it more difficult to say which is the cause and which is the effect.

Perhaps it is not out of place to mention an extraordinary case, an attractive, healthy-looking athletic girl of about 22, who was sent to me soon after I commenced practice. She suffered from intractable colitis, so severe that she frequently passed casts. I myself saw one that was over a foot long. Treatment by means of zinc ionisation was given without benefit. There was no question that she suffered acutely, not only from the colitis but also from the shock of the ionisation, which was considerable. She was brought into a nursing home because of the shock and collapse following each treatment. One day there was another type of shock, however, for she was caught taking an extremely powerful purgative! The whole condition was self-induced, solely, so far as we could judge, in order to evoke sympathy. The history showed that she had been very constipated as a schoolgirl and probably she had found that diarrhoea evoked more interest than constipation, so much interest in fact that she was willing to undergo torture to obtain it. Perhaps, had she not found this way of gaining attention, she would have discovered another, but the case has always stuck in my mind as an illustration of the danger of calling undue attention to the bowels.

Our scanty and unreliable clinical knowledge of colitis makes the correct interpretation of the X-ray pictures, not only of the gross shadows of the food in the large intestine, but more especially of the mucous membrane patterns, merely a matter of surmise. I think we should be well advised if we held our hand in diagnosis from the mucous membrane pattern until we have a really satisfactory background of observation on normal subjects. From my very small experience in this direction I am quite satisfied that we have a long way to go before we can place any reliance on mere changes in mucous membrane patterns in the large intestine, apart of course from the few definite diseased conditions which are fairly well recognised.

There is no characteristic X-ray appearance of the indefinite conditions that are classed under the name of colitis, even in the gross shadow of the outlined large intestine. One by one the signs described have been refuted until the novice is utterly at sea. The ribbon sign, an entire absence of haustral segmentation in the well-filled intestine, was shown to be quite inconstant, present at one time and absent at another. It is of course always seen for a short time after an enema, before the haustral segmentation reappears (Plate fig. 260). Crane's string sign was for a time regarded as the one reliable diagnostic point, but even this now appears to be far less reliable than was claimed, and in fact some observers, including myself, do not believe that it has diagnostic significance unless it is definitely confirmed at a subsequent examination (Plate fig. 259). The irregular disposition of the colonic contents and the absence of haustra are no longer accepted as indications of colitis. Some observers regarded the traces left adherent to the mucous membrane either after natural mass move-

PLATE XVIII

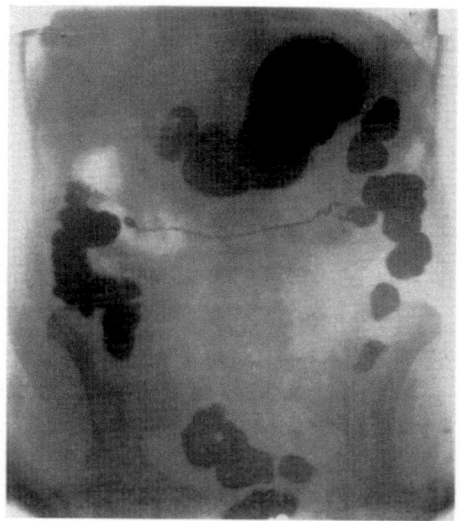
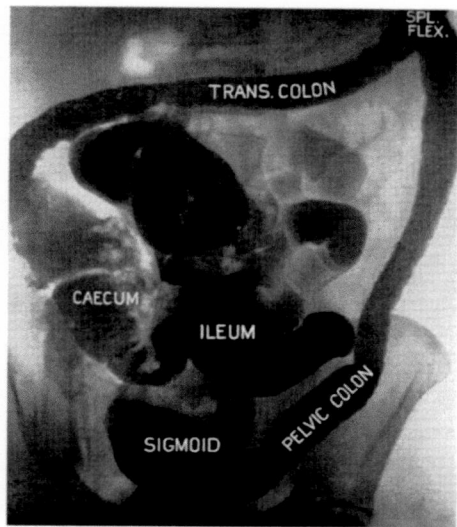

Fig. 259

Fig. 260

Fig. 259. String sign of mucous colitis exhibited in the transverse colon. Film made on the day following the opaque meal. The appearance is due to the mixture of the barium with the tenacious mucus. The string sign is most frequently observed in the last portion of the transverse and the upper two-thirds of the descending colon. (Contributed by A. W. Crane.)

Fig. 260. An enema has flowed through the whole length of the colon, giving the appearance of a ribbon, and into the small intestine.

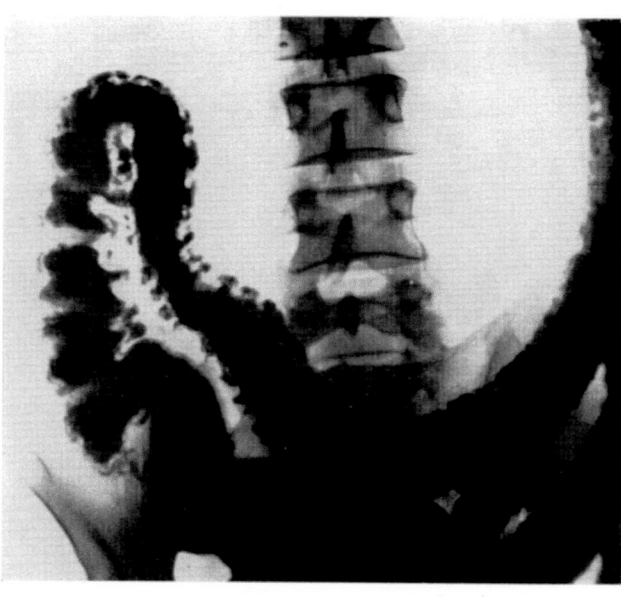
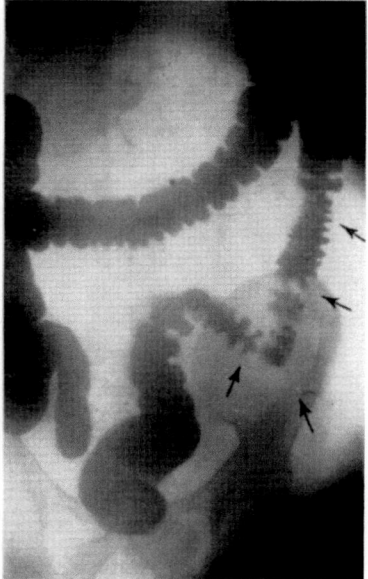

Fig. 261

Fig. 262

Fig. 261. An advanced case of ulcerative colitis. Blood and mucus were abundant in the stools and histologically the bowel wall showed extensive oedema with areas of ulceration extending through the mucosa to the submucous layer. (Contributed by S. D. S. Park.)

Fig. 262. Colonic spasm associated with kinking (angulation). (Contributed by J. L. Kantor.)

ment or, better, when the patient has been to stool after an opaque enema, as a sign that the mucous membrane was unhealthy and did not clear itself normally. I doubt very much if this is of the slightest importance, especially after enemata.

Sections of large intestine were deemed to be in a spastic condition because they were narrowed, and some observers still speak of spastic constipation as if it were a clinical entity, presumably dependent on an unhealthy area of mucous membrane. If the colon were in spasm, the contents would, on the gradient theory, be expelled either up or down from the affected area. The whole of the large intestine is in a constant state of tonic contraction and I doubt the importance of these narrowed areas that are seen from time to time both in unhealthy and healthy subjects, unless perhaps they indicate a slightly increased localised tonic action of a section of the musculature. More probably, however, they are merely due to unequal distribution of the colonic contents.

Taken all in all, and of course apart from the definite pathological conditions, I am very sceptical of the radiological and clinical diagnosis of colitis. Mind and body are so closely linked that action and reaction are in many cases inseparable and we should do well to avoid giving credence to radiological signs that may perhaps be merely comparable to a facial expression induced by someone treading on the patient's toe. The vagaries of the large intestine in their very close relationship with the mind are a subject that would well repay radiological study, but the difficulty of obtaining observations on normal subjects and the time required are so great that this branch of clinical radiology will probably remain in the same unsatisfactory state as the clinical diagnosis of neurasthenia.

The following case, for which I am indebted to Dr E. W. Twining, illustrates this point. The observation on the formation of the *point d'appui* is also of interest:

A lady, aet. 49, suffered from very persistent and intractable colic and diarrhoea for 5 weeks: stools loose, with no blood or mucus, almost continuous by day, and frequent motions during the night. She had a pronounced dread of cancer. Barium enema showed nothing abnormal in the lumen of the colon, but immediately it was filled, a large mass movement took place which voided the enema into the funnel placed 1 ft. above the patient. This occurred on each of four occasions on which the colon was filled. The mass movement always originated at the hepatic flexure; as the contraction wave passed slowly along the transverse colon towards the splenic flexure the patient complained of colic, which became intense as the contraction wave reached the splenic flexure.

The patient was assured that there was no suggestion of cancer, and from that day the bowel action became regular and there was no sign of the so-called "colitis".

Let me not be misunderstood. There is such a thing as definite colitis and in advanced cases the various radiological signs, such as those of Stierlin, Kienböck, Kantor and Crane, are to be found. Very occasionally an advanced case of ulceration is met with (Plate fig. 261) in which the actual ulcer craters are filled and an appearance somewhat comparable with diverticulitis is seen. My point is that these signs must not be taken by themselves apart from a careful consideration of the clinical picture, for they are not reliable. The radiologist must throw the burden of diagnosis on the physician. He should take warning from the condition of "hilum phthisis", for which thousands of healthy people were condemned as consumptive less than twenty years ago solely on radiological grounds: the appearance of root shadows that are now known to be within the limits of the normal. The clinical diagnosis of tuberculosis was not strong enough to refute radiological misinterpretation. The recognition of the early signs of colitis is not one of the high lights of radiology or of clinical medicine.

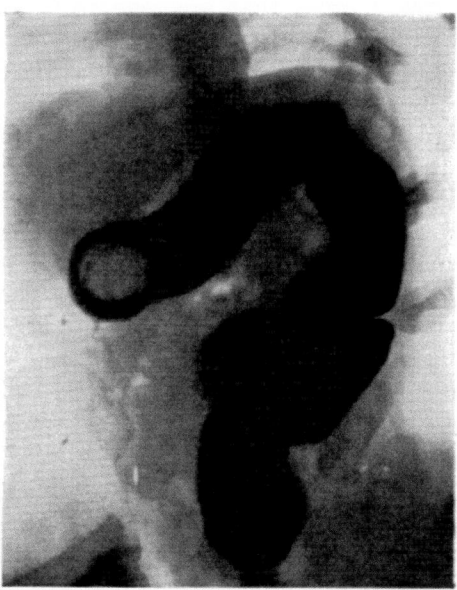

Fig. 263. Intestinal intussusception in an infant two years old, demonstrated by a barium enema. Note the characteristic "filling defect" in the transverse colon, caused by the invagination of the caecum and ascending colon into the transverse colon. (Contributed by A. Howard Pirie.)

The clinical diagnosis of the milder types of colitis is even weaker, for there are no physical signs and no constant gross changes in the faeces. Moreover, some subjects have considerable mucus in the stools quite apart from disease, and even more disconcerting is the fact that patients' statements on the subject of diarrhoea are not as reliable as they might be: some exaggerate wantonly, others are bad observers, and only a small number seem to tell a story that is in strict accord with radiographic findings and with the reports of nurses when the patient is placed under careful observation.

INTUSSUSCEPTION

Acute intussusception is not likely to be met with in an X-ray department, but relatively chronic cases may be diagnosed. Two are recorded by Davis and Parker (108); in both, polypoid lymphosarcomatous growths were the exciting cause and palpable tumours were present. By means of the enema fairly definite appearances were made out (Fig. 263). Their summary of conclusions is:

The barium enema early in the course of the affection is characteristic. There is a momentary obstruction to the flow of the barium, but by change in position, manipulation and maintenance of pressure, barium can be made to pass around the intussusceptum, leaving a central gas-filled filling defect.

The barium enema is equally characteristic after the formation of adhesions. There is then a complete obstruction to the flow of the barium, the head of the enema having a characteristic "U" or cupola shape, a filling defect not commonly observed in other lesions causing obstruction. The apex of the intussusceptum may contain gas.

The motor meal study may show:

(*a*) An apparent absence of one segment of the bowel—usually the caecum or ascending colon.

(*b*) A thin track of barium as it passes through in the intussusceptum.

(*c*) An annular filling defect at the neck of the intussusceptum.

DIVERTICULITIS

The terms diverticulitis and diverticulosis are in use to describe an inflamed and an uninflamed condition respectively. In view of the following, this nomenclature does not seem to be correct.

In 1889 T. Buzzard wrote (72):

"I was anxious to find out what was the significance of this termination "itis", which we so freely use, and I tried to get references to it. I looked in vain in the Greek classics, and could not find it in the Greek lexicon at all. It is evidently of comparatively modern origin. I spoke to a Greek friend of mine and he could not help me, but what is more important he put me into communication with Professor Kontos, of Athens, who I understand is considered, both in Germany and in Greece, to be the highest living authority on Greek philology. Professor Kontos was kind enough to interest himself in the question and to make a communication to me.... This is a very literal translation, but it is to this effect:—'Arthritis and nephritis, and pleuritis and splenitis, and all such things are literally epithets or adjectives, and the word nosos—disease—is understood. The disease about the ribs is pleuritis, just as the disease about the joints is arthritis, and nephritis is the disease about the kidneys'. It appears from this that the word 'neuritis', for example, is an adjective with the word 'disease' understood, and that all that is meant by neuritis is disease affecting the nerve, as myelitis would be disease affecting the marrow or spinal cord, and that the idea of inflammation with which it has come to be associated is simply an invention of much later date, for which there is really no authority whatever, and that we should be perfectly right in the future, etymologically correct, in using the term neuritis for a condition which may present no signs of what is ordinarily called inflammation."

Colonic diverticula were first described by Cruveilhier (106) in 1849 and by Virchow (320) a few years later. Little, however, was written on the subject till the beginning of this century. Telling (310) was one of the first to point out the importance of the condition. Radiographically it was recognised in 1914 by Le Wald (326), working for Abbe, and shortly after by Case (86, 87), and since that date a number of important radiological papers on the subject have appeared.

Diverticulitis is a symptomless condition, but the pockets are subject to inflammatory changes, perhaps due to the lodgment of faeces or concretions. In the course of routine X-ray examination diverticula are found quite frequently. The cause of their formation is unknown and various theories have been propounded, one of which suggests that they are due to the deposition of fat between the peritoneal coat and the muscular wall, thus weakening the support from the peritoneum. Certainly, as Telling pointed out, the frequency with which diverticula are covered by the fatty epiploic appendages is striking.

The Pre-Diverticular Stage

George and Leonard (128) suggested that a pre-diverticular stage might be recognised:

"Particularly along the descending colon and sigmoid one occasionally finds a peculiar serrated appearance. This may extend over several inches of gut and is associated with more or less narrowing of the lumen. These serrations are small, close together, and with a rather sharp point, presenting at times a sawtooth appearance.... The serrations do not change in size or shape. Furthermore, palpation under the fluoroscopic screen usually shows us that the intestine is more or less like a rigid tube.... One infers that the serrated appearance is due to inflammatory thickening and induration of and about the intestinal wall, secondary to the presence of diverticula, the diverticula themselves not being visible."

As Case (86) has pointed out, this description is very similar to that given by Spriggs and Marxer (303), who definitely described a stage preceding the development of pouches as minute hernial sacs between the muscular fibres (Plate fig. 264). They maintain that there is a previous inflammation causing a concertina-like appearance. What appears to be radiographically a somewhat comparable condition has been described by Muir (257) under the title of "The Irritable Colon". It is characterised by pylorospasm, fixation of the appendix and stasis in the terminal ileum, with exaggerated segmentation in the colon.

My experience in the study of colitis is not wide enough to justify dogmatism. It is a chronic condition and reliable deductions can only be made from a series of examinations of a number of cases in an institution in which patients reside for prolonged periods. The average radiologist sees his patients but once or twice, and has little, if any, opportunity to follow up and see whether or not his interpretations have been correct. I may be wrong, but I prefer to neglect such appearances. Diverticula are symptomless unless infected, and perfect health is

Plate XIX

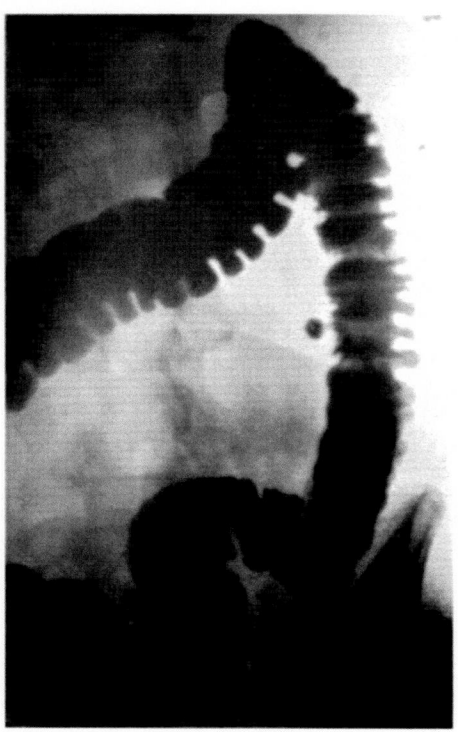

Fig. 264. Irregularity of the wall of the descending colon, described as the pre-diverticular stage of colitis. In this instance, one well-formed diverticulum was present. (Contributed by E. I. Spriggs.)

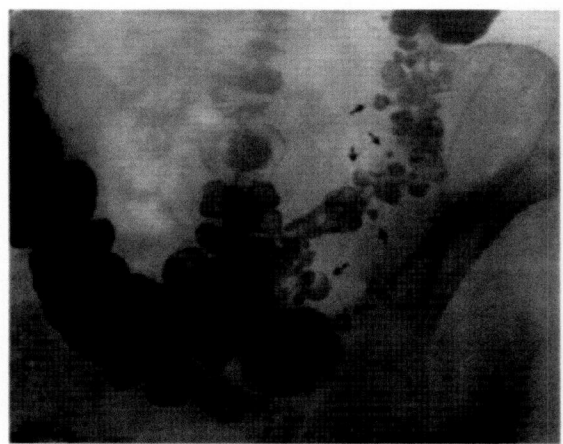

Fig. 265. Diverticulitis of the pelvic portion of the large intestine.

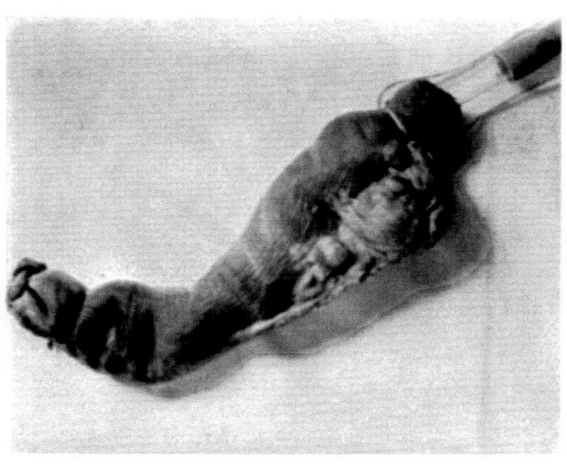

Fig. 266. Photograph of specimen with multiple diverticula. Several of the diverticula had pedicles. (Cf. Fig. 267.) (Contributed by J. T. Case.)

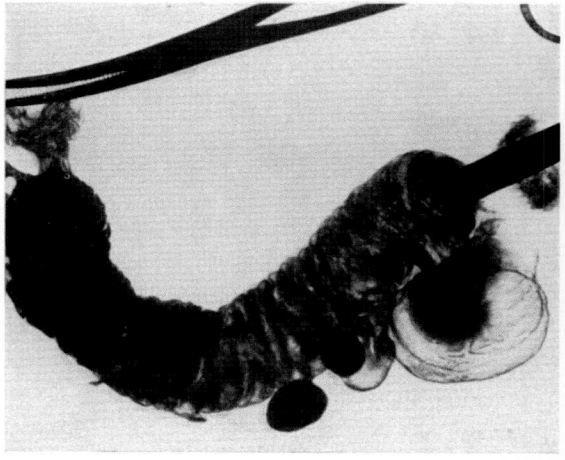

Fig. 267. Radiograph of the specimen shown in Fig. 266 after injection with opaque salt solution. (Contributed by J. T. Case.)

compatible with numerous well-marked saccules. The radiologist may discover the pre-diverticular stage or even definite diverticula, but it is not necessarily wise to allow the patient, or even his physician in some cases, to know what has been found, unless there are definite symptoms. There is such a thing as judicious reticence. To tell a patient and his doctor that all is well may not be spectacular, or popular with some patients or doctors, but surely the radiologist's chief function in the examination of the alimentary tract is to relieve the patient's mind, to lift the fear that is nearly always present: the fear that some slight disturbance of function is the first indication of serious disease. In a recent case, radiographs were brought to me for an opinion. They showed changes similar to those seen in Plate fig. 264, but with no sign of diverticula. Colitis and diverticulitis had been mentioned. Re-examination after a holiday was suggested and, when the further observations were made, the colon was apparently perfectly normal. The radiologist informed the patient of the findings and, I gather, the patient is now perfectly well.

The Diagnosis of Diverticulitis

The diagnosis of diverticulitis depends on the demonstration of the pockets. These fill with the opaque food far more readily than with the enema (Plate figs. 264–267). Why this should be is not clear, but I have frequently failed to demonstrate diverticula with the enema, and conversely, the enema seldom revealed diverticula that had not been filled by the opaque food. Re-examination after an enema has been voided will, however, sometimes show diverticula that were not seen when the bowel was filled.

The most frequent seat of diverticula is the lower part of the descending colon and the upper sigmoid. They appear as small currant-like shadows protruding from, and sometimes connected by a neck to the shadow of the food in the lumen. They may be single, but more often there are numerous small saccules, and in some cases they can be found scattered along the whole length of the colon. Naturally, only those that are on the profile of the colon are seen until the bowel is emptied. Some of the pockets may retain the opaque food for days, and when the bowel is empty look like scattered seeds, the size of peas, along the course of the colon. Presumably the pockets are always filled by faecal material and it is curious that the opaque food should displace this. Possibly the barium cakes in the pockets.

Whenever symptoms are present, the observer should palpate carefully to see if any of the diverticula are the seat of localised pain on deep pressure. When inflammatory changes take place, the diverticula may perforate, sometimes without warning. Lockhart-Mummery and Graham Hodgson [220] maintain that diverticula when once formed tend to increase both in size and in number, but that in the absence of inflammation they are not likely to cause symptoms. These writers, however, believe that perforation may occur without inflammatory changes, and therefore regard diverticulitis as a serious condition even in the absence of symptoms. On the other hand, Spriggs estimates the risk of perforation at about 1 per cent.: this figure is based on a study of 410 cases. More often, however, surrounding fibrosis occurs and may be so dense that the mass, at operation, may easily be mistaken for malignant disease. It seems likely that cases in which colostomy has been performed for malignant disease and yet the patient has survived for many years were really diverticulitis. Therefore in every case of suspected carcinoma of the colon, particularly of the sigmoid, it is advisable to search for the presence of saccules in other parts.

POLYPOID CONDITIONS

Various types of polypi may be revealed by the intensive study of the mucous membrane, but they are rare. Heredity is said to play a part, as in other polypoid conditions. In one of my cases, the whole of the descending colon appeared on successive days like a band covered with a thin wash of opaque salt, showing fine regular streaks with a few indefinite cross lines (Plate fig. 268). The clinical picture was that of severe colitis that had resisted treatment. There was diarrhoea, much mucus, and tenderness over the descending colon. The section of intestine, when removed, showed the whole mucous membrane evenly covered with a fine villous type of polyp. There was no healthy mucous membrane left, from the splenic flexure down to the sigmoid.

Wesson and Bargen (334) have classified polyps of the large intestine, distinguishing between inflammatory pseudopolyps and true polyps. They say that the incidence of carcinomatous change in adenomatous polyps is directly proportional to the number present, the probability of cancer approaching 100 per cent. in cases of multiple adenomatosis. Such conclusions, however, can hardly apply to the polyposis which seems to be so prevalent in Egypt (p. 231) and other countries where intestinal parasites are common.

Polypoid and other conditions may be beautifully demonstrated by injecting air per rectum (Plate fig. 269), a method that was, for a time, employed as a routine by Case in 1912 and also by myself and others.

CARCINOMA OF THE LARGE INTESTINE

New growths may occur in any part of the large intestine, but are most frequent at the junction of the descending colon and sigmoid, in the rectum and at the splenic flexure. Radiologically there appear to be two main types of growth. The annular is a densely fibrotic ring that may give the first indication of its presence by causing obstruction. If it occurs in a region where palpation is possible it can be felt as a sausage-shaped mass. The soft, proliferating type gives

PLATE XX

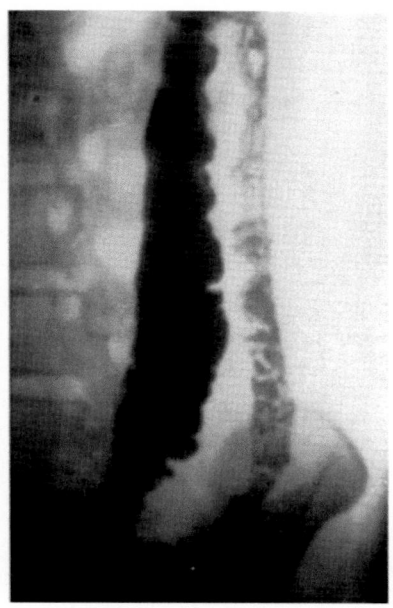

Fig. 268. Villous type of colitis. The whole of the descending colon was lined with a carpet of evenly distributed stringy villous shreds.

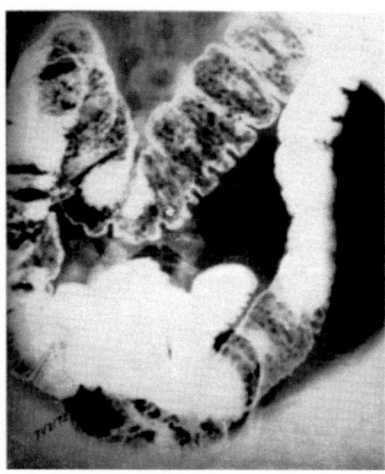

Fig. 269. Polypoid condition of the large intestine shown by a combined technique of air and opaque salt injection. (Contributed by H. M. Weber.)

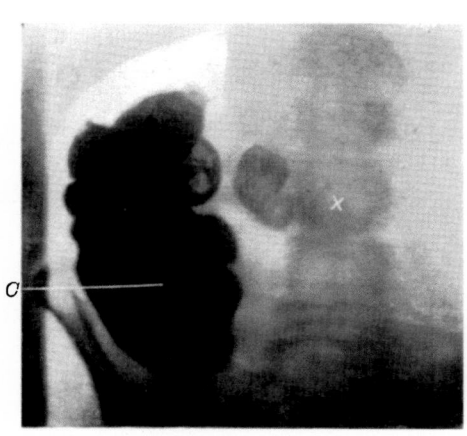

Fig. 270. Dilated caecum in a case of neoplasm of the splenic flexure of the colon. C, Caecum.

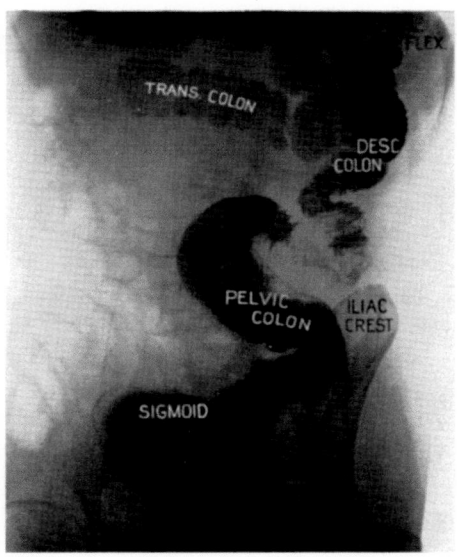

Fig. 271. Growth of descending colon demonstrated by enema. The sausage-shaped mass was readily felt.

rise to early ulceration and a more papillomatous type of growth in the lumen of the gut, with rapid extension to surrounding parts.

In the early stages of any disease involving the mucous membrane of the intestinal tract, there is always a tendency to local irritability, and the affected part is usually empty: only in the later stages can the opaque food be relied upon to show the diseased area satisfactorily. Thus, when the obstruction is at the splenic flexure, the caecum is often markedly distended (Plate fig. 270) and practically no shadow is seen in the transverse colon. In fact, such an appearance should

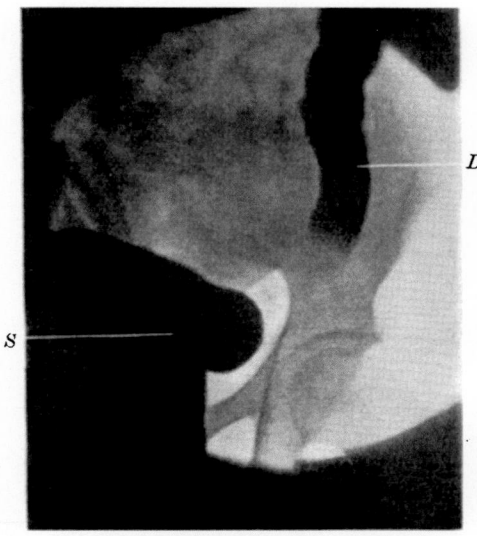 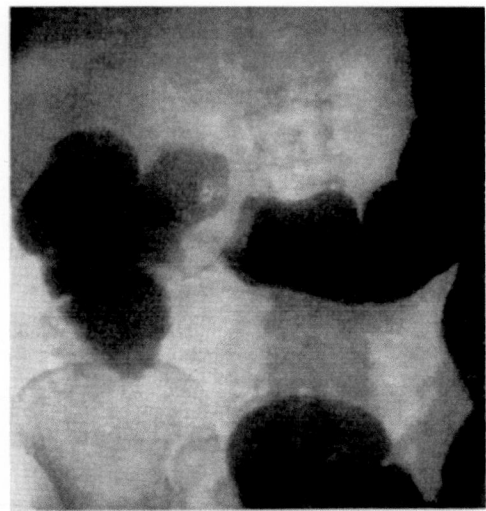

Fig. 272. Growth of the pelvic colon. In this case the growth was quite small and was almost limited to the mucous membrane, but the associated spasm was so marked that it looked as if a much larger extent were involved. *DC*, Descending colon. *S*, Sigmoid.

Fig. 273. Growth near the hepatic flexure demonstrated by enema. (Contributed by F. Haenisch.)

always make the observer suspicious. The main line of attack in all these cases must be the barium enema (Plate fig. 271, and Figs. 272 and 273), the meal being of great assistance in showing the normal, but of comparatively little value in revealing the abnormal in the early stages. Both methods should therefore be used, but even so a certain number of lesions will escape detection.

When the colon only is suspected, the best plan is to vary the routine and instruct the patient to take an opaque meal at bedtime the night before the first examination; this will often outline the greater part of the colon as far as the splenic flexure. The stomach should be examined in every case, but the enema should be given before sufficient food has passed out of the stomach to interfere with the view of the colon. The enema will join the shadow in the splenic region so that the whole colon can be examined at once. When, however, part of the food has passed on and lies in the sigmoid it is much wiser to defer the enema examination till the following day in order to have an unobstructed and uncomplicated view of the enema shadow.

Indications of Growth

A much dilated rectal ampulla very strongly suggests a growth low down in the sigmoid. Why the rectum should be dilated *below* the growth is not known,

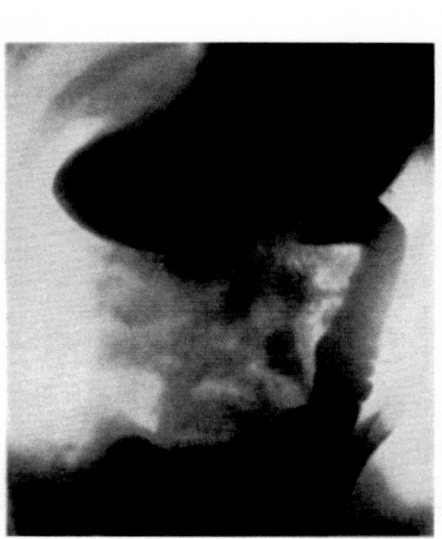 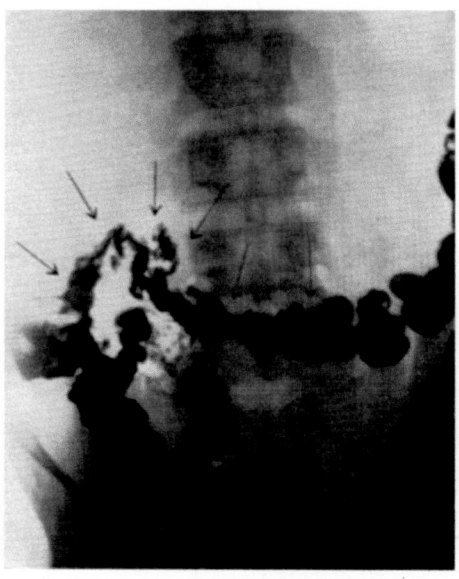

Fig. 274   Fig. 275

Fig. 274. Gastro-colic fistula due to the perforation of a carcinoma of the transverse colon into the stomach. The stomach has been filled from a barium enema. (Contributed by W. D. Dickson.)

Fig. 275. Tuberculosis of the transverse colon. (Contributed by A. Howard Pirie.)

but it is a valuable sign, because the lesion is often in a position in which its shadow is exceedingly difficult, if not impossible, to see satisfactorily. In such cases the surgeon should be asked to use the sigmoidoscope.

The points on which carcinoma is diagnosed are (1) obstruction, which is due to carcinoma in a large percentage of cases, and (2) filling defects. In the advanced cases there is no difficulty. The opaque enema is seen finding its way through the irregular canals in the papillomatous type of growth, or passing in a fine stream through the more fibrotic annular growths. By manipulation the radiologist ascertains whether the bowel is fixed or not, and by tactile sense he determines the presence of thickening and perhaps the extent of the growth.

Unfortunately only a small length of the colon can be palpated, for the upper part of the descending colon passes under the costal margin, and growths in the splenic flexure are common. For these he has to depend entirely on the filling defect, and in order to see the whole splenic flexure he must rotate the patient to the right.

Carcinoma involving the hepatic flexure is comparatively rare, and I have only seen a few cases of malignant disease of the caecum and ascending colon. Growths of the transverse colon usually also involve the greater curvature of the stomach and occasionally perforate into it (Fig. 274).

The diagnosis of early malignant disease is by no means easy, because the colon is so irritable and so liable to spasm. It is sometimes quite impossible to tell whether a filling defect or even an obstruction is due to spasm or to growth. If the observer is in any doubt he should insist on re-examination.

Differential Diagnosis

The conditions with which malignant disease of the large intestine may be confused are: (1) old diverticulitis with adhesions, (2) adhesions, (3) tuberculosis. In diverticulitis the appearances may be identical with those of neoplasm and the only diagnostic point would be the presence of diverticula in other parts. Extensive adhesions may give rise to difficulty but the clinical history should give the clue, and in tuberculosis there is likely to be other obvious evidence of the disease in so advanced a case. Hyperplastic tuberculosis (p. 305) may be found in the colon as well as in the caecum (Fig. 275); it may have been the condition really present in some of those cases of supposedly malignant disease where life has been prolonged indefinitely by colostomy.

HIRSCHSPRUNG'S DISEASE: IDIOPATHIC DILATATION OF THE COLON

This condition may affect the whole or a part of the large intestine; when the sigmoid only is involved the term megasigmoid is used. It is rare, and I have seen very few cases in recent years. The aetiology is unknown; achalasia has been suggested. Hurst suggests that many cases are due to progressive disease of Auerbach's plexus and compares the condition with achalasia of the cardia (p. 209) and with idiopathic dilatation of the ureter. In some of the cases I have seen, the dilatation was the result of obstruction. The mother of a child had noticed that an enema was only effective if a catheter had previously been passed and gas withdrawn from the rectum; this suggested an air-lock due to kinking, and radiological investigation supported this view. After a preliminary colostomy, some of the redundant sigmoid was removed; no organic lesions or bands were seen. The patient made a complete recovery. An equally satisfactory result was obtained by similar treatment in a second case.

The opaque food shows a wide, long, looped and folded inert colon with few haustral segmentations and usually much gas. The enema flows freely, and very large quantities are needed to fill the colon. An attempt should not, however, be made to fill it when once the condition has been recognised, as the barium is very difficult to evacuate satisfactorily and might cause obstruction. A curious feature of this condition is that the opaque enema usually flows freely but the purgative enema often fails. This fact suggests to me that the cause may be an abnormally long sigmoid with a tendency to kinking.

CHAPTER XIX

THE GALL-BLADDER

(In collaboration with Dr L. A. Rowden)

The gall-bladder is so closely related to the intestinal tract that diseased conditions in it are apt to give rise to gastric symptoms. Hence, an opaque meal examination that fails to reveal the source of the gastric symptoms should be followed, if it has not been preceded, by a gall-bladder examination.

The first X-ray plates on which gall-stones were shown were taken by Carl Beck in 1899, and the first exhibited in this country were the work of Thurstan Holland. Among the early investigators the names of Köhler, Cole, Case, Pfahler, and particularly Knox, will always be remembered. The most extensive treatise on the subject, however, was the book published in 1922 by George and Leonard (129). Their results were obtained by straight radiography, the direct method. From the study of physiology, however, an indirect method of investigation, cholecystography, "the dye test" or the Graham test, was evolved in 1924 by Graham and Cole (139). The history of gall-bladder radiology therefore falls sharply into two periods: before and since the introduction of this indirect method.

In the days when the direct method was the only line of attack, the chance of obtaining information depended entirely on pathological changes in density. In the indirect method, the gall-bladder is visualised by means of a radio-opaque substance excreted through the liver. The indirect does not replace the direct method but is merely complementary to it. The films taken by the direct method are now called the control films.

ANATOMY AND PHYSIOLOGY

The traditional descriptions of the gall-bladder, like those of the stomach, suggest a definite size, shape and form. "It is four inches in length, one inch in breadth at its widest part, and holds eight to ten drachms." Its position also is definitely described, but is in fact very variable (cf. pp. 100 and 334). Although muscle is described in the walls, the student frequently fails to realise that the muscle is there for a purpose, that the walls do in fact contract and relax, and that even the mucous membrane of the gall-bladder and of the ducts has a definite muscularis mucosae and is therefore equipped for independent movement.

The gall-bladder has an incomplete outer serous coat, derived from the peritoneum. Inside this is the fibro-muscular coat, a thin but strong layer that is the framework of the sac. It is composed of dense areolar tissue containing smooth muscular fibres, both longitudinal and circular, but these do not form separate strata. It is loosely attached to the mucous membrane, which is composed of high columnar epithelium, is pitted in a honeycomb manner, and feels like velvet pile. It is interesting to note that gall-stones do not seem to form in the pits. This perhaps indicates that in life either the muscularis mucosae obliterates the pits or they are constantly changing. Towards the neck of the gall-bladder the mucous membrane is gathered into some 5–12 folds that are

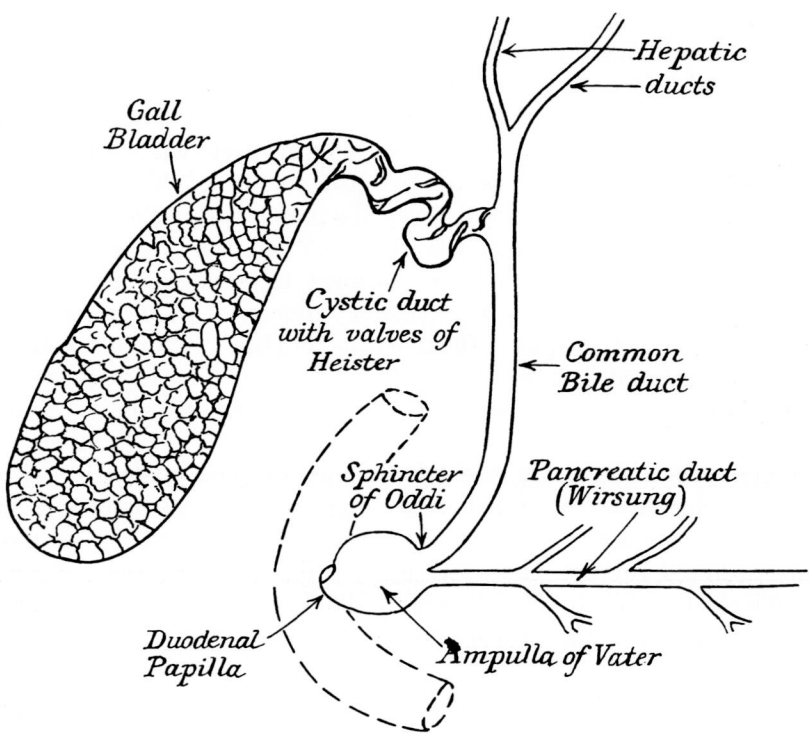

Fig. 276. Diagram of the biliary passages. Sometimes the cystic ducts and the pancreatic duct do not join but open separately into the duodenum.

placed rather obliquely and are known as the valves of Heister. They appear to provide a screw-like valve. As the muscularis mucosae is prominent in and about these folds, it seems likely that they may play more than a passive valvular part in the filling and emptying of the gall-bladder. Gall-stones are apt to lodge between them and may act like a ball-valve. Near the neck of the gall-bladder are a number of large saccular glands, resembling those in the mucous membrane of the common bile duct. The disposition of the biliary passages is shown in Fig. 276.

Bile is excreted continuously by the liver, passing through the hepatic and cystic ducts, where it is rendered more fluid by the secretion of the walls. The function of the gall-bladder, so far as it is known, is to act as a reservoir and concentrator of the hepatic secretion. During fasting the flow of bile is slowed, and most of it enters the gall-bladder and is retained there, being highly concentrated by osmosis and diffusion: up to eight times that in the bile ducts. An increased secretion of bile does not necessarily mean an increased flow into the intestine. Two factors are concerned in bile expulsion: the pressure in the common bile duct and the resistance of the sphincter of Oddi, and normally both are operative together. The former is raised by increased secretion or by contraction of the gall-bladder, and at the same time the sphincter of Oddi is said to relax, and there is an increased discharge of bile into the duodenum, partly from the gall-bladder but mostly direct from the liver. The control mechanism appears to be the combined function of the vagus (motor to the gall-bladder and inhibitory to the sphincter) and of the sympathetic, which has exactly opposite functions.

The liver is one of the organs of excretion of the halogen constituents of the body: chlorine, bromine and iodine, of which the atomic weights are 35·46, 76·92 and 126·92 respectively. Salts of chlorine are normally present in the bile in very large quantity; although they are so highly concentrated, their atomic weight is so low that they will not cast a shadow. Bromine and iodine salts are absent, or only present in very small quantities, under normal conditions. It was argued that if bromine or iodine salts could be rendered non-toxic and given in sufficient quantities, they would be excreted by the liver and concentrated to such an extent that the gall-bladder would be rendered radio-opaque. After much animal experimental work, tetrabromophenolphthalein and tetraiodophenolphthalein were prepared in non-toxic form for human investigation. The two compounds are used in the form of their sodium salts, which are relatively less toxic than the hydroxyl compounds. The tetraiodophenolphthalein sodium salt contains 58·6 per cent. weight for weight of iodine and the corresponding bromo compound 47·2 per cent. weight for weight of bromine. The iodine compound thus contains a higher proportion of the opaque element; in addition the atomic number of iodine (atomic No. 53) is higher than that of bromine (atomic No. 35) and indicates a still greater opacity for the iodine compound. The iodine salt is therefore obviously the one to use, but is very difficult to render non-toxic. It has the added advantage that it tends to increase the flow of bile. When given intravenously, 0·2 per cent. is found in the bile ducts and it attains a concentration of 0·6 per cent. in the normal gall-bladder. A density such as this renders the bile in the gall-bladder sufficiently opaque to throw a shadow. This is, in outline, the principle of the indirect method of investigation, or cholecystography.

Constituents of Bile

The bile is composed of numerous constituents the concentration of which varies in different parts of the tract. The following table is taken from Starling's *Physiology*, 1920, p. 760:

From a biliary fistula (Yeo and Herroun), in 100 parts		From the gall-bladder (Hoppe-Seyler), in 100 parts	
Mucin and pigments	0·148	Mucin	1·29
Sodium taurocholate	0·055	Sodium taurocholate	0·87
Sodium glycocholate	0·165	Sodium glycocholate	3·03
Cholesterol		Soaps	1·39
Lecithin	0·038	Cholesterol	0·35
Fats		Lecithin	0·53
Inorganic salts	0·840	Fats	0·73
Water	98·7		

The important constituents of bile are the cholesterol (a fat-like, pearly substance, a monatomic alcohol, $C_{26}H_{44}O$), and the lecithin (an allied fatty substance, $C_{44}H_{90}NPO_9$), which are held in solution by the inorganic salts. The pigments are merely waste products from the disintegration of haemoglobin. "The digestive function of bile therefore lies in its power of serving as a vehicle for the suspension and solution of the interacting fats, fatty acids and fat-splitting ferment" (Starling's *Physiology*, 1920, p. 763).

Gall-stones are formed from the concentration and imbalance of these constituents in the gall-bladder. When the gall-bladder functions poorly, either as a result of the sedentary habits of the patient or because the mucous membrane is not working satisfactorily, it becomes a blind end, and in it the bile stagnates, becomes inspissated, and is concentrated to such an extent that the cholesterol may actually separate out and form stones. If this happens, the cholesterol will always tend to deposit on any particle of foreign matter that may be present. Cholesterol stones are often found to contain a minute calcium centre which, presumably, formed one of a few grains of gall-sand before the cholesterol was deposited on it.

PATHOLOGY

The mucous membrane may be the seat of inflammatory changes, either catarrhal or suppurative, that put it out of action. Complete or partial recovery may take place, leaving degenerative changes of lesser or greater extent. In the most severe cases the mucous membrane is completely destroyed and nothing is left but a fibrous layer that becomes part of a general fibrosis affecting the whole wall of the sac.

Stones in the gall-bladder are relatively common, the incidence varying in different countries. Out of 4616 autopsies at St George's Hospital, gall-stones were recorded in 268 (5·8 per cent.), and this appears to be about the average figure for this country. In the United States the percentage is rather lower, and in Germany it appears to be considerably higher: nearly 10 per cent. Gall-stones are more frequently found in women than in men. The predisposing causes, according to Rolleston and McNee (285), are stagnation of bile and infection. Stagnation may be brought about by sedentary habits, obesity and constipation, and by any interference with diaphragmatic respiration, e.g. pregnancy and tumours. Ninety per cent. of women in whom gall-stones are found have been pregnant, but stones are relatively rare in women who have not borne children. Some workers, such as Mann and Higgins (232), basing their conclusions on animal experiments, have suggested that the emptying of the gall-bladder is delayed or actually does not take place at all in the later stages of pregnancy. The human gall-bladder certainly seems to behave erratically at this time. In a series of thirty-nine such cases (Levyn, Beck and Aaron (218)) the gall-bladder was visualised in nineteen. There was no delay in the appearance of the shadow and, apart from the deformities and distortions of the gall-bladder that might reasonably be expected in the circumstances, nothing abnormal was noted.

At one time it was held that stagnation of the bile in the gall-bladder was the primary, and possibly the only cause, but later it was recognised that any condition which might predispose to infection also played a large part. The extensive history and literature on the subject are summarised by Rolleston and McNee, who maintain that gall-stones may be either (a) aseptic or (b) inflammatory in origin.

The aseptic type is essentially connected with the over-concentration of cholesterol in the gall-bladder. This substance is absorbed from the intestine, circulates in the blood (mostly as esters of higher fatty acids) and is excreted by the liver into the bile as pure cholesterol. It is well known to surgeons that the mucous membrane of the gall-bladder and bile ducts may be found infiltrated with cholesterol-esters, but whether these are being secreted or excreted is not clear. It seems to be reasonably well established that under certain conditions, presumably those associated with stagnation, the cholesterol concentration increases to such an extent that the bile solidifies, sometimes as large single stones, sometimes as multiple small stones. An extraordinary number may be present: 20,000 have been recorded. It is a curious fact that when a large number are present, they are strikingly uniform in size.

Whether these cholesterol stones are pure or formed on some minute nucleus is not certain. The inflammatory exudate poured into the gall-bladder is rich in calcium salts and in many of the specimens radiographed a minute calcium centre can just be detected; micro-organisms or a fragment of cell detritus may form the nucleus of others (cf. Plate fig. 278g). Micro-organisms have been cultured from the centres of stones.

The commonest type of stone resulting from stagnation and over-concentration is formed chiefly of cholesterol. This is the type found in stout women of middle age and sedentary habit. There are also lime salt stones, mostly composed of calcium carbonate. These may be laid down either pure or in combination with cholesterol. Under normal conditions, the various inorganic salts in the bile are in solution. What the changes are that convert them into insoluble form is not known, but the change, whatever it may be, is associated with degeneration in the mucous membrane and, in general, is the result of inflammatory conditions. Whereas the cholesterol stone casts a very faint shadow, less than that of the normal tissues, lime stones throw quite heavy shadows, comparable to those of renal calculi. Very frequently a layer of lime salt is deposited on a cholesterol stone. This gives a ring shadow and some of the illustrations of excised gall-bladders show cholesterol and lime deposited in alternate layers (Plate fig. 278 *d* and *f*). This formation indicates successive attacks of inflammation leading to degenerative changes: in the intervals, when the cholesterol is deposited, the gall-bladder is functioning inadequately, so that the normal fatty constituents are over-concentrated.

Most radiologists have at one time or another had the embarrassing experience of failing to detect in films of the gall-bladder region large stones which, when placed under the fluorescent screen, even under a subject's body, gave quite heavy shadows. The explanation is of course perfectly simple: the gall-stone threw a shadow of exactly the same density as that thrown by the surrounding tissues. Fig. 277 shows radiographs of two large gall-stones in a glass. They give very heavy shadows, but when the glass is filled with water their

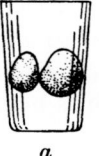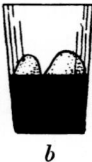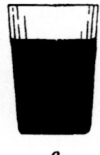

a   *b*   *c*

Fig. 277. *a*. Tracings from radiographs of two large gall-stones in a tumbler. *b*. Tracings from radiographs of water poured in till the glass is half-full. *c*. The stones are covered by the water; their shadows are of equal density to that of the water, and therefore do not show.

shadows are completely lost in that of the water: they merely replace an equal quantity of water of approximately the same density. Hence, in the body, it is inherently impossible to detect such stones by ordinary radiography, no matter how perfect the technique may be. Only about 10 per cent. of gall-stones contain lime salts in such quantity that they are more dense than the surrounding tissues and therefore give a shadow. If the stone is more or less uniformly impregnated with lime salts, it will give a solid shadow that is readily detected. If, however, the lime is deposited as a layer on a cholesterol centre, it will give a ring shadow. If, for some reason, only a part of the cholesterol centre is covered, a crescentic or new-moon shadow results. Such shadows are not readily diagnosed and are apt to be mistaken for calcification in rib cartilages. In the relatively heavy shadow thrown by cholecystography, gall-stones of low atomic weight, e.g. cholesterol, will show as less opaque areas. Lime salt stones, therefore, can be detected by direct radiography and cholesterol stones by cholecysto-graphy.

If the gall-bladder is normal and healthy, no technique will show its outline unless, perchance, there is some air in the adjacent colon to give the necessary contrast. But a diseased gall-bladder may be so sclerosed that, with good technique, its outline becomes visible; in fact, George and Leonard laid down long ago that the detection of the gall-bladder outline on an X-ray plate was evidence of an unhealthy condition. They maintained that with their technique they could show 98 per cent. of pathological gall-bladders. Few other workers, however, attained an accuracy as high as 50 per cent., but this was before the introduction of the Potter-Bucky diaphragm and other advances in tech-nique. With the very marked increase in detail and contrast that has come within the last few years, the gall-bladder outline is seen much more frequently, and many workers, notably Courtney Gage (125), maintain that this sign is not necessarily of pathological significance.

Fibrosis may be so extreme that the gall-bladder becomes an almost solid tube with a relatively small lumen. Moreover, occasionally, lime salts are deposited in the walls and give irregularly crescentic, new-moon shadows which, like those of irregular lime deposits on cholesterol stones, closely resemble calcification in costal cartilages. Under such conditions, the gall-bladder will show quite obviously in the direct radiograph. A gall-bladder that does not fill in chole-cystography is either pathological or for some reason is not receiving bile.

A STUDY OF EXCISED SPECIMENS

Perhaps the best introduction to the radiographic study of this subject is an analysis of a small series of radiographs of excised gall-bladders. Dr Rowden has studied over a hundred of these that have been placed at his service, by Lord Moynihan and others, untouched and merely ligatured off before excision. The technique for the radiography of these specimens is, of course, very different from that applicable to the living subject. Very soft radiations are employed and far greater detail is possible. These pictures give the key to the problems of this work and are well worth study. They also tell something of the history of the formation of the stones. In the first four cases the diagnosis of gall-stones was made on the control films, i.e. by the direct method. In the other cases, no radiographic evidence of the stones was obtained and the diagnosis of a pathological condition rested on the fact that the salt was not detected in the gall-bladder, or that gall-stones gave negative shadows with cholecystography.

Plate fig. 278a. A gall-bladder containing many stones of varying consistency. The large ones are composed of dense lime salts throughout but are surrounded by a zone of cholesterol which has also been laid down on a number of minute lime salt centres, i.e. gravel. In this case there have been repeated inflammatory attacks, leading to degenerative changes in the mucous membrane and, as a result, the larger opaque stones were formed together with some gravel of a similar composition. The diagnosis of repeated attacks is based on the laminated appearance of some of the stones, with a suggestion of thin layers of cholesterol between the deposits of lime. Between the attacks, the inflammation settled down; the mucous membrane was injured but not put out of action. The gall-bladder was not functioning properly; the bile was inspissated and stagnant, and cholesterol was deposited on these centres until the gall-bladder was almost filled with stones. This interpretation is supported by the history of the case and also by the fact that the mucous membrane was apparently healthy when the gall-bladder was opened. The large stones were readily detected on the control radiograph—the direct method—but no trace of the others was seen. No cholecystography was made, but if any opaque salt had entered the gall-bladder it would have cast only a poor shadow because there would have been room for so little bile. The heavy shadows would probably have been obliterated, but the smaller, almost pure cholesterol stones might have been detected as mottled clearer areas in the gall-bladder shadow.

Plate fig. 278 b. Three large stones of different types contained in a gall-bladder with fibrotic, atrophied walls. There was no true bile at all in the gall-bladder, and cholecystography would have given a negative result. The upper stone was recognised on the control radiograph and the lower one could just be detected as a "ring" shadow. Probably the upper stone was the first laid down, very likely after an inflammatory attack that left the mucous membrane unhealthy. There was then stagnation in the gall-bladder, the cholesterol centres of the two lower stones were laid down and an incomplete layer of cholesterol was deposited on the upper stone. Subsequent inflammatory attacks led to the deposit, around the cholesterol, of lime salts that gave the outer ring.

Plate fig. 278 c. Two medium-sized gall-stones of soft, unequal consistency. The upper one, lodged between the valves of Heister, is a cholesterol stone with an irregular deposit of lime salt on the surface, soft and sandy in consistency. The lower one has lime salts deposited above and below, i.e. the fibrosed gall-bladder had already contracted down to this stone when the inflammatory attack occurred that gave rise to this deposit. The walls of the sac were dense and fibrotic, and there was no bile in it. In this case the stones were recognised on the control film but the shadows were not typical. The gall-bladder was probably shut off by the upper stone and the lime salts were deposited after a severe attack that put the mucous membrane completely out of action and led to sclerosis of the walls.

Plate fig. 278 d. A small fibrotic sac containing four stones, each of which has a lime salt centre, a cholesterol investment and a thin lime salt outer wall. Cholecystography did not show the gall-bladder and the direct radiographs showed the stones as faint new-moon shadows. The history is probably one of an inflammatory attack after which the nuclei were laid down. Then followed a period in which, the wall being injured, the contents were stagnant and the cholesterol was deposited. Then followed another inflammatory attack and, as the result, the lime salts on the surface were added.

Plate fig. 278 e. A large gall-bladder almost completely filled with stones, only three of which show clearly, even in the excised specimen. Of these three, two are of pure cholesterol, coated with a thin layer of lime salt. These were the first laid down, and all the others were subsequent, including the large transradiant one that has no lime

PLATE XXI

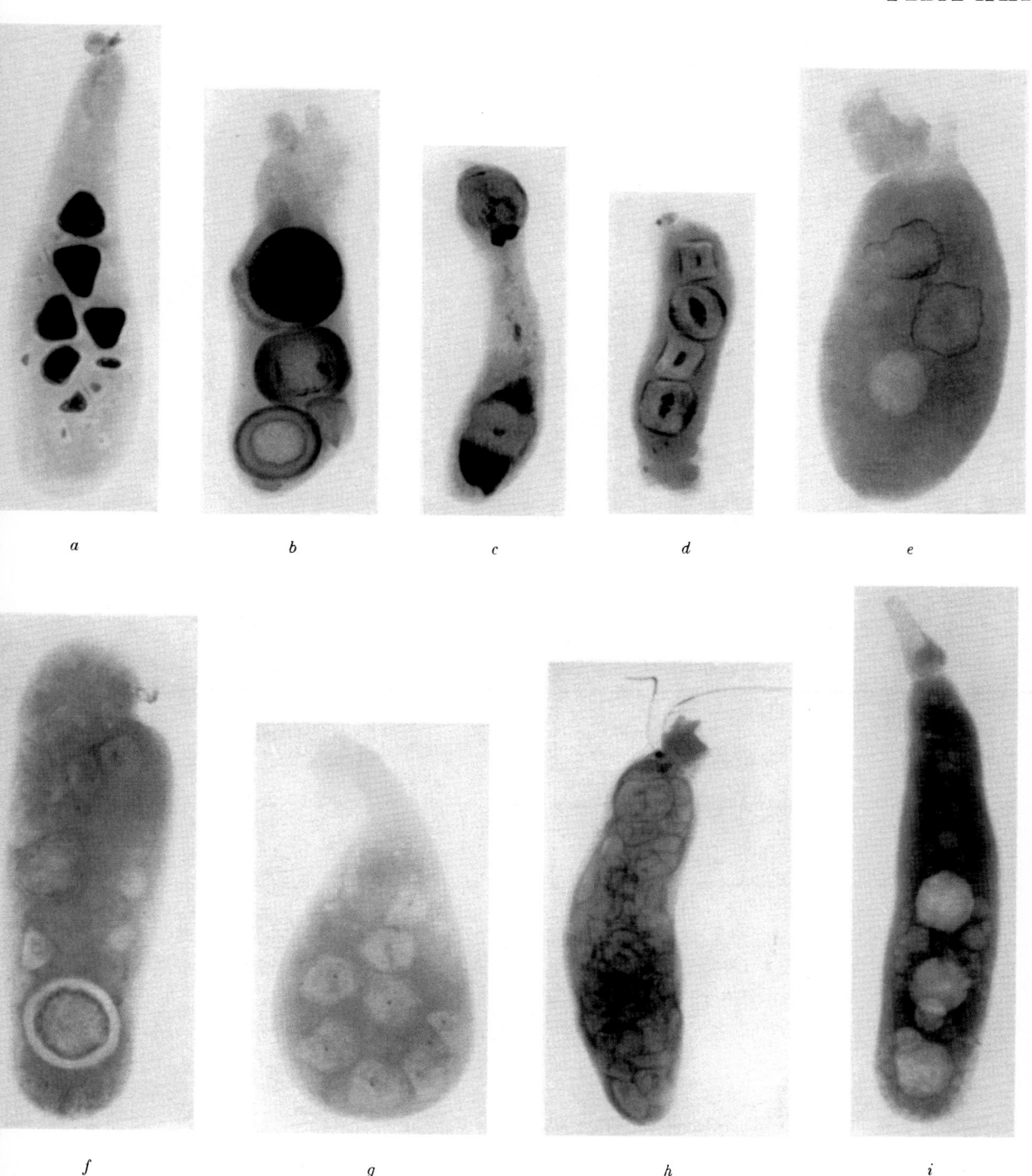

a

b

c

d

e

f

g

h

i

Fig. 278. Radiographs of excised gall-bladders. See text, pp. 325 to 327.
(Contributed by L. A. Rowden.)

deposit. The indications suggest damage to the mucous membrane after the first two were formed and the subsequent deposit of other stones until the gall-bladder was completely filled. The control film failed to reveal the thin lime deposit on the stones. The gall-bladder could not be filled by cholecystography, as the walls were somewhat fibrotic and the gall-bladder was not functioning. There was therefore no indication of the presence of stones from the X-ray examination.

Plate fig. 278f. A gall-bladder filled with many cholesterol and two large composite stones. The structure of one of these is clearer than that of the other. A ring of lime salt surrounds the cholesterol and is in turn encased by it. These two cholesterol-centred stones were formed before the others; and lime deposit was laid down on them. Then there followed a period of inactivity in the gall-bladder; the cholesterol stones were formed in large numbers and the outer casing of cholesterol was laid down on the large stones. The mucous membrane was rather fibrotic but not entirely unhealthy.

Plate fig. 278g. In this specimen the mucous membrane was entirely healthy in appearance. About ten gall-stones were present and each had a minute lime salt centre. In this case there has possibly been an infection, e.g. typhoid, and gravel has been deposited about bacilli. Organisms have been cultivated from such stones. Recovery has been satisfactory but inactivity in the gall-bladder has led to the deposition of the cholesterol on these centres.

Plate fig. 278h. A gall-bladder with a dense atrophic wall and atrophied mucous membrane. It contained a multitude of stones, all made of cholesterol with just a trace of lime salt covering. It seems likely that there was a severe inflammatory condition from which the mucous membrane did not recover. The gall-bladder was thrown out of action at once and the inspissated bile soon deposited stones that filled the whole sac. Had the gall-bladder continued to function there would have been a more definite lime deposit over all the stones and probably an outer casing of cholesterol. The fact that there was something wrong could only be recognised by the failure of the gall-bladder to fill. Although the wall was so dense, it did not throw a shadow that could be detected.

Plate fig. 278i. In this specimen the mucous membrane was healthy and all the numerous stones of various sizes are of pure cholesterol. With cholecystography the large stones were detected; the gall-bladder did not give a good shadow because it contained so little bile, the cavity being occupied by the cholesterol stones. In such a case it is not possible to be sure whether the poor shadow is due to imperfect filling or to the presence of numerous cholesterol stones.

From the examination of several hundreds of gall-bladders removed surgically, it was found that gall-stones are single in 15 per cent. and multiple in 85 per cent. of cases. The more numerous the stones, the more probable is it that some of them will show calcium deposit. Of 100 excised gall-bladders that were obviously pathological, 70 per cent. for one reason or another could not conceivably have given a shadow with cholecystography; e.g. the cystic duct was obstructed, the gall-bladder was a fibrotic sac completely filled with stones, or the mucous membrane was completely atrophied.

PREPARATION OF THE PATIENT AND ADMINISTRATION OF THE SALT

The evolution of the technique to obtain the most satisfactory results with cholecystography has been gradual. At first the most reliable results were obtained by intravenous injection, but this had the disadvantage of involving a minor operation and in most clinics it has given place to the oral method of administration, which has now become so satisfactory that the intravenous method is reserved only for those cases in which the stomach is in such an irritable condition that the salt cannot be retained. To test the reliability of the oral method Kirklin (199) examined 250 patients in whom it had failed or given only a very faint gall-bladder outline. When the drug was given intravenously to these patients only 1 per cent. showed normal gall-bladder filling. He states that this is the usual ratio and he has therefore discarded the intravenous method as a routine.

The essential point in the success of cholecystography is that the salt shall be absorbed in sufficient quantity. This cannot happen if there is vomiting or catharsis. The method of administration should therefore aim at avoiding these troubles.

The Oral Method

Many variations of technique have been recommended; we are aware that the following is not in accord with standard practice, but we claim that it gives entirely satisfactory results.

Forty-eight hours before the test, a purgative is given, preferably colocynth and hyoscyamus, or a pill containing podophyllum, which tends to stimulate the liver and empty the gall-bladder. On the following day the control films are taken (the direct method of examination). At least two are exposed, with slight variations of kilovoltage. These should be carefully examined before any further procedure is undertaken, in order that the nature of any doubtful shadows may be cleared up. If necessary, films are exposed in the lateral position, and occasionally a fluoroscopic examination with palpation may be helpful. In some cases, perhaps 10 per cent., this may be all that is necessary and no cholecystography will be needed.

The patient should go into a nursing home after this preliminary, or control, examination and in the evening should have a full meal. Kirklin (199) insists that this meal should be as fat-free as possible. As the result of extensive tests, he claims that if fatty foods are allowed, a very definite number of normal gall-bladders will not be visualised. In fact, during the comparative trials he made, he found that the number of non-filling gall-bladders and incorrect deductions rose by 25 per cent. He therefore eliminated all fat from this meal and his accurate diagnoses rose to well over 90 per cent. as checked by operation. His arguments are so convincing that we have no hesitation in recommending that the meal immediately preceding the giving of the salt should be fat-free. Half an hour after the meal, the patient is given a drachm of sodium bicarbonate in a quantity of water to neutralise the free acid in the stomach.

The salt is then given. The keratin-covered capsules, that were at one time advised to avoid gastric irritation, are not now recommended, as they are apt to deteriorate and sometimes remain undissolved in the intestine. Dr Rowden employs ordinary No. 3 gelatine capsules, which he himself fills in order that he may be certain that the rather unstable salt is fresh and that it has not had time to affect the solubility of the capsules. With this technique it is rare to find much salt unabsorbed, and undissolved capsules are never seen. The quantity of salt used is up to 4 g., according to the weight of the patient, and this goes into twelve or sixteen capsules. The patient lies on the right side as far as possible and takes about four capsules every quarter of an hour, washing them down with water. As the stomach empties most rapidly from a half to one and a half hours after a full meal, the capsules will probably pass into the small intestine unruptured and thus obviate any tendency to nausea and vomiting. If the capsules do rupture in the stomach, some of the salt is likely to be precipitated by the gastric juice and become insoluble. After the drug, Dr Rowden gives one-sixth of a grain of morphia, in the form of a tablet placed under the tongue. With this technique restlessness is prevented and vomiting is uncommon and, in any event, generally does not occur until the salt has left the stomach. The morphia has the added advantage that it retards the action of the bowels and thus promotes absorption. If the films show more than a very small amount of the salt passing through the intestine, it is evidence that the absorption is incomplete: either the salt or the technique is unsatisfactory.

Many workers prefer to administer the drug in fluid form. The salt is mixed up in a glassful of grape juice, orange juice or even ordinary effervescent mineral water, and is not distasteful to most patients. Kirklin uses a uniform quantity for all patients, i.e. 4 g. dissolved in 30 c.c. of distilled water. This is mixed with any of the above excipients and the whole dose is given immediately after the fat-free meal.

In a recent paper on cholecystography (201) he says that the intravenous method has been superseded in North America by the oral method, since the latter is easy, safe and efficient. The salt is given in solution to ensure absorption and in a palatable vehicle, after a full meal so that it does not cause nausea, vomiting or purging. Grape-juice is agreeable to most patients and well disguises the taste. Fats are withheld temporarily. The test has been applied to over sixty thousand patients at the Mayo Clinic and has proved extremely reliable.

In most cases the drug begins to be excreted into the gall-bladder in about fourteen hours, and to be fairly well concentrated two hours later. Arrangements should therefore be so timed that films are taken at fourteen and eighteen hours. There does not appear to be any advantage in radiographing either before fourteen or after eighteen hours, unless for special reasons. After the first film has been taken, showing that the gall-bladder is receiving the salt, Kirklin recommends very strongly that a full meal, rich in fats, shall be given. The object of this is not to determine the rate of discharge, which has no clinical significance, since any gall-bladder which can accept the salt is capable of discharging it. The value of the fatty meal is that it produces more active concentration and contraction of the gall-bladder, and so gives information as to the contractile power and shows up a gall-bladder that is inherently non-contractile. Moreover, by concentrating the shadow it renders stones and papillomata more clearly visible.

The Intravenous Method

The preparation for the intravenous injection is the same as for the oral. Up to 4 g. of the salt, dissolved in distilled water, is usually injected into the median basilic vein in front of the elbow. It is wise to withdraw a little blood into the syringe to make certain that the needle is in the vein, for considerable damage may be brought about if the injection flows into the tissues. As the absorption is more rapid than by the oral method, the gall-bladder is outlined earlier and the films are exposed at eight, ten and twelve hours.

Cholangiography

Saralegui (289) has described a technique of injecting the biliary ducts with thorotrast after operation. The salt is injected warm through a drainage tube under fluoroscopic control. No ill-effects ensue and calculi are clearly revealed —in some cases when they have not been discovered at operation.

Radiographic Technique

In no sphere of radiology is the highest standard and most meticulous accuracy of technique more important. Slip-shod and thoughtless methods that produce any type of radiogram will not suffice. Accuracy of results can only be obtained by an absolutely standardised technique which can be repeated at will. For various reasons, mostly inherent in the apparatus, this was until recent years only possible in the hands of very highly skilled radiologists who specialised in this work. To-day, there is no reason why any worker should not develop a satisfactory technique provided he has reasonably adequate apparatus at his disposal. The greatest difficulty in standardisation with which the radiologist has had to contend in the past has been the fluctuation in the voltage of the supply. Nowadays, the addition of a stabiliser will remedy this, and he can be sure that, with a certain setting, he will obtain a definite and uniform result which can be repeated at any time, and varied within the narrow range that makes for success or failure in patients of varying radio-density, for even patients of the same size are not necessarily of equal opacity. Hence, for the first films that are exposed, some variation, either in the time of exposure or in the kilovoltage, should be a standard routine, and a note should be made of the setting which gives the best diagnostic result, so that it can be employed in all subsequent exposures in this case. In general terms, that setting will be most satisfactory which gives just sufficient penetration with the minimum kilovoltage. Instantaneous exposures would be an advantage but all that is necessary is that there shall be no movement during the exposure, which can therefore be as long as three seconds. The photographic technique must be standardised.

Certain small points are important in the actual taking of the radiograms. The patient must lie on his face, and if he is not made comfortable he is apt to be unsteady and to move. His head should be on a pillow and turned to one side, and

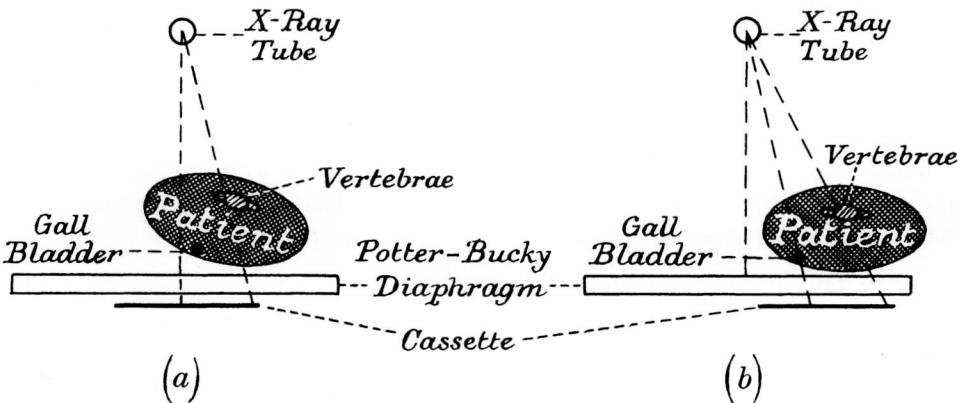

Fig. 279. Diagrams to illustrate position for obtaining obliquity: (a) by rotating the patient; (b) by decentring the patient and the cassette.

he should have a pillow under his legs. He must stop breathing during the exposures; some patients have to be taught to do this, and before a film is exposed the radiographer should invariably see that the patient is able to check his respiration entirely when so instructed. Even intelligent people sometimes have to be made to keep the mouth closed and to pinch the nose in order to stop respiration.

The phase of respiration is also important. Most patients find it much easier to hold the breath and keep absolutely still in *unforced expiration* than in the phase of strained full inspiration which is so commonly employed. A compressor band across the back is very helpful and should always be used.

In order to be certain that the shadow of the gall-bladder is not overlapped by that of the vertebrae, it is customary to rotate the patient slightly (Fig. 279a). This, however, is not necessary, except with the curved type of Potter-Bucky diaphragm, for the same object can be attained by decentring the patient and the cassette laterally (Fig. 279b). If costal calcification gives shadows that overlap the gall-bladder, the patient and the cassette can be moved downwards away from the central ray. This method of obtaining slight obliquity is much preferable to rotating the patient, as the position can be reproduced easily and exactly.

Since the position of the gall-bladder varies considerably, it is customary to use 12 × 10 films for the first exposures, but when its position is known, 10 × 8 films are employed, with a small cone diaphragm localiser which, even with the Potter-Bucky diaphragm, improves the quality of the film. Radiographs taken in the lateral position are occasionally of value in the rare case of more or less solid lime-salt stones. Gall-stones that only show faintly in the ordinary films will not be detected at all in lateral films. Fluoroscopy, combined with palpation, is also occasionally of value in the same class of case.

THE DIAGNOSIS OF GALL-STONES

The illustrations in this chapter are of selected cases, chosen because the points are readily seen. In practice, the average shadow on which a diagnosis is made is much less distinct and the films must be examined with meticulous care. Such films, however, are not suitable for reproduction and the beginner must realise that he cannot often expect to see such definite outlines.

A. *The Direct Method* (Plate figs. 280–282)

Interpretation of gall-bladder films calls for the best possible conditions, both of illumination and of time and concentration. There is a tendency to overlook the importance of careful and systematic examination of the control films. Some radiologists merely glance at them, relying on cholecystography to give all the information. A great deal can be learned from the direct films, but they need careful study. Sometimes the indefinite shadows of mixed stones that are just detected on the direct films are completely lost in cholecystography, for they are just too dense to show as less transradiant areas.

The control films should also be studied for any indication of the gall-bladder outline. This may be shown up by air in the intestine, but if it can be detected apart from air, there is very strong presumptive evidence that the gall-bladder is pathological. Areas of calcification in the rib cartilages should be noted and, if possible, other films should be exposed in such a way that these shadows will be thrown away from the gall-bladder.

The pure cholesterol stone is so much less dense than the surrounding tissues that large ones may occasionally be detected as less opaque areas by direct radiography. The ring shadow cast by a layer of lime salt deposited round a cholesterol centre is almost typical, but I have seen renal stones that gave the same type of shadow. About 10 per cent. of gall-stones contain sufficient lime salt to give a recognisable shadow. A small proportion are so dense that they are easily seen on the fluorescent screen. They may be mistaken for *renal calculi*

PLATE XXII

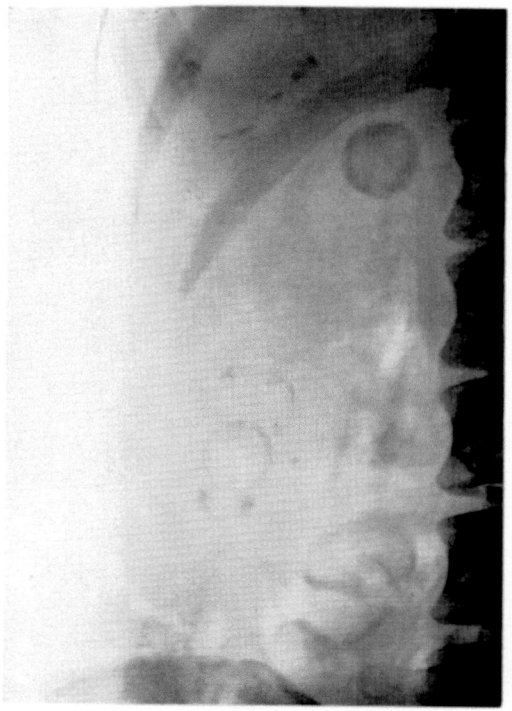

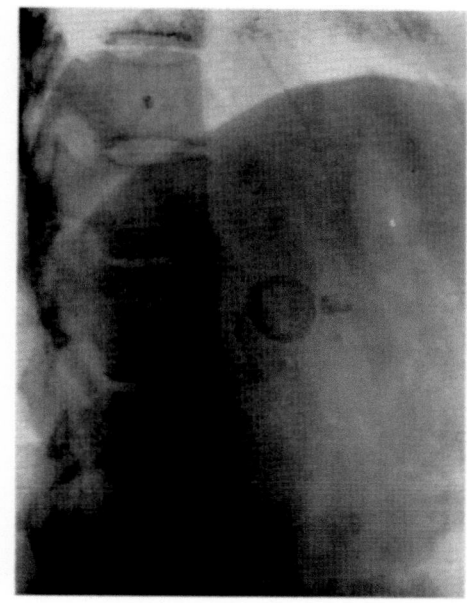

Fig. 280

Fig. 281

Figs. 280, 281. Radiographs showing ring type of shadow seen in the antero-posterior and lateral views without cholecystography. (Contributed by L. A. Rowden.)

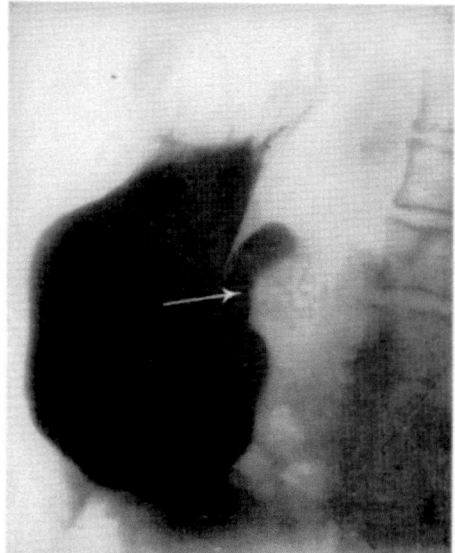

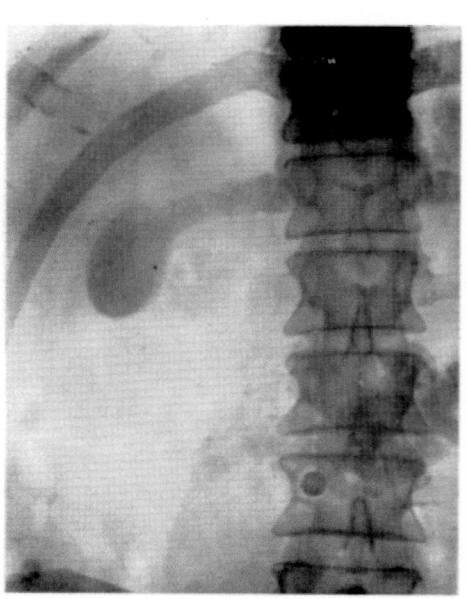

Fig. 282. Collection of negative type of stones in lateral view without administration of the dye. Apparently each of the numerous stones is coated with lime salt. (Contributed by Arial W. George.)

Fig. 283. Gall-bladder shown by cholecystography. (Contributed by L. A. Rowden.)

but, if they are visible on the screen, it is easy to make the differential diagnosis by palpation, for the gall-stone is relatively near the anterior abdominal wall and is quite freely movable. A lateral radiograph will show it well in front of the vertebral column, whereas a renal stone lies farther back and its shadow is superimposed on that of the vertebrae. A film taken in the prone position will give a smaller shadow than one taken in the supine position, for the stone will be nearer to the film. Conversely, the renal stone will be larger in a film taken with the patient lying on his face. Another method of obtaining the same information is to localise the stone by the ordinary triangulation method. Those who have had war experience will probably find this less confusing. But perhaps the most satisfactory technique is to expose two films, one in full inspiration and the other in full expiration, and note the relative movements of the renal outline and the shadow of the stone.

Calcareous glands are not frequently met with in the gall-bladder region. They are usually in the mesentery and freely movable. The calcification is irregularly disposed and spotty. The position of the shadow, even without compression, is not constant and the shadow may even have disappeared out of the picture when another film is exposed.

Dr Rowden has examined 50 *rib cartilages* post mortem, and finds that their shadows never curve upwards but invariably downwards. In incompletely encased gall-stones the convexity is very frequently upwards. But the main diagnostic point is the movement of rib shadows on respiration.

Pancreatic stones are very rare and I should imagine that, although difficult to differentiate from renal stones, their position far back in the abdomen would negative the diagnosis of gall-stone.

A number of other conditions might be mistaken for gall-stones but are usually easily excluded, e.g. foreign bodies, opaque objects in the clothing, faecal masses and cutaneous papillomata.

B. *Cholecystography* (Plate figs. 283–284)

The pre-requisites for satisfactory filling of the gall-bladder by cholecystography are

(1) That the salt circulates in the blood in sufficient quantity.

(2) That the liver is functioning actively and excreting the salt.

(3) That the mucous membrane of the gall-bladder is sufficiently healthy to concentrate its contents.

(*a*) If the gall-bladder fills and concentrates the salt satisfactorily,

(1) the liver is functioning,

(2) the cystic duct is patent,

(3) the gall-bladder mucous membrane is at least more or less healthy.

(*b*) A faint but definite gall-bladder shadow indicates

(1) that the liver is functioning,

(2) that the cystic duct is not occluded,

(3) that the gall-bladder is either packed with stones or capable of dealing only with a small quantity of bile and incapable of concentrating it.

One of the chief troubles in interpretation is to determine whether or not a weak gall-bladder shadow is due to defective filling. It is quite likely to be due to insufficient absorption of the salt: perhaps the patient has vomited, or there is diarrhoea, or the salt is not satisfactory and is seen in unduly large quantities in the intestine. In all such cases a confirmatory examination should be undertaken after an interval of a week.

(*c*) If the gall-bladder does not fill and the salt is not found in excess in the colon and the radiologist is confident of every detail of the technique, there is almost certainly a pathological condition. This may be hepatic disorder, in which case jaundice would be likely; obstruction of the cystic duct; or a definitely pathological gall-bladder that is neither receiving nor concentrating the bile. Brailsford[67] has exposed an important fallacy. For some unknown reason the gall-bladder fails to fill in a certain number of cases of gastric and duodenal ulcer and the diagnosis of gall-bladder disease is incorrect. He argues from the cases he reports that every failure to obtain a satisfactory gall-bladder shadow should be followed by an opaque meal examination.

The density of the shadow obtained by cholecystography varies within wide limits but, in general, the densest concentration is noted in thin subjects and, unfortunately from the radiologist's point of view, the shadow is weakest and least concentrated in stout subjects. Perhaps there is a definite association between obesity and the power of the gall-bladder to concentrate the bile.

The size of the gall-bladder as seen by cholecystography does not vary very greatly. It is seldom larger than a hen's egg and the usual size is about that of a pigeon's egg. Very small ones are not frequent and are usually pathological; even if they do accept the dye they take such small quantities that it does not cast a recognisable shadow. The large type of gall-bladder is not seen because it is usually associated with cystic duct obstruction and the bile that carries the salt does not get into it.

The shape and position vary considerably. In tall, thin women it tends to be elongated and to occupy a lower position than that described in the anatomical text-books. It may even be found below the crest of the ilium and overlapping the sacro-iliac synchondrosis, very occasionally to the left of the vertebrae. In short, thick-set men it is more globular and may be found as high as the 11th or even the 10th rib (cf. p. 101).

Cholesterol or other stones of lesser density than the concentrated salt in the gall-bladder, if sufficiently large—say a quarter of an inch in diameter—will

PLATE XXIII

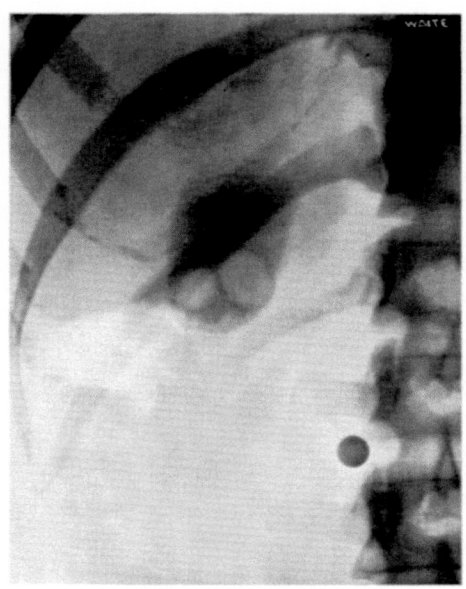

Fig. 284. Gall-bladder with indirect cholecystography, with two large cholesterol stones showing as clear areas (negative shadows). (Contributed by L. A. Rowden.)

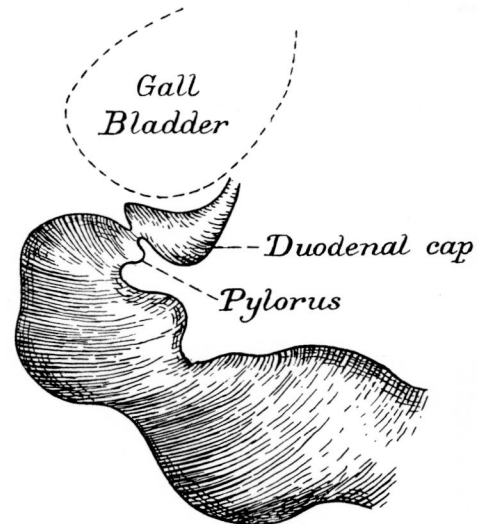

Fig. 285. Diagram showing the type of deformity due to pressure of the gall-bladder on the duodenal cap.

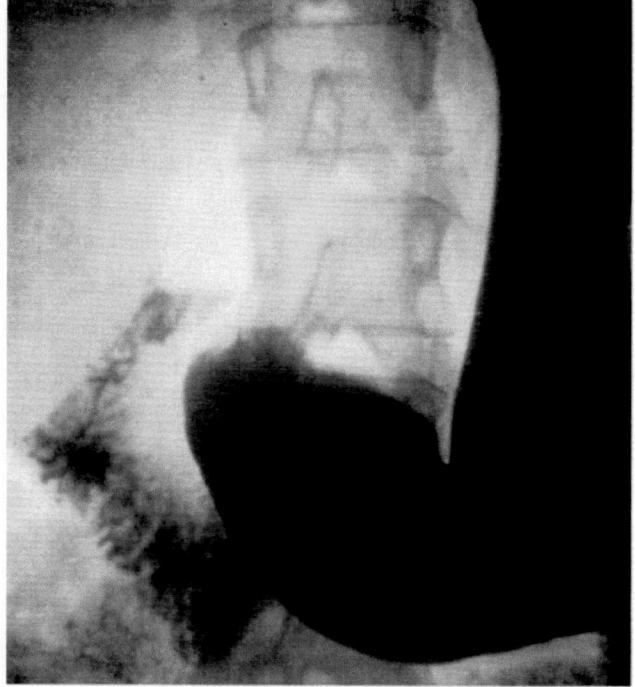

Fig. 286. Dunce cap effect. (Contributed by L. A. Rowden.))

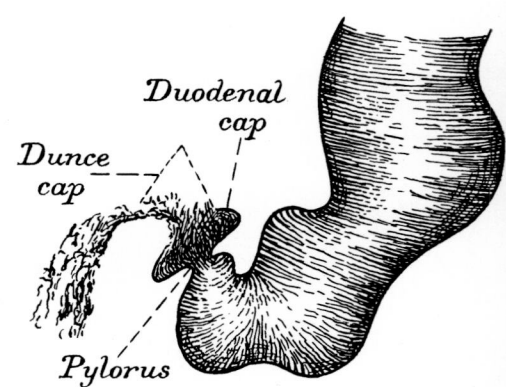

Fig. 287. Diagram to illustrate the dunce cap effect: a tag of duodenum is drawn up by an adhesion from the gall-bladder. In this a pocket of air is held.

appear as lighter areas in the midst of the gall-bladder shadow. These are often called "negative shadows", a term that we dislike but for which we have no alternative. The presence of numerous non-opaque stones occupying the greater part of the gall-bladder is indicated by a mottled appearance with fairly sharply defined outlines, i.e. the gall-bladder is fairly well defined although its contents do not give a heavy shadow. In such cases, the control films will possibly reveal a very ill-defined and almost imperceptible shadow of the gall-bladder and its contents. Stones that contain considerable proportions of lime salt will be more readily detected on the control films and are more likely to be completely obliterated by the salt in the gall-bladder.

Bubbles of air in the intestine may simulate filling defects in the gall-bladder shadow but are not likely to occupy the same position in other radiographs. Knutsson (209), however, has reported two cases in which perforation of a duodenal ulcer gave rise to an occluded collection of gas that was superimposed on the gall-bladder shadow. In one of them it led to a very excusable error in diagnosis.

The Significance of Gall-stones in a Gall-bladder that is functioning satisfactorily

The powers of recovery in the gall-bladder appear to be considerable. In the past there has been a definite tendency in surgical and radiological literature to regard the presence of stones in the gall-bladder as a definite indication for operation. It seems to us, however, that if cholecystography gives a satisfactory filling there is very strong presumptive evidence that the gall-bladder is functioning quite satisfactorily, whether it contains stones or not; the stones are merely indications of past irregularities and do not necessarily call for operative treatment. We suggest that the presence of gall-stones of any kind associated with good filling constitutes an indication for medical treatment, with periodic radiographic control tests. The stones are doubtless a source of danger in that they are foreign bodies which are apt to aggravate any inflammatory or other disturbance, but this does not constitute a sufficient justification for operation without a clinical history of repeated attacks.

INDICATIONS FROM THE OPAQUE MEAL

Gastric disturbances are common in disorders of the gall-bladder. Duodenal irritability is frequent and delay in the stomach is also noted but, apart from the following occasional signs, nothing definite is found.

The gall-bladder is in close relationship with the duodenum and if enlarged it may press upon the cap and produce a rather characteristic deformity (Plate fig. 285).

Adhesions about the gall-bladder may also produce distortions of the duodenum that are very similar to the persistent deformity of duodenal ulcer and cicatrisation; in fact, unless the crater of the ulcer can be recognised, it is often impossible to distinguish one from the other. By palpation, it may be possible to show that the duodenum is unduly fixed towards the gall-bladder region. A deformity that Dr Rowden has likened to a dunce's cap (Plate fig. 286) is produced by an adhesion dragging up a tag on the upper surface of the junction of the first and second parts of the duodenum. This is seen as a conical air space above the site of the duodenal cap.

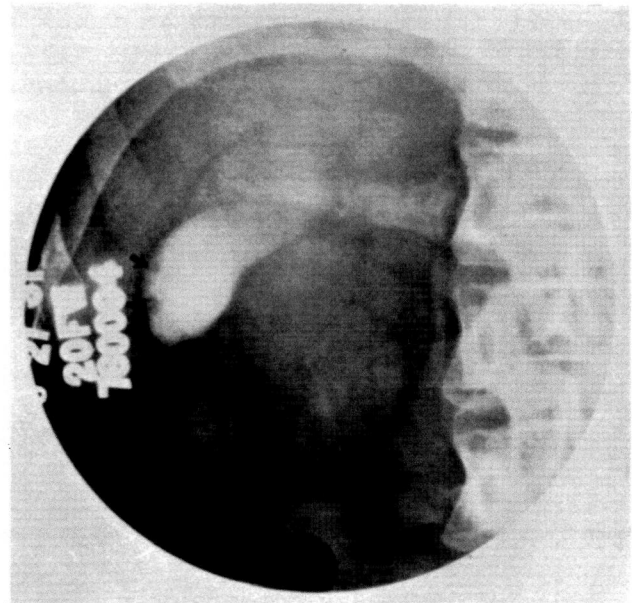

Fig. 288. Two papillomas cf the gall-bladder. (Contributed by B. R. Kirklin.)

The transverse colon is also sometimes tucked up to the gall-bladder by adhesions, a fact that can be detected by palpation.

OTHER CONDITIONS OF THE GALL-BLADDER

Papillomata of the gall-bladder are probably not very rare, but have only recently been recognised. A typical case is shown in Fig. 288. Caylor and Bollman[93] have shown that gall-bladders with hypertrophic rugae, which are frequently associated with papillomas, produce the greatest concentration of bile.

Primary carcinoma of the gall-bladder is rare. Dr Rowden has only met it twice. In one of these cases two large stones were detected by the direct method, and in the other the gall-bladder failed to fill with cholecystography. In neither was there any radiographic indication of the growth. Walters and Olsen [328] have reported fifty cases of papillary colloid adenocarcinoma of the extrahepatic bile ducts. They were of two types, squamous cell carcinoma and adenocarcinoma. It appears from these figures, therefore, that primary carcinoma arising in the biliary passages is perhaps not so rare as we are accustomed to believe.

Duodenal ulcer perforating into the biliary passages, producing an internal biliary fistula, is very rare. I have seen no case myself but have been shown three by different observers in this country (cf. p. 249). Gråberger [138] describes a case and gives a number of references to others that have been published.

APPENDICES

APPENDIX I

THE ORGANISATION AND EQUIPMENT OF AN X-RAY DEPARTMENT

As a chapter on apparatus and organisation seemed necessary but did not find a suitable place in the text, it has been relegated to this appendix, which is abstracted, with additions, from a paper written by request for the Rockefeller Foundation, and published by them in "Methods and Problems of Medical Education, XIIth Series, 1929".

General principles have become standardised, but apparatus still goes out of date very rapidly. For instance, coil sets are now entirely obsolete and the mechanical rectification of transformer sets has given place to valve rectification; the self-protected type of hot-cathode tube has displaced the older types, and it and its leads are now nearly always made shock-proof by being enclosed in earthed metal casings. Moreover, "deep" X-ray therapy has now found its place in every properly equipped department—sometimes, most unfortunately, when the adequate supervision of an experienced radiologist is not available.

The Essentials of an X-ray Department

A radiologist seldom has a free hand in planning an X-ray department. Most installations are limited by economic conditions such as finance or available space. Certain points are obvious to the radiologist but are not appreciated by the layman, and frequently not even by his medical colleagues. If money is presented or collected for an X-ray department the managers naturally wish to accept it, and are apt to overlook one or more of the following three essential conditions:

1. A properly trained radiologist is absolutely essential; no elaboration of equipment can fulfil its purpose without such a man.

2. The radiologist must have adequate facilities of space, apparatus and time in which to do the work.

3. The department must be planned and equipped with a view to the work it will be called upon to handle.

That these three cardinal points are not fully appreciated is very evident. One often finds a competent radiologist forced to work in unsafe conditions and with equipment utterly inadequate for the work. On the other hand, one is sometimes confronted with a beautifully equipped department which, owing to the absence of a competent radiologist, is of hardly any value. In many instances, also, apparatus has been installed that is quite unnecessary, e.g. an expensive localiser for foreign bodies in the eye in a small country cottage hospital, where perhaps one such case would be seen in five years!

Provisions for a Radiologist

The problem of providing a radiologist is frequently a very difficult one, particularly in the smaller centres where there is a population of 10,000–20,000. There is not, and probably never will be, sufficient work for a whole-time specialist, and it usually happens that one of the staff of the local hospital, a general practitioner, undertakes the work. The outfit is used not only for the hospital cases but also for the convenience of the local practitioners, and it serves a useful purpose, up to a point which depends on the efficiency and self-sacrifice of the man who undertakes the work. More often than not, in this country, this man does the work in an honorary capacity or for some small honorarium which offers no inducement to equip himself for his responsibilities in an adequate manner, even if he has the necessary time and energy at his disposal after he has done that part of the day's work on which he depends for his livelihood. The arrangement of making a small charge for radiographs in public institutions is a thoroughly bad one, for the public imagines that it is paying for a very different class of service from that which is actually rendered. Without a medical man specially trained in X-ray interpretation,* the utility of the department is limited to the simplest applications of the science. Managers of small hospitals accept these small fees as a relief to set against the heavy working expenses. They do not take into account the capital outlay and other standing charges that are borne by the institution. The moral effect of a small charge for X-ray pictures made in public institutions makes progress impossible. No radiologist could make a living in competition with such a system, for, in private practice, the overhead charges of capital and rent, in addition to working costs, make low fees an impossibility. It is therefore very highly advisable from every point of view, especially when private patients are seen in public institutions, that a reasonable fee should be charged for all private work that is undertaken. Unless this is done, it is impossible to provide a satisfactory reward for the radiologist, who must put in a great deal of time, not only in the actual work but travelling to meetings and to see the work in other centres. It is only by so doing that he can keep up to date. The most satisfactory solution is to employ a well-trained radiographer,† who will make the X-ray plates, and to pay an

---

* Diplomas in medical radiology are granted by the Universities of Cambridge (9 months), Liverpool (6 months) and Edinburgh (9 months), and by the Conjoint Board (9 months). They are post-graduate courses and are open to all who hold a medical qualification approved by the responsible committee or board.

† The Society of Radiographers (c/o The British Institute of Radiology, 32 Welbeck Street, W. 1) undertakes the training and examination of candidates for membership in the society. Successful candidates are entitled to the M.S.R. Certificate. A course of training is also supplied by Guy's Hospital. This does not in any way qualify the radiographer to undertake the purely medical work of interpretation, and, in fact, there is an undertaking to refrain from attempting to do so.

honorarium to an experienced visiting radiologist who should attend as necessary for the screen examination, reporting and supervision. For private cases, ordinary consulting-room fees should be charged and divided between the radiologist and the hospital in such a way that the working expenses are covered. It is a first principle that no hospital which depends upon charitable or State contributions should make profit from medical services rendered to any patient. In a number of cases the hospital takes one-third and the radiologist two-thirds of all fees that come above the estimated working and overhead expenses.

For certain specialised branches, particularly those in association with tuberculosis schemes, the most satisfactory method is that the X-ray work should be centralised and that one of the medical officers should take a diploma in radiology and become responsible for this very important side of the work.

Staffing an X-ray Department

The staff required for an X-ray department is suggested in Table I. These are my own ideas and many will criticise them, some from the point of view of generosity, others claiming that the staff is insufficient. The point that must be kept in mind, however, is that the X-ray department is a means to an end and not the end itself. Its function is to supply X-ray information as and when necessary for the needs of the hospital and not as and when convenient to the members of the radiological staff. Consequently, no matter what arrangements are made, the work must be done in rushes at times, and it is for these times that the department must cater or risk holding up the work of the hospital.

The staff must be permanent and, in order to avoid monotony, assistants should if possible work round the different duties so that they become interchangeable. This is a feature of especial value during holiday months. In some hospitals the matron is inclined to attempt to give some training in the X-ray department as a routine procedure, the nurses doing this work for perhaps three months, by which time they have probably just learned how to keep out of the way of those who are doing the actual work. Temporary assistance hampers the work and leads to unnecessary "repeats" and a general low standard.

The problem of staffing an X-ray department is a universal one. The following is from the pen of Case:*

"There are in the United States and Canada something like 2000 hospitals of fifty beds or more. Are there available 2000 physicians with special training in roentgenologic work to take charge of the roentgen-ray services in these hospitals? In the evident absence of any such number of available roentgenologists, it is recognised that in small hospitals, especially those situated in the smaller communities, no physician is

* "The fundamental requirements of an efficient roentgen-ray service in hospitals." *Journal of the American Medical Association*, 1924, LXXXII, 2071.

available, however ideal it would be to have one. The staff members send their patients for roentgenologic study, each reading his own film records, and making his own fluoroscopic studies, if, indeed, any are made.

"It is manifestly impossible and unthinkable to permit or expect anyone but a physician to undertake the interpretations of the roentgen-ray findings with any hope of transmitting to the clinician all the help which the roentgen-ray is capable of giving.... the usefulness of anyone but a graduate physician for roentgen-ray interpretation is steadily decreasing. Even in the small community, where nowadays each physician makes his own interpretations, it would be not only ideal but in thorough sympathy with the principle of hospital standardisation and mutual co-operation between physicians thereby involved, if the agreement could be reached that one of the physicians in the community should devote special attention to roentgen interpretation and act as consultant in this capacity....

"A hospital of 150 beds or more should not be considered completely staffed without a physician-roentgenologist who devotes full time to his work. He may devote his services to more than one hospital, but his major time and thought should be devoted to perfecting himself in his roentgenologic work and to reaching out into new lines of roentgen-ray development. He may spend only a few hours a day in the hospital and the rest of his time in his office outside the hospital; or the hospital may wisely arrange for his private work to be conducted in the institution. Still larger hospitals should have the full-time services of a physician-roentgenologist. Especially in this type of institution the roentgenologist may advantageously combine his roentgen-ray work with radium therapy and the various surgical procedures that are more commonly involved in the application of radium."

TABLE I. *Staffing an X-ray Department*

Duties	Large General Hospital with Teaching School	Large General Hospital	General Hospital up to 200 beds	General Hospital up to 60 beds	Cottage Hospital
General organisation and teaching	2 honorary medical officers	1 honorary medical officer	1 honorary medical officer	1 honorary medical officer	1 honorary medical officer
Fluoroscopic examinations					
Reporting	2 junior medical officers	1 junior medical officer			
Prescribing treatment					
Physics of the X-ray department	1 physicist (part time)				
Radiography	3 radiographers	2 radiographers	1 radiographer	1 radiographer	
Repairs to apparatus	1 mechanic				
X-ray treatment, ordinary	3 assistants	2 assistants	1 assistant		
X-ray treatment, intensive					
Developing, etc.	1 photographer				1 nurse who is trained in radiography
Prints, lantern-slides	1 photographer (with librarian duties)	1 photographer			
Clerical work (museum)					
Clerical work (routine)	3 clerks	2 clerks			
Responsible for the department	1 sister	1 sister	1 sister	1 nurse	
Attending to patients	2 nurses	1 nurse			
Cleaning	1 charwoman	1 charwoman	1 nurse		
Porterage	1 porter	1 porter			

The first object must be to attempt to classify the institutions in which X-ray departments are necessary, and indicate the general outline on which a suitable department should be planned and organised.

Commencing with the smallest radiological unit and working upwards, we have:

1. The cottage hospital and its private counterpart—the room of the practitioner who does some radiology in addition to other medical work.

2. The small hospital of anything up to sixty beds and its private counterpart—the consulting rooms of the radiological specialist.

3. The middle-sized hospital of 200–300 beds with its counterpart—the small clinic of two radiological specialists working together.

4. The large general hospital and its counterpart in private practice—the radiological clinic.

5. The large general hospital to which a teaching school is attached.

In addition, there are the departments in the hospitals for skin, teeth, urogenital and orthopaedic surgery, and last, but not least in growing importance, the tuberculosis dispensaries. With these, however, I do not propose to deal, except to emphasise the importance of supplying adequate ventilation for all X-ray rooms, particularly those devoted to screen examinations of the chest. The possibility of infection is greatly increased in a small unventilated room.

Housing the Department

There are three factors that play a big part in the planning of a new department: (1) the estimated cost, (2) the space available and (3) the fact that, no matter how small the outfit installed, it will be expected to fulfil all the functions of an extensive equipment. The cottage hospital usually recognises its limitations and knows that it is not capable of undertaking every class of work, such as major operations, yet the X-ray department, once installed, is expected to deal with anything and everything. Hence the outfit in a small hospital has to perform many functions, with the result that, in order to fulfil all requirements, it consists of a series of compromises and additions, "gadgets" by which alone it is able, with considerable waste of time, to meet most demands. It is analogous in fact to the amateur's workshop which is used for carpentry, metal-work, forge, and every other job of the handy man, from snobbing boots to making a wireless outfit. The efficiency of the small workshop and the small X-ray department depends first on the ingenuity of the worker in making the best of difficult circumstances and of a shortage of the special tools, and secondly on the fact that he is engaged on only one kind of work at a time. In the small cottage hospital compromise and makeshift are unavoidable, for, in spite of the inadequacy of the equipment, the outfit may be called upon to do practically anything within the whole range of radiology. Fortunately, however, another factor comes in, i.e. the small number of cases dealt with and the consequent time available for re-arrangement of apparatus.

For the cottage hospital, therefore, one room for all X-ray purposes and its adjacent dark room may fulfil the requirements.

When, however, we come to the small general hospital of sixty to one hundred beds with an out-patient department, radiographic and treatment work will each be in progress the greater part of the day, necessitating separate rooms. Possibly two sets of apparatus for treatment will be required. Coming to the larger general hospital, with its more numerous out-patients, we find sub-division is again necessary for, on the radiographic side, the work goes on so persistently that there is no time for the fluoroscopic examinations to be done in the same room. Hence a screening room must be added. In addition, it will be necessary to add more accommodation for X-ray treatment, and possibly four sets of apparatus will have to be installed for the purpose.

The provision of accommodation for intensive X-ray treatment (deep X-ray therapy) must be considered. It is an axiom that no intensive X-ray installation should even be considered in a hospital where the whole-time services of a well-qualified medical X-ray officer are not available. Until such time as we know more of the value and risks of maximum doses of radiations of extreme penetration, this treatment must be under the closest supervision of a medical officer. The provision of this type of apparatus in small hospitals, especially when there is not a thoroughly efficient medical officer in charge, is certain to lead to disastrous results, such as have already brought discredit on one of the very few forces that we can call to our aid in the war against malignant disease. In my view, not only in the interests of public safety but also in the interests of radiology, this form of treatment, and, in fact, of all X-ray treatment, should be under licence of some kind—as it already is in France and Italy.

The last class of department is that necessary for a teaching hospital, in which there is not only the large volume of routine work of the general hospital, but in addition a continual demand for the special work that is essential in a hospital where every new idea must be tested out, where the medical and surgical staffs are, or should be, engaged in original investigation in which the assistance of the X-ray department may be essential, where records are of the utmost importance both for teaching and investigation, where undergraduate students have to be given some grounding in the elements of radiology, and where it may be necessary to instruct the radiologists of the next generation. In short, it is a department where there will be constant inquiries and visitations in addition to the daily work—yet the routine work must go forward all the time. Moreover, if good work is to be done, the observer must be quite free from all these interruptions, for screen examinations and reporting are just as exacting as the most intricate surgical operation. The same concentration is necessary to secure good results. In fact, it is necessary to arrange the work so that one of the medical officers will be available to deal with all the inquiries from colleagues and students, and can demonstrate cases when necessary in a room where all the data and pictures for teaching purposes are at hand. For the sake of the collaboration which is so essential for the efficiency of X-ray work, the interest of colleagues must be studied and encouraged.

In the early days one set of apparatus had to be adjusted for all purposes, from the search for a pin to the treatment of cancer. In the cottage hospital this still applies. It means, however, that only a small number of cases can be dealt with if they vary much in character. The larger departments differ only in the fact that the numbers dealt with make it necessary to multiply the units, and since the units are multiplied, they are adapted permanently to one or other of the various types of work they will be called upon to perform, i.e. the compromise and makeshift that are necessary for an "all purpose" unit should disappear exactly in proportion to the number of outfits that are installed to cope with the work.

The desideratum list of rooms in a large X-ray department is as follows, and probably, as the work of an X-ray department increases, further sub-division will be necessary, especially in the larger teaching hospitals.

1. Ordinary radiographic room.
2. Second radiographic room for screening fractures and other special work.
3. Fluoroscopic screening room. If there is a large bulk of abdominal and chest work, a second screening room will be necessary.
4. Special room, a room where special cases (urography, ventriculography, etc.) can be carried on without interfering with the routine of the department.
5. Dark rooms.
6. Ordinary treatment rooms.
7. Intensive treatment rooms.
8. Medical officers' room.
9. Office.
10. Plate viewing room.
11. Nursing staff room.
12. Room for examining patients.
13. Film store-room.
14. Service room.
15. Waiting-hall.
16. Dressing rooms.
17. Workshop.
18. Lavatories.
19. Large demonstration room.

The following table will give an approximate idea of the way in which the work can be condensed into smaller space according to the size of the hospital.

TABLE II. *The Housing of an X-Ray Department*

(The figures in parentheses indicate the approximate floor space in superficial feet.*
No allowance is made for passage floor space.)

Large Hospital with Teaching School	*Large General Hospital*	*Hospital up to 200 beds*	*Hospital up to 60 beds*	*Cottage Hospital*
X-ray treatment (ordinary) (500)	X-ray treatment (ordinary) (400)	X-ray treatment (ordinary) (250)	X-ray treatment (ordinary) (150)	
X-ray treatment (intensive) (500)				
Radiographic room (ordinary) (250)	Radiographic room (250)			X-ray room (250)
Radiographic room (special) for screening (200)				
Screening room (ordinary) (350)	Screening room (350)	Radiographic room (250)	Radiographic room (250)	
Screening room (for serial plates, etc.) (170)				
Demonstration room (600)				
Medical officers' room (200)	Medical officers' room (130)			
Examining room (120)				
Office (180)	Office (130)			
Nurses' room (sewing, etc.) (180)		Office (130)		
Plate viewing room (130)				
Plate store-room (180)	Plate store-room (130)			
Service room (100)				
Laboratory (200)				
Dark rooms (350)	Dark rooms (250)	Dark room (100)	Dark room (100)	Dark room (80)
Waiting room (400)	Waiting room (350)	Waiting room (300)	Waiting room (150)	
Lavatories	Lavatories	Lavatories	Lavatories	
Workshop (150)	Workshop (150)			

* The following figures are quoted from the Report of the American College of Surgeons on Hospital Standardisation (1925):
Minimum floor space required: (a) For hospitals of from 50 to 100 beds, at least 400 sq. ft. (b) For hospitals of from 100 to 150 beds, at least 650 sq. ft. (c) For hospitals of 150 beds and up, 1200 to 3000 sq. ft.

Position of the X-ray Department

The position of an X-ray department in a hospital should be carefully considered. In order to save transport it should be so placed that it is central in relation to the departments from which most of the work will come. An analysis of the diagnostic cases in the Manchester Royal Infirmary in 1925 shows as follows:

Medical wards	...	...	...	...	2,089
Surgical wards	...	...	...	...	2,265
Out-patients	...	...	...	...	2,605
Accidents	...	...	...	...	4,091
Sundry	...	...	...	...	315
					11,365*

But even more important is a position convenient for the clinical staff of the hospital, for only by the closest possible co-operation with the clinician can the maximum efficiency of an X-ray department be attained. It seems to be fairly obvious that both from the administrative and the scientific and social intercourse standpoints, the proper position for an X-ray department is that which is most central.

Size of Rooms

The rooms should be as large as possible, within reason. An indication of the sizes suitable is given in Table II. The floor spaces suggested are, if anything, the minimum size, and I advise an addition of 30 per cent. if practicable. They should be lofty, dry, and well ventilated. Cellars are seldom, if ever, suitable.

A northern aspect for the windows of those rooms in which the medical officer works is an advantage in that the light is not so strong and it takes less time for his eyes to get into condition for screening.

Floors

The best material for floors is wood blocks. Boards, also, are quite satisfactory, but do not look well. Linoleum and rubber linoleum are not successful, as the castors of apparatus and beds sink into these materials. Concrete and other composition floors are not advisable owing to the increased danger of electrical shocks.

* The following are the figures of the total admissions to the hospital for the same period:

In-patients	...	...	...	11,047
Out-patients	...	...	...	17,722
Casualties	...	...	...	26,347
				55,116

In rather more than one in five of all admissions, therefore, the assistance of the X-ray department was called for in diagnosis. In the U.S.A., so far as I could judge, the proportion was on the whole higher, there being a strong tendency to refer every case to the X-ray department before any attempt was made to arrive at a diagnosis by clinical methods—an unfortunate tendency that is constantly increasing in this country also.

Ordered Sequence of Rooms

More often than not an X-ray department has to be fitted into an existing building, and it may be difficult to arrange the rooms, and the work within them, in a well-ordered sequence. This is a very important point and one which means much in efficiency, since the work moves smoothly forward all the time, and little going to and fro is necessary. Consequently a comparatively small department may be able to deal with a much larger number of cases than a bigger one in which this principle has not been considered. For example, in the old department at the Manchester Royal Infirmary the rooms all opened off one narrow "blind" corridor which was always blocked by waiting beds, and the work was carried on under great difficulties although dealing with comparatively small numbers. An outlet at the far end of this corridor would have made it possible to deal with fully half as many cases again.

Protective Material for Walls and Floors

It used to be held that the partition walls of an X-ray department, and also the floors and ceilings, if situated above or below occupied rooms, needed consideration even if these rooms were only used for diagnostic purposes.* Such protection is, however, superfluous except for the safety of photographic materials in the dark room. For this purpose three-pound lead is ample protection. The protection of the walls of cubicles in which X-ray treatment is carried on is another matter and is of course essential. The details of the protective values, method of building walls, etc., were given in the first edition of this book but are now omitted as they are readily available elsewhere.

Windows

The windows should be of ample size, for light and fresh air are essential for the health of the workers. Ordinary window glass, even the thinnest, is opaque to ultra-violet radiations, consequently that small quantity of ultra-violet radiation which reaches the earth is cut off. It is stated that by the use of vita glass these rays are not shut out and physical alertness and efficiency are promoted. It is a small matter, but one which may be of value in adding to the safety of the workers in X-ray departments. The cost is not prohibitive.

---

* Cases are recorded of supposed injury to patients in wards above and below X-ray departments, though I have never come across an instance and cannot credit the reports. Since the quantity of the rays varies inversely with the square of the distance, it would take approximately thirty-four hours' continuous running to produce a skin reaction at a distance of 10 ft. under ordinary *therapeutic* conditions with a unit skin dose that takes seven to eight minutes at 8 in. at 110 K.V. Probably this time would be at least doubled if we took into account the filtration value of the patient, the floors and the ceilings. Under present-day *radiographic* conditions we estimate that, without any filtration or interposition of the patient, it would take 10,000 to 15,000 average radiographic exposures, given within a few days, to produce a skin reaction at this distance—in fact, it becomes a *reductio ad absurdum*.

In darkening the radioscopic, radiographic and dark rooms, sliding or folding shutters are the most effective method of making a room light-tight, but the same purpose may be accomplished by roller blinds such as are used for large shop windows. They are, however, heavy and clumsy to work (unless electrically operated). Moreover, it is not easy to make them entirely light-tight, unless there is a generous overlap for the casing. In a number of the Continental clinics all the shutters are operated synchronously by an electric motor.

Roller blinds, made of stiff linen painted black or of thin "American cloth", sliding in deep grooves (2 in.), are fairly satisfactory for the purpose, but holes develop in time and, if the window is not well fitted, a strong wind is apt to blow the blinds out of the groove. These blinds may usefully be strengthened with transverse wooden laths. This type of blind is not suitable for a window that is more than four feet wide, but of course a wide window may be divided.

Ventilation

The ventilation system in a department is of primary importance to the health of the workers.

Fans should be provided in all working rooms, and in addition extracting fans will be necessary in the screening, radiographic and treatment rooms if the work is likely to be at all heavy. A ventilating system by which the whole of the air is changed fairly rapidly is the ideal method. Personally, I mistrust the extraction system of ventilation. In practice the air seems to run in channels and the general effect is not satisfactory unless subsidiary fans are used to stir up the air in the room. In one department that I know well, although the air is said to be changed 11 times an hour, the stuffiness of the atmosphere is such that I always felt tired when working there. In the screening rooms the windows had to be opened from time to time to clear the air. A simple desk fan of the revolving type makes all the difference in such circumstances. I have found the use of such a fan invaluable in averting the ill-effects of prolonged screen examinations.

Doors

The doors of all working rooms must be wide enough to take a bed. Sliding doors are more satisfactory than hinged doors, and if quarters are at all cramped they are a necessity. They are not, however, easy to make light-tight.

Decoration

High tension electrical currents used to charge all the particles in the air and either attract or repel them, with the result that not only the apparatus itself but also the surrounding walls were blackened, and the particles were so driven into them that there was no form of wall covering that would resist. Varnished paint that could be washed down lasted better than paper or bare paint, but the most effective method of finishing the walls in the neighbourhood of the apparatus was with tiles. The decoration of X-ray rooms should be light and cheerful; there is no need for sombre colours which are depressing and which quickly look dirty and tawdry. The introduction of shock-proof apparatus and cables now eliminates the problem of decoration, for the atmosphere is no longer charged and there is no blackening of the walls in the region of the apparatus.

The Dark Room

The common idea that any hole will serve for a dark room is entirely wrong. Someone has to work in such a room, probably for long hours, therefore it should be reasonably large, preferably high, and provided with good windows, so that the atmosphere may be as healthy as possible for the worker. A fan of the extracting type is not essential, though it is highly advisable, but an ordinary fan is an indispensable part of the equipment. The room must of course be rendered light-tight, but blackening of the walls and ceilings does not effect this purpose; all that it does is to absorb and deaden any stray light that may get in. There is no reason why a dark room should be decorated in more sombre colours than any other room in the department, but varnished and other reflecting surfaces should be avoided.

Organisation of the Dark Room

The ordered sequence of dark-room work is a very important point. The unexposed films are issued in their envelopes or in loaded cassettes and placed in the hatch to the radiographic room, through which, when exposed, they come back with the name written in white chalk on the back. They are unwrapped on the same dry bench as that used for loading. If space is available, it is advantageous to have a "dry" and a "wet" dark room. The films are placed in their hangers and passed in order through the developing, rinsing and hypo tanks—all these being placed in one larger outer tank filled with water that is kept at a temperature of 65° F. by hot pipes. In very exceptionally hot weather, ice has to be placed in this outer tank. Next, they pass into a washing tank, above which is a viewing box on the wall, so that the wet films can be inspected without wetting the floor. Nevertheless, duck-boards are desirable for the comfort of the assistant, who does so much standing in front of the tanks. The most satisfactory way of attaining this is to provide for them when the floor is laid down, by a sunk and drained section into which the duck-board is fitted flush with the floor. An open trough drain around the developing and washing tanks is a useful precaution against spilling and overflowing. When washed, the films again pass along to a drying rack, an adaptation of the hanging type of kitchen clothes-hanger, placed over a large sink—a relic of plate days but still useful for this and other purposes. The films dry overnight and most of the work is reported on the following day. In damp weather the films may still be wet after twenty-four hours, and a drying cupboard expedites matters. If the films are to be sent out of the department on the day of examination, an efficient and well-heated drying-chamber, with extracting fan, is essential. In a recent paper (53) I showed that very rapid drying of films is possible under experimental conditions. Films were completely processed in fifteen minutes, the actual drying being accomplished in less than five minutes. Much experimental work has been done in attempting to turn these experimental results to practical account, and a drying chamber that will pass films through within ten minutes has been made and in its experimental state seems to be satisfactory. The advantages of rapid processing and delivery of dry films are very considerable from every point of view: patients can be dealt with at once instead of returning, possibly from a distance, when the result of the X-ray examination is known; the doctor can deal with the case at once and is saved the necessity of going over it again when the films are available; for the same reason it may actually save hospital days; but perhaps the most important point is the fact that the approach of the radiologist to a dry finished film is of a different order from the relatively casual way in which he is apt to look at wet films, giving only too often a rapid glance and a lightning diagnosis in place of the detailed and respectful study that should be given to every radiograph. The practice of reporting on wet films should be abolished, no matter how urgent the case may be. This can only be done, however, if a really rapid X-ray service is established.

The lighting of the dark room has been much improved in recent years. With the advent of special yellow-green glass, high-powered electric lights can be used with safety. Formerly one small glimmer of light over the developing tanks was all that was allowed. To-day there are three of these new lights all placed fairly high, one in the middle of the room, one over the loading bench, and one over the developing tanks. This gives ample light and is perfectly safe for X-ray films, in spite of its appearance, although it fogs the high-speed plates of ordinary photography in a few seconds. For those who are accustomed to the old conditions of a dark room, this lighting, by which they can see the writing on the films or the time on a watch in any part of the room, comes as a revelation. It certainly helps in the efficiency of the work and facilitates the care that should be lavished on the delicate and expensive intensifying screens. In the latter respect alone it is a great economy.

The safety of a dark-room light cannot be gauged by the senses. It should be tested by exposing one of the ordinary films for two or three minutes on the bench on which the films would be handled in the ordinary routine work. This test should be made in every dark room. It was a shock to the writer to find how very faulty was the feeble ruby light with which he worked at one time. Since writing the above, being troubled by fogged plates, we re-tested one of these new so-called safe-lights, recently purchased from another source. We found that it was hopelessly defective, causing appreciable fog in a few seconds, even at four feet distance. The heat of the lamp had affected the colour screen.

Recovery of Silver

The surplus silver on the X-ray films is dissolved out by the sodium hyposulphite (fixing) solution, and this silver can be recovered. It is, however, a process of precipitation and must be done out of doors, owing to the large quantities of H_2S given off. The hypo, remnants of printing papers and other scraps are all placed in a tub and to this is added commercial sodium sulphide in the proportion of one pound to a gallon of hypo. After the precipitate has settled, the liquid is drawn off and the process is repeated until a sufficient quantity of the "sludge" is collected. This is then dried and sent to the refiners for recovery of the silver. In a large department the amount of silver recovered is considerable.

Printing and lantern-slide making from X-ray negatives present no special difficulties and require no special provision except the reducing camera and the necessary illumination.

Layout of Apparatus

Each department will present its own problem of apparatus and if there is not an experienced radiologist in charge one should be consulted. The installation should not be left to the instrument-maker, no matter how good his reputation may be. It is for the radiologist, who knows the practical working, to lay out the department in conjunction with the instrument-maker, who will draw plans to show how he proposes to place the apparatus. For those who cannot realise from a plan the size and capacity of a room, it is very helpful to cut out pieces of paper to scale, representing various pieces of apparatus, and place them in position on the plan. It will sometimes give the solution to difficulties, and show where space is ample or apparatus is too crowded.

There is no reason why transformers and other generating apparatus should not be placed in a dry room either below or above the department. This plan saves space, and also solves some of the difficulties of ventilation. It has the disadvantage, however, that the apparatus is out of sight. A cupboard built out through the wall is a very good solution of the problem, since it can be easily ventilated. The problem of polluted air from high voltage electricity is, however, no longer of importance, since all modern apparatus is shock-proofed.

Main Current

A power supply that does not fluctuate is essential. A separate cable from the main supply is highly advisable if lifts or other heavy intermittent drains on the supply are taken from the same cable; the fluctuations render satisfactory and uniform working conditions impossible. Even when all precautions are taken variations may occur. On one occasion during the summer, when there is normally a very small demand, the advent of a sudden storm rendered the town almost dark, with the result that, as the generating station was quite unprepared, the voltage fell to such an extent that all X-ray work had to be discontinued. Such happenings, in a minor degree, are very frequent in smaller towns.

If there are two sources of power available, it is advisable to have both brought to the department, and, if the department is a large one, it is well to divide the load between the two stations and to have an arrangement by which the whole of the work can be switched on to one or other of the stations in case of breakdown.

Wiring

That all the wiring for the department should be centralised on one switchboard is, of course, common-sense practice. In addition, it enables those who are responsible to switch off and leave everything safe when the department is closed. On more than one occasion damage has been done by unauthorised persons gaining admission to the department and trying their hand on whatever switches they could see. The risks of such thoughtless interference are considerable and are avoided by switching off and putting out the pilot light on the main board, which should be placed close to the entrance to the department. I have had the experience of finding the switches on control boards put on while the current has been switched off, and on one occasion, when the main switches were put on in the morning, a deep therapy apparatus started functioning to such effect that a tube was ruined!

When the department is planned, the general outline of the instrumentation should have already been decided upon and the place for each large piece of apparatus drawn to scale on it in order that the wiring may be installed during building operations. The introduction of insulated cables for the high tension current has revolutionised the layout of departments and has completely eliminated the dangers of electrical shocks. All tubes and accessible cables should be shock-proof. There is, however, no reason why inaccessible portions of the high tension system should be so dealt with, and an overhead tubular system of connecting rods with shock-proof cables leading down to the tubes is quite satisfactory and eliminates considerable expense, especially in regard to change-over switches to supply different tubes from the same apparatus. In one new department, the overhead system, although shock-proofed, is carried in a false roof.

Finality is not yet in sight in regard to X-ray departments and, although equipment is gradually becoming more or less standardised, a few years may bring unexpected changes. Therefore, all wiring should be made as accessible as possible—preferably on the roof of the cellars below. A wiring plan should be framed and fixed beside the main switchboard.

Plugs

Plugs, preferably of the type which cannot be withdrawn without switching off the current, should be fixed at each point where instruments or viewing boxes are likely to be placed. These plugs should be of a standard uniform size for all positions, irrespective of the use for which they are intended. The difference in cost for fitting a smaller type is one which is dearly bought by the inconvenience of finding that, in emergency, a viewing box beside the X-ray couch cannot be used because the plug will not fit.

Earth Wires

Earth wires should be brought to each point at which a tube stand, couch or screening stand is likely to be placed. Flush earthing plugs, recessed into the floor, are by far the most satisfactory means of making connections to apparatus. A fixed contact is, of course, safer, but less convenient.

Telephone and Bells

Telephones in the office and elsewhere are essential. Extension into the radioscopic room is of value because the radiologist then does not have to leave the darkened room and spoil his accommodation. In a large department a loud speaker type of telephone from the radiographic rooms to the dark room is of great service and saves much passing to and fro to enquire.

Signal bells should be provided to every treatment couch.

Lighting

All electric lights must be kept at a safe distance from the high tension conductors of the X-ray installation. In addition to the danger of earthing, the high voltages induced by the high tension current will wreck the lamp filaments. If there is any doubt as to the position being safe for a lamp, a test should be made with a carbon filament lamp. If, on switching on the high tension current, the filament is seen to oscillate, the position is certainly one which a metal filament would not stand. Four feet distance is normally sufficient to obtain safety. If, however, for any reason it is necessary to have a light nearer than this, the bulb can be protected by enclosing it in an earthed wire cage. The lighting cables can cross the line of the high tension conductors fairly close—12 in. in a radiographic room, 24 in. in a deep therapy room—but they should not run parallel with them, otherwise induced voltages will result in broken lights.

In each room that will be used for fluoroscopy points for red lights should be provided. These should be so placed as to give good illumination of the meters on the switchboard, and, in addition, they should provide sufficient light on the table on which the notes will be made. The control for these lights should be conveniently placed for the use of the observer.

In the dark room, both safe-lights and ordinary lights are suspended, the safe-lights being placed over the developing tanks and working benches. Points should also be provided for a viewing box over the washing tank and for the illumination of a reducing camera.

OFFICE WORK

Efficient office work, with a satisfactory system of indexing and filing, is essential in an X-ray department. Each worker develops his own system according to local conditions, and sometimes the indexing and filing system grows to such dimensions that it breaks down because of the labour involved. For those who are starting, I would strongly advise against any complicated system. Begin with a simple one which can be expanded as necessary. If an elaborate system is installed and fails, it may wreck the simpler basic system on which it was founded.

Charts are used for showing graphically the work done during each month. We have records of the monthly totals of treatments and diagnostic cases extending back over nearly twenty years and, among other benefits, they were of great value in demonstrating to the management the necessity for new premises.

In private practice there is the additional office work of accountancy, and it is exceedingly helpful if a costing scheme is carried out. It entails considerable extra clerical work, but in my opinion it is well worth it.

Office work, therefore, is no small detail. It is of vital importance not only to the X-ray department but also to the whole of the medical and surgical services that look to the department for assistance.

It is obviously impossible for clinicians to come to the X-ray department for consultation over the films of every case, and just as impracticable for the radiologist to obtain this necessary consultation by visiting his colleagues. Hence routine co-operation must be in writing, the clinician giving as much help to the radiologist as he can by the information furnished on the requisition cards (Fig. 289), while the radiologist responds with his reports, which are duplicated.

It is much more satisfactory that the X-ray department should be responsible for the keeping of the films than that they should be included with the clinical notes. This latter system may be good in looking up one individual case, but for all other purposes, particularly research of various kinds, the information obtained by centralised filing of all X-ray records in the X-ray department altogether outweighs in value this one good point, which is theoretical rather than real, since films are so easily mislaid or abstracted in the wards. Moreover, if the notes are bound, this method of keeping all records together breaks down entirely. Filed in the X-ray department, they are readily available when and where they are most often wanted, i.e. where they can be compared with those taken when the patient comes for re-examination.

FILING AND INDEXING

In a hospital department every requisition form for an opaque meal examination should be filled up in the wards on the authority of or preferably by the hand of the honorary physician or surgeon. If this rule is not enforced many cases will be sent quite unnecessarily by the house surgeon before any adequate clinical examination has been made. The requisition card should contain a space for "clinical diagnosis", and no case should be accepted by the radiological department unless this is filled in. It should be definitely understood that this diagnosis is merely a tentative opinion for the guidance of the radiologist who, in the press of hospital work, cannot possibly go into the clinical side of the case. The satisfactory filling-in of the heading "clinical diagnosis" is the least the clinician can do by way of co-operation and assistance to the radiologist in the essential work of building up a diagnosis.

In private practice the patient's doctor usually supplies adequate notes of the case and to these the radiologist adds his own notes. The simplest method is to put all the letters and notes of each patient into a separate folder. These are filed numerically and a separate alphabetical card index is kept, bearing the name of the patient and his file number.

In many hospital departments elaborate questionnaires are in use. These are all so detailed that, in my experience, they are seldom filled in. Out of curiosity, I counted the number of questions on one of these forms from a well-known American clinic. After the name, etc., the form requires no less than 135 items of information under 15 heads for the stomach and gall bladder, while the synopsis allows for a further 40 and the barium enema for a further 65! The great disadvantage of such forms is that they tend to fix the observer's attention on answering the questions rather than on studying the patient.

It is necessary in hospital work to have a really satisfactory indexing and filing scheme. The one which we have had in use for many years has the merits of comparative simplicity and efficiency. It stands the crucial test of the holiday season, when so many schemes break down or become unreliable. In fact it is so reliable that other members of the staff find it their most rapid means of obtaining the salient points about old cases, for the requisition card has been filled in by themselves and bears the tentative clinical diagnosis and, on the back, not only the radiological report but also the operative findings.

No.

History:

Museum No.

Plate File.	Region	Angle.	Plate File.	Region	Angle.
1			4		
2			5		
3			6		

Report:

Date .... 192 .... Physician or Surgeon ....

Patient's Name .... Age ....

Address .... Ward ....

Clinical Diagnosis ....

Gen. Supt.'s Signature: ....

Has there been { Operation? .... / Previous X-Ray Examination? ....

Requirements ....

Bed, Walking or Chair Case ....

INSTRUCTIONS. .... Signature.

Screen examinations of chest and abdominal cases on Monday, Tuesday, Wednesday, and Thursday at 10 o'clock.

Preparation of Patients.

(1.) Urinary examinations. Clear bowels as if for operation.

(2.) For abdominal examinations, stomach, intestines, etc., with bismuth. Give purgative the night but one before the examination (not the previous night) and enema on the morning of the examination. Light breakfast at 5-30 a.m., and nothing unless a little milk until patient returns to the ward. Patient takes his ordinary diet till examination is completed, and no purgatives are to be given.

All medicines containing bismuth or iron to be discontinued a week before the examination.

Clothing of Patients.

For all chest and abdominal examinations the patient must be supplied with X-Ray gown, shoes, stockings, and dressing gown.

NOTES OF THE CASE TO BE SENT DOWN WITH THE PATIENT.

(23) 10,000. 17/10/27.

Fig. 289. Requisition Card. (6 × 4 inches.)

Requisition cards (Fig. 289) are dispersed to all the wards and are sent down each day to the department. Should there be too many requisitions, an appointment card (Fig. 290) is given, and the instructions for preparation printed on the card are varied accordingly. Our own porter brings the cases down from the wards; this regulates the numbers and keeps up the supply. Before this was arranged we were constantly either waiting for patients or the whole department was filled with bed cases, who might have a long, cold wait for their turn.

The cards are accepted by the department secretary who

(1) Enters the name, private address and ward in the register book (Fig. 293).

(2) Puts the serial number from this book and the last two figures of the year on the requisition card, e.g. 1223/31. These figures also go on all films of the case.

(3) Enters on a separate alphabetical card index the name and serial number of the patient, e.g. Jones, John, 1223/31.

In most large departments this number is also radiographed on to the plate when the exposure is made. We have not found this necessary, and the practice has the objection that, unless the numbers are fairly large, they may not be

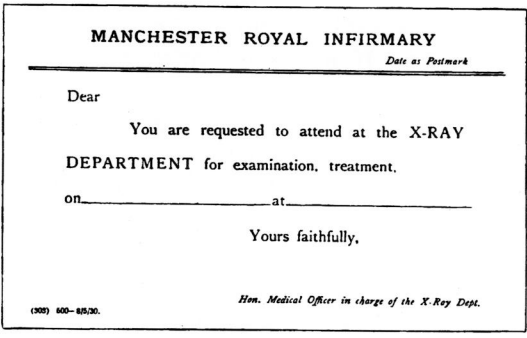

Fig. 290. Appointment Card.

sufficiently exposed on the edge of the plate. They are unsightly, and sometimes interfere with a part of the image that may be of importance. Our practice is to write the name of the patient in pencil on the film in the dark room; and it is the duty of the office staff to sort out the films and write in the name, number and date in Chinese white, after the films are dry.

The number and the size of all films used and clinical and radiographic notes are entered on the back of the requisition card and the films (each of which bears the name and number 1223/31) are filed numerically and also according to size. Thus all the 12 in. × 15 in. films are in one drawer and all the 12 in. × 10 in. films in another, and so on.

For the convenience of the radiologist who is doing the gastro-intestinal observation, we have a blank gummed slip of the same size attached to the side of the requisition card. On this he makes his notes of the examination.

The register book is essential, and it was around this book that our system was built up. It is the key to the number on each card and is also very necessary for office purposes. In it are entered those details from which the returns are made, i.e. the daily number of patients and the sizes of the films used in each case. If this register is properly kept, the stock-taking of films becomes a very small piece of work, which can be done in a quarter of an hour. Incidentally, the register is particularly useful if a member of the medical staff wishes to turn up a case the name of which he does not remember, but which he knows "came from Ward No. 4 and was done on such a day". A glance down the names entered on this date shows from which wards the patients came, and the case with its register number is usually found quite easily.

Or if the records of John Jones are wanted and we only know that he was under a certain physician at an approximate date, a glance down the columns of the daily register book gives the clue to the number, and the registration card can be found at once. On it we find a copy of the actual report, a duplicated carbon print of the report that has gone to the wards, and the number and size of the films exposed. If, for example, we note 2, 15 in. × 12 in., 3, 10 in. × 8 in., we look in the 15 in. × 12 in. and 10 in. × 8 in. drawers and find the films bearing the number 1223/31 in their proper place, perhaps lying between numbers 1220/31 and 1227/31 if the intervening numbers happen to have been small parts, such as fingers, taken on smaller films. Some workers prefer to keep all the films of each case together, but in practice our method works admirably and does not waste time, because it is so much easier to go through a file of films that are all of one size. This would not apply if separate folders were used for each case, but uniformity is essential in a filing system and it is wasteful of space and material to file, for example, finger radiographs in folders suitable for gastro-intestinal work.

After the report is dictated it is not only typed on to the report sheet (Fig. 291) but is duplicated on to the original requisition card. A gummed follow-up slip (Fig. 292) is attached to reports on cases that are likely to come to operation.

No complications have been allowed to enter into this system and it gives only the bare essentials. It does not answer such questions as how many gastric ulcers have been diagnosed. Information of this type would involve further index entries under headings of "Disease", etc. for which we have not the staff available. So far as the system goes it is as nearly perfect and as nearly fool proof as any that I have come across. It has not been changed, even in detail, either by myself or my successors in the last twenty years.

The reports, together with the films, are sent out as early as possible each morning, the reports being the first duty of the radiologists on arrival. They are distributed by our own porter, who obtains the signature of the ward sister or staff nurse for their receipt, a simple and obvious device that has saved much argument. We know by the signature that the report has been received and we know where the films are, and there they remain so long as the patient is in the ward. Thereafter they are due back in the department and are collected by our porter from each ward and checked off in the same receipt book. It is surprising, but they do in fact all come back, thanks to the co-operation of the nursing staff. Some are damaged by careless handling, but it is very seldom that any are missing.

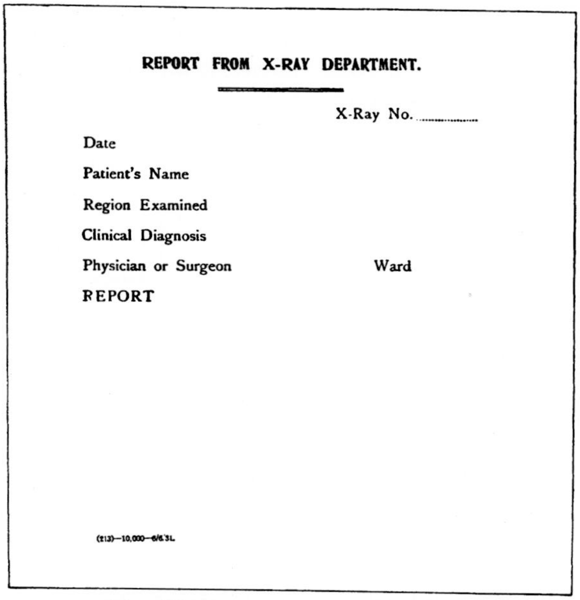

REPORT FROM X-RAY DEPARTMENT.

X-Ray No. ....

Date

Patient's Name

Region Examined

Clinical Diagnosis

Physician or Surgeon Ward

REPORT

(213)—10,000—6/6/31L.

Fig. 291. Report sheet. (6 × 5 inches.)

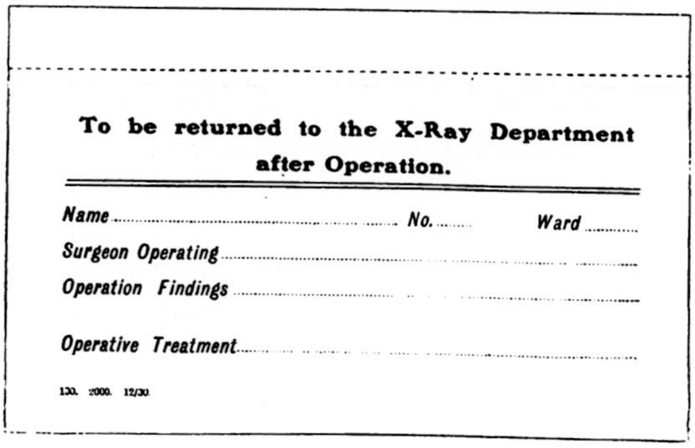

To be returned to the X-Ray Department after Operation.

Name .... *No.* .... *Ward* ....

Surgeon Operating ....

Operation Findings ....

Operative Treatment ....

130. 2000. 12/30.

Fig. 292. Follow-up slip. ($5\frac{1}{2} \times 3\frac{1}{2}$ inches.)

Teaching and Museum Films

In some hospitals surgeons make their own collection of films for teaching purposes, and in one large teaching hospital that I know all the best material in the institution is in the hands of one surgeon. This is not right, and can be avoided by increasing the dark room staff so that prints or lantern slides can be provided whenever required. A library of lantern slides is, by mutual consent, available to any member of the staff. The making, maintenance and indexing of such a library is no small matter in a large teaching hospital, but is well worth the trouble, not only from the point of view of the staff but also from that of the radiologist, who can make of all this material a very valuable common ground on which he can keep in touch with the work and interests of his colleagues. If a member of the staff requires lantern slides for his own use, a charge is made, but if they are for the lending museum, the cost is borne by the institution. Lantern slides of special importance are, if possible, made before the films are

Date 193	Register No. of Exam.	Name	M	S	OP	AR	CB	Eye H	St M H	Chrti H	Ear H	Physician or Surgeon	Screen or Film	Region Radiographed	Bt forward Received / Carried forward	Films received and used				
																15"×12"	12"×10"	10"×8"	8½×6½"	6½"×4½"
														Brought forward...						
														Carried forward...						

Fig. 293. Headings from register book. Columns 4 to 12 indicate the ward from which the case is referred.

sent to the wards, but in any case important films are fixed in special paper folders marked "For museum, please handle with special care", and are seldom damaged.

When films are returned to the department, they are all filed in the drawers of the metal cabinets except those that have been ear-marked for the museum. These are filed separately in boxes that are indexed pathologically, and a corresponding reference is made on the registration card. From these, lantern slides and prints are taken as necessary. In the ideal department of a teaching hospital, the lantern-slide collection and its indexing would be on a very large scale. Ours is an ordinary working department, but the filing and indexing system functions and, if funds and space permitted, could easily expand on its present organisation into an ideal one.

APPENDIX II

THE RADIATION RISKS OF THE ROENTGENOLOGIST

AN ATTEMPT TO MEASURE THE QUANTITY OF ROENTGEN RAYS USED IN DIAGNOSIS AND TO ASSESS THE DANGERS*

By A. E. BARCLAY, M.D., D.M.R.E. (CAMB.),*
AND SYDNEY COX, B.SC.

This paper was written before the introduction of the international r unit. In revising it as far as possible without re-writing we have, whenever practicable, expressed the unit skin dose in terms of the r unit. The following table shows the correspondence between the r unit and the unit skin dose at various kilovoltages.

Kilovolts	Filtration	Physical Dose estimated with back-scatter	Physical Dose estimated without back-scatter
80–100	None	470 r	450 r
150	5 mm. Al.	600 r	530 r
180	0·5 mm. Cu.	900 r	675 r
200	1·5 mm. Cu.	1100 r	900 r

For the purposes of this paper the value of 450 r per U.S.D. has been taken. Until further data have been obtained it is obviously impossible to translate U.S.D. into terms of r units after the beam has been filtered through various thicknesses of lead. It should be noted, however, that for an increase in the penetration of the beam there is a corresponding increase in the number of r equivalent to the U.S.D.

It is obvious that man can tolerate some quantity of radiation without ill effect. In this paper we attempt to arrive at a figure that will represent a safe daily limit of exposure to X radiation.

To obtain exact information as to the actual quantity of radiation, either primary or secondary, produced in the diagnostic services of a roentgen-ray department is obviously impossible owing to the number of variables. Believing, however, that an approximation would be of value, we have attempted to reconstruct the old conditions and also to assess the quantities of the radiations that are nowadays produced under average working conditions and to express these quantities in terms of the only known factor that bears any relation to the human body, i.e. the unit skin dose (U.S.D.).

* Reprinted and revised, by permission, from *Amer. Journ. Roent.* 1928, XIX, 551.

Assumptions

Many assumptions have to be made which may not be scientifically accurate but which involve a margin of error that is probably negligible by comparison with other variables that complicate the problem. For instance, we are assuming that the rate of discharge of the electroscope is the same for a given quantity of radiations within the limits of the range of wave lengths that are employed in roentgenography, roentgenoscopy and light roentgen-ray therapy (minimum peak of 0·089 Ångstrom units), an assumption that medical workers accept in therapeutic work over a wider range of voltages with no serious effects on their patients in the way of unexpected reactions.

We are also assuming for the purpose of these investigations that the secondary radiations have the same characteristics as the primary beam, and that their effect on the electroscope and on the skin is the same.

Basic Standard—The Unit Skin Dose

For the whole of this work we have started from the unit skin dose measured at the half distance (4½ in.) without the interposition of any filter at all. For the measurement of the unit skin dose (which took eight minutes at 9 in.) a number of readings with the pastilles of Sabouraud and Noiré were made to confirm our standard technique on the light or ordinary roentgen-ray therapy apparatus (16 in. coil working at a sphere gap peak reading 0·089 Å., 6–7 in. point to point). This is the accepted standard setting in the department where the readings were made, but the variations of main current are such that, in testing for these readings, we obtained peak records of as low as 0·113 Å. under what were supposed to be normal conditions. In actual practice, the therapeutic results are satisfactorily uniform, i.e. the unit skin dose does not vary to any very great extent, and unexplained or unexpected reaction is unknown. The measurements of the discharge of the iontoquantimeter were made, however, when the readings gave 0·089 Å. as peak with 1·8 to 2 ma. We took the unit skin dose produced under the above conditions as our standard.

Instrumentation

The instrument used for the measurements was an iontoquantimeter (Schall's manufacture). In order to make it more sensitive the aluminium ionisation chamber was eventually replaced by a round cardboard box (size: 5 in. length × 5½ in. diameter) coated inside with aluminium paint and varnished outside with shellac. The electrode itself was increased in size by the addition of a brass rod (size: 3½ in. × ¼ in. diameter). With these modifications we found that the sensitivity of the instrument was so much increased that we could obtain a sufficiently rapid reading of the discharge due to the secondary radiations whenever these were present in fairly large quantity. We also fitted this ionisation chamber with taps, enabling us to fill it with methyl bromide for increased sensitiveness.*

Calibration of the Instrument

Other factors being constant, we assumed that the intensity, i.e. quantity, of the primary radiation varied inversely with the square of the distance. Using this factor for calibration purposes, we found that with our large ionisation chamber our iontoquantimeter was 78 times more sensitive than the original instrument.

When we filled the chamber with methyl bromide, there was a further increase of sensitiveness, between 20 and 25 times, depending on the density of the gas in the chamber—a factor that necessitated calibration each time we filled the instrument with gas. With this sensitive instrument we obtained our readings of the smaller quantities of secondary radiations, and the residue of the primary beam that had found its way through several layers of lead foil.

With these degrees of sensitiveness, we obtained our readings in periods of time that made it unnecessary to make any allowance for natural leak. We had therefore succeeded in calibrating our iontoquantimeter and could read its discharge to scattered and secondary radiations in terms of the unit skin dose.

Known Conditions of Tolerance to Roentgen Rays

Certain facts are known concerning the tolerance of the human skin to roentgen rays.

(1) The skin can only tolerate a certain quantity of radiations without ill effect. This quantity is the unit skin dose. At 80–100 KV. this represents 450 r.

(2) Given a period of rest (six weeks is the usual period allowed), the skin will again stand the same dose, but this tolerance diminishes if exposures are repeated.

(3) One-half U.S.D. can be given on three successive days, i.e. a total of $1\frac{1}{2}$ U.S.D. (675 r), without producing any greater reaction than with a single U.S.D. given at one sitting.

(4) With doses at three or four day intervals, between $\frac{1}{3}$ (150 r) and $\frac{1}{2}$ (225 r) U.S.D. has been given for months without any ill effect on the skin.

Absence of ill effects in unprotected roentgen-ray workers of long standing gives definite indication that large quantities of radiations can be tolerated without injury.

* It was sufficiently delicate to indicate quantities which corresponded to what we later on deduced as our safety limit.

For these suggestions and for facilities for carrying out the preliminary tests, we are indebted to Prof. W. L. Bragg and his department at the Manchester University. The actual measurements were made at the Manchester Royal Infirmary and in a private clinic in Manchester.

There is no question as to the cumulative effect of roentgen-ray doses of a certain magnitude, but it is evident that the time interval between the doses is a very potent factor. We might put it that the larger the dose, the longer the interval, while the smaller the dose, the more frequently can it be repeated without fear of cumulative effect and actual damage to the skin structures.

Workers in old roentgen-ray departments have been exposed for years to a daily dose that must in the aggregate amount to a vast quantity of radiations. For one operator, who is still in charge of roentgen-ray therapy, we have worked out the figures, reconstructing the conditions as accurately as possible for the years 1917 to 1922. Neither in this period nor since has she been ill or shown any indication of either direct or remote effect from the enormous quantities of radiation in which she existed during those six years. On reconstructing the conditions,* we find from electroscopic readings (which not only take in the secondary rays, but also the primary beam arising from the stems of the anti-cathodes which extended outside the tube boxes) that she sustained a *daily* dose of at least $\frac{1}{140}$ or 0·007 U.S.D. (3·15 r) for each working day.

During the war, all roentgenologists were exposed to vast quantities of radiations, not only because of the nature of the work but also because the protective devices were so very defective. Of all this exposure it is obviously impossible to form any estimate, but we have measured up the additional exposure sustained by one roentgenologist in the private work (chiefly therapeutic) which he carried on at the same time. Practically every afternoon he sat at his desk while patients were being treated for an average of one hour within 4 to 5 ft. of a Coolidge tube (operated at a 6 in. point to point spark-gap with 1·8 ma.) carried in an open wooden box with lead rubber lining of approximately 0·75 mm. lead value. Taking an average for *this exposure alone*, we find that he was subjected to a daily dose of primary and secondary radiations amounting to about $\frac{1}{440}$ or 0·0023 U.S.D. Added to this was all the exposure he received in military and other hospital practice. It is probable that this worker received a daily dose that was very far in excess of the 0·007 U.S.D. (3·15 r) above recorded.

It is clear, therefore, that the time during which the subject is exposed to the rays is of as much importance as the total quantity to which the skin is exposed, i.e. an enormous quantity can be tolerated provided it is divided into small enough doses and the intervals are not too close together.

* In this period she had charge of three 16 in. coils, housed in a basement room (size 18 × 13 × 10 ft. high), and she spent practically the whole of her time at a desk in the corner beside the one window. The only protection afforded was the lead rubber of the open wooden boxes in which the Coolidge tubes were housed. Under these conditions she gave 43,456 treatments of an average length of twenty minutes each in the six years.

*Deduction of a Safety Limit—*0·0014 U.S.D. (0·63 r) *Daily*

We therefore have two definite figures of the quantity of radiations tolerated over long periods without known ill effect, i.e. one case of 0·007 U.S.D. (3·15 r) daily for six years, and another of 0·0023 U.S.D. (1·035 r), which was only a fraction of the total dose. These quantities are exceedingly small, yet the protection of these two workers was possibly no less inadequate than that of any others at this period.

Using these two observations, could we arrive at a figure as being safe, and one that can be tolerated day after day without risk? We suggested that a protection scheme that reduces the *possible* incidence of rays on the operator to a daily dose that is in the region of $\frac{1}{25}$ of that which had been known to be tolerated without ill effect (0·007 U.S.D. (3·15 r)), must be well within the limits of safety. We therefore took as our arbitrary standard 0·00028 U.S.D. (0·126 r) as our safe limit for daily exposure. We now maintain that we placed this figure unnecessarily low and that 0·0014 U.S.D. (0·63 r)—i.e. $\frac{1}{5}$ instead of $\frac{1}{25}$—is a more reasonable figure (see p. 35). Provided that confirmation of these figures can be had from other workers, we believe that a *possible* small daily exposure of this magnitude would be absolutely harmless and could be used as a basis of safety for all workers who are in any way exposed to roentgen radiations of medium wave lengths.

The question of *idiosyncrasy* will of course be raised. While admitting that there may be such a thing as variation in human tolerance, we believe that the limits of variation are comparatively narrow, amounting to only a small fraction of the total dose given. If it were not so, the almost mathematical certainty with which the well-organised and controlled clinics deal with ringworm would not be possible. The margin that divides success from disaster in these cases is a narrow one, and disaster would be frequent and not an almost, if not quite, unknown happening. MacKee[1] states that the use of the word idiosyncrasy has disappeared in direct proportion to the knowledge of technique and of those factors such as irritants which accentuate the action of rays.

The lighting up of the roentgenoscopic screen and the effects on ordinary duplitised roentgenographic film of the quantities of radiations approximating to our daily safety limit form a rough guide for the worker.* For this purpose we reproduced the conditions under which the radiologist worked. An ordinary standard Eastman film was exposed in the position in which he sat at his desk and iontoquantimeter readings were made at the same time in the same position. The film was developed in the tank under standard conditions at 65° F. It will be noted that the quantity of radiations indicated by the heaviest

---

* Dental films are coated on one side only. If these are used for testing, two of them superimposed give the same readings as duplitised films.

blackening of the film was tolerated by this worker for years without any ill effect on the skin or cutaneous structures—this, however, does not argue that he did not, unwittingly, take grave risks.

From our measurements we conclude that the maximum blackening of a film either carried by or placed in the position of the worker for the whole of a day's work should never exceed that indicated by the shade produced in twelve minutes on our scale, since this corresponds roughly to the safety limit.

On the scale reproduced in the original paper were given:

(1) The time during which the film was exposed.
(2) The quantity of radiations measured by the iontoquantimeter.
(3) The corresponding blackening of the film.

Applying the safety limit to roentgenography

The problems we have to face are therefore (1) how to arrive at a measurement of the quantity of radiations that can reach an operator during diagnostic roentgen-ray work, and (2) how to determine the amount of protection necessary to reduce this quantity to 0·63 r as the maximum possible daily exposure. With this end in view, we have made numerous readings of both the primary and scattered radiations under average conditions of roentgenography and screening. It does not follow that the results we have obtained are necessarily correct for other installations, but we believe that the conditions of our tests in a busy department are quite average technique and that our deductions, subject to corroboration from other sources, can be of use to others, even if the conditions vary materially from our own. It is to cover possible variations that we have made so wide a margin (i.e. $\frac{1}{5}$ of the dose we know to have been tolerated).

Records of the chief roentgenographic room of the Manchester Royal Infirmary show that this room deals with a daily average of 22 patients, using 35 films (maximum 50 patients with 80 films exposed). The total daily average time of operation of the roentgen-ray tubes is two minutes thirty-five seconds (3875 milliampère-seconds). The maximum daily operation of the tubes recorded over several weeks' work was four minutes four seconds. This figure is surprisingly small, but it shows an average of 4·4 seconds per exposure, which is accounted for by the large number of abdominal and other heavy cases in which the Potter-Bucky diaphragm is used.

Two tubes are used in this room, i.e. a gas tube and a hot cathode tube. On comparative readings under working conditions (0·124 Å., measured with 10 cm. sphere gap, and 25 ma.), we found that the gas tube was 10 times and the hot cathode 11 times more active in discharging the electroscope than the control tube which was giving our unit skin dose in eight minutes under standard conditions.

From this we calculated that the actual quantity of radiations produced in this room each day during the average exposure of two minutes thirty-five seconds would be 3·4 U.S.D. under standard conditions, i.e. 9 in. from cathode.

Only a thoughtless and negligent roentgenologist would to-day allow a roentgenographic assistant to be in the direct line of the rays. Common sense indicates that the tube, even if protected, should be directed away from the operator. Nevertheless, let us assume that the operator is entirely unprotected and in the direct line of the rays during the whole of the exposures. Then the following table shows the effect of the protection value of distance from the roentgen-ray tube and also of interposing various thicknesses of lead.

The Effect of Distance and Filtration on the Intensity of Radiations used in Radiography

Distance from X-ray tube	Direct radiation, possible daily maximum	Effect of lead filter					
		¼ mm.	½ mm.	¾ mm.	1 mm.	1¼ mm.	1½ mm
9 in.	3·4 U.S.D.	—	—	—	—	—	—
4 ft.	0·120	0·0042	0·0012	0·00042	0·00019	0·00009	0·00005
6 ft.	0·053	0·0016	0·00053	0·00019	0·00008	0·00004	0·00002
8 ft.	0·030	0·0011	0·00030	0·00011	0·00005	0·00002	0·00001
12 ft.	0·013	0·0004	0·00013	0·00005	0·00002	0·00001	0·000005

It seems, therefore, that the following thicknesses of lead or their equivalent are sufficient to give protection with an adequate margin of safety even for a roentgenographer who persistently, and in ignorance, works *in front of the anti-cathode* and therefore in the direct line of the primary beam:*

0·5 mm. lead is sufficient at a working distance of 12 ft.
0·75 mm. lead is sufficient at a working distance of from 6 ft. to 8 ft.
1·0 mm. lead is sufficient at a working distance of 4 ft.

Secondary Radiations

If, however, the operator is behind the anti-cathode, as he should be, he is only exposed to secondary radiations. These also we have measured.

The quantity of secondary rays varies with the type of tube box used and the size of the aperture. For our tests in the roentgenographic room the tube was in an open lead glass bowl, with the cathode stem projecting, and a wide open aperture. The conditions were those of actual practice, except that we had no patient, and only the couch top on which to scatter our primary beam.

The total quantity of secondary rays produced in a day's roentgenographic

* These figures were applicable for our old figure of 0·00028 U.S.D. There is therefore a margin of × 5 for the new safety limit.

work is very small. In the room in which we made these tests (size $18 \times 16 \times 12$ ft. high) we obtained readings with the sensitised iontoquantimeter indicating that the total quantity was 0·0006 U.S.D. (0·27 r) for a day's work at 8 ft. from the tube, this being the ordinary position of the operator, for whom we had, of course, provided a well-protected shelter when the department was built.

On another outfit and under rather different conditions we have made a number of measurements while patients were being treated, to determine what proportion of these secondary and other rays came from the patient and what proportion by escape of rays through the open top of a most inadequate and antique tube box.

These figures were complicated by the primary rays arising from the cathode stem, which extended outside the tube box. Our figures showed the following:

20 per cent. originated from scattered and secondary rays from the open top of the tube box.

30 per cent. originated from the cathode stem protruding beyond the protection.

50 per cent. originated from the patient.

With a deeper tube box and one that was large enough to take in the active length of the anti-cathode stem, i.e. a half of it, these figures would be greatly changed; a much higher proportion of a smaller total would be due to secondary radiation from the patient. The self-protected tube cuts out the first two but does not influence the last.

The conditions of these experimental tests were as nearly as possible actual working conditions, and we believe that these do not differ materially from the accepted practice in other centres.

Deductions for Roentgenography

We are therefore of the opinion that for roentgenographic work:

(1) Distance from the active tube, whether adequately protected or not, is the essence of safety.*

(2) The tube box for roentgenographic work need not be of greater protective value than 1 mm. of lead to give perfect safety even to an ignorant operator

---

* The possible danger to patients and others in rooms below or above a roentgen-ray department is frequently raised. Taking 12 ft. as the probable distance from the tube to the endangered person in the room below we find that 3·4 U.S.D. at 9 in. is reduced to 0·013 U.S.D. at 12 ft., i.e. if there was nothing but air between the tube and the endangered person it would take seventy-seven days to deliver a U.S.D. But practically all these rays will be filtered through a patient's body and the floor materials, i.e. at least equal to 1 mm. lead. The probable time of a U.S.D. must therefore be in the region of 130 years! Out of curiosity we placed photographic films in the basement below various installations and all of them were unaffected in a month. We applied the same test to the basement directly below the deep therapy apparatus. Just the very faintest change could be detected after a month's exposure, but the floor of these rooms is ferro-concrete. A very rough estimate indicates a period of perhaps four years for one U.S.D. under our deep therapy apparatus at 12 ft

who works with the anti-cathode directed towards him, and who may be forced to work within 4 ft. of the tube.

(3) It is unnecessary to use a completely enclosed tube box, since the total quantity of secondary rays produced is practically negligible, and total enclosure only reduces it by 50 per cent.

(4) If a protective screen for the operator is used, $\frac{1}{8}$ mm. lead will cut down any scattered or escaping radiations by roughly 80 per cent. and is therefore ample for the purpose.

(5) It is unnecessary to incorporate protective material in the walls or doors of a roentgenographic room of reasonable size, i.e. any room that is suitable for this class of work. Even a dark-room wall next to a roentgenographic room needs only about 0·5 mm. lead to save risk of fogging.

Applying the Safety Limit to Roentgenoscopy

Quantity of Radiation employed

It is comparatively easy to obtain approximate figures for roentgenography, but for roentgenoscopy and its accessory service of plate-taking during screen examinations it is not possible to arrive at anything more accurate than a rough estimate. The novice not only makes prolonged screen examinations, but uses a wide-open diaphragm quite unnecessarily. The expert makes his observations rapidly and always uses the minimum diaphragm opening, and it cannot be too strongly emphasised that the use of the smallest practicable pencil of rays is the controlling factor that limits the risks of the observer.

Taking the screening service of the Manchester Royal Infirmary, we have a weekly average of 58 gastro-intestinal examinations, 30 chest cases and 3 foreign bodies. Our proportion of screen work, and time absorbed in screening each case, is probably well above the average.*

Working then on this basis, which is a very liberal one and is, purposely, generous on any doubtful points, we have a daily period of thirty-two minutes

---

* The following are the figures on which these results are based. The times were obtained by observation of several workers doing the routine examinations. A recording clock was placed in the circuit of the roentgen apparatus and the figures give the average readings.

1st day gastro-intestinal examinations				26 at 4 minutes each
2nd	,,	,,	,,	21 at 2 minutes each
3rd	,,	,,	,,	10 at 1 minute each
4th	,,	,,	,,	1 at 1 minute
Chest cases	...	...	...	... 30 at 1 minute each
Foreign bodies ...	...	...	...	3 at 1 minute each

To the exposure in screen examinations is added the following for exposures during the taking of films in the course of the examinations:

91 films, average $\frac{1}{8}$ sec. exposure = 12 sec. total.

The average intensity of this is 10 times our screening, and under the conditions of our work equals two minutes' screening.

during which the observer will be in front of the active roentgen-ray tube. Working at 0·124 Å. and 4 ma. the tube was found to be 4·4 times more active in discharging the electroscope than the control, which gives the U.S.D. in eight minutes at 9 in. Therefore, if we measure the quantity at 9 in. from the tube used in roentgenoscopy, we have 17·6 U.S.D. per daily exposure of thirty-two minutes. But since the minimum possible distance of the observer from the tube is 20 in. this quantity is cut down to a maximum of 3·6 U.S.D. daily.

At our minimum possible working distance for screening, i.e. 20 in., this quantity becomes:

0·111 U.S.D. when 0·25 mm. lead or its equivalent is interposed.
0·036   ,,   0·5 mm.   ,,   ,,   ,,
0·006   ,,   1·0 mm.   ,,   ,,   ,,
0·0014 ,,   1·5 mm.   ,,   ,,   ,,
0·00039 ,.   2·0 mm.   ,,   ,,   ,,
0·00013 ,,   2·5 mm.   ,,   ,,   ,,

It appears, therefore, that a completely enclosed tube box of 2 mm. lead equivalent is adequate to give the necessary degree of protection.

The same figure of protective value is the obvious one, if it is practical, for the lead glass of the fluorescent screen, but there is no need to leave any margin of safety since, in screening, there is necessarily a patient in position, and the protective value of this added filtration is in itself usually equal to 0·5 mm. lead for abdominal examination and 0·25 mm. for the chest.* Moreover, the distance is never anything like 20 in. in practice. It is very seldom so little as 30 in. and more usually nearer 36 in. between the target and the observer.

Secondary Radiations in Roentgenoscopy

To arrive at an estimate of the quantity of secondary radiations the measurements were necessarily an approximation based on electroscopic readings taken during actual examinations.

Other things being equal, the quantity of secondary radiations depends on the size of the beam of primary rays used in the examination, i.e. on the skill or

---

* A roentgen film fixed to the lead glass of the screen during a heavy day's work should be developed and compared with a scale. The lead glass used by the writer is only equal to 0·5 mm. lead, yet the films of his tests are very little blackened. This is probably because he uses a small diaphragm. Although our figures show 2 mm. lead as the correct protective value, we are confident that, even when there is possible incompetence, a very much smaller protective value is adequate for perfect safety except in those departments where the work is incessant with 30 or 40 screen examinations a day. High value protective lead glass is very expensive and for movable screens for couch use is so heavy that it hampers work. For this purpose, at any rate, we are confident that 0·5 mm. value is sufficient, for the observer's face is seldom in the direct line of the rays, as he is standing to the side of the couch and does not, as a rule, get his face right over except when searching for, say, a foreign body.

otherwise with which the operator controls the diaphragm. We purposely used a large diaphragm opening during these tests, i.e. produced more secondary rays than we should do under normal working conditions.

Using a fluorescent screen that is adequately protected with lead glass against the direct beam, the electroscope shows that the quantity of secondary radiations is much more abundant at the sides than directly in front of the fluorescent screen. This fact adds to the safety of the operator when the patient is standing before the screen.

The reverse is the case, however, when he examines a patient lying on the couch, for all the stream of secondary rays coming from the patient strikes his own chest and abdomen.

Using a tube box of 3 mm. lead protection, but with a wide-open diaphragm, we have made measurements at the point where the observer would be standing during an examination of a patient on the couch.

Allowing that half of the total screen examination (thirty-two minutes) is done on the couch, we get sixteen minutes as a daily maximum of screening with the patient lying down. From our measurements with the iontoquanti-meter we calculate that this would give 0·27 r from the secondary rays during the sixteen minutes' exposure beside the couch. Even without the quantity to which he is exposed in front of the upright screening stand, this is about half the value of the safe limit that we have laid down (0·63 r). Neither the protective material of the tube box nor the use of a lead screen on the side of the couch can give adequate protection, for practically all this radiation comes from the patient's body and strikes the observer's chest and abdomen. The only way to guard against this would be side flaps on the fluorescent screen, which would be impossible since palpation could not be employed. We therefore regard the wearing of a thin protective apron as very highly advisable, though not absolutely imperative, for all couch-side screening work. The electroscope indicates that even so little as $\frac{1}{8}$ mm. lead equivalent is ample for such aprons, since it reduces the possible incidence of the rays to a fraction that is far below the danger limit.* If anyone doubts the dangers of screening beside a

* Roentgen-ray-proof aprons of the ordinary type hang unused in roentgen departments from year's end to year's end because of their weight. From our measurements it seems quite obvious that the heavy protection afforded is unnecessary and unpractical. Some years ago we had a new type of apron made out of a single sheet that covers back and front down to the thighs, and consequently is balanced on the shoulders. It is slipped over the head and is left open at the sides. There is no protection for the arms. Smocks of this type affording 0·25 mm. lead protection (cutting off about 97 per cent. of the scattered radiations) weigh 9½ lb. We ourselves use the same article made in $\frac{1}{8}$ mm. lead, and this weighs only 4½ lb. We are quite satisfied that it gives ample protection for our conditions— it nearly obliterates the illumination of the screen from the scattered rays. The absorption figures show that it reduces these by about 88 per cent. Tests with dental films under these smocks confirm this view (Fig. 16, p. 42).

couch, let him note, with the screen, the secondary radiation coming towards him from the patient's flanks when he has the diaphragm wide open. It is also instructive to note how effective is $\frac{1}{8}$ mm. lead in cutting off the rays which produce this illumination. Even more telling is the blackening of a dental film which has been worn in a waistcoat pocket by the observer who does the work.

Deductions for Roentgenoscopy

Distance, the fool-proof safety factor, cannot be utilised in roentgenoscopy. Moreover, the observer is in the direct line of the rays. Nevertheless, roentgenoscopy can be rendered safe, provided:

(1) That the tube is completely enclosed in protective material of not less than 2 mm. lead equivalent.

(2) That the diaphragm is of not less than 2 mm. lead equivalent and of the adjustable rectangular type.

(3) That the lead glass of the screen, or an outward extension of similar protective value, be large enough to catch the whole of the primary beam when the diaphragm is fully open. Theoretically it should be of the same protective value as the tube box and diaphragm. In practice, however, thanks to the protective value of the patient's body and the fact that the distance is at least 30 in., we do not consider more than 1 mm. lead necessary for reasonable safety, even if the observer remains in his place while roentgenograms are being taken (as the writer has always done).

When using a totally enclosed tube box the dangers in front of the upright screening stand from secondary radiations are very slight, if not negligible, as compared with those to which the observer is exposed when he examines patients on the couch. Protective screens on the side of the couch only reduce the secondary radiations by a fraction, i.e. the massive screens fixed to the side of the couch are valueless as a protection against secondary radiations and superfluous for primary radiations if the tube box is of the totally enclosed type and of adequate protective value. With the iontoquantimeter placed in the position of the observer, its rate of discharge is cut down 8 times, i.e. 88 per cent. of the radiations are cut off, by surrounding it with a light lead rubber apron of $\frac{1}{8}$ mm. lead equivalent. Two layers of loose blanket reduced these secondary radiations by 10 per cent., which we interpret as the protective value of the observer's clothes.

It is not necessary for the safety of passers-by or even those who may constantly work on the other side of the wall to incorporate protective material in the walls of roentgenoscopic rooms. If a dark room is next door it is advisable to add some protection to the walls for the safety of the film stocks.

The protection of the observer's hands during screen examinations has been dealt with elsewhere (2).

BLOOD CHANGES

For many years past, roentgenology has been regarded with suspicion as a possible source of danger. The death of every roentgenologist is called in question and natural causes are only accepted grudgingly. There is a lurking fear that these rays may yet bear death in forms that we do not understand. We look for circumstantial evidence of data in common between those deaths that do occur—every unexplained feature is whispered about as probably "due to his work", "not unlike the death of So and So". Surely the time has come, after all these years of suspicion, to investigate things with an open mind. For instance, so far as we know, only one death is supposed to have been due to aplastic anaemia resulting from roentgen-ray work, all the others having occurred in radium workers. To infer, if not actually to state that roentgen rays and aplastic anaemia are in the relation of cause and effect in this case is at least unjustifiable, for not only were the conditions of work far from ideal in every particular but, in addition, there was a known chronic infection. How many of the blood changes that were found, say, eight years ago have turned out to be anything serious? Have any of these changes been found when reasonable ventilation and other conditions were the lot of the worker?

The effect on the blood of massive doses of high-voltage roentgen radiations and of radium even in small quantities is quite definite, but we have considerable doubt whether the comparatively infinitesimal quantities of radiations to which the roentgen-ray worker is exposed in the course of his diagnostic work can have any influence in producing serious changes in the blood.

Mottram's striking paper (3) in 1920 on the blood changes in those who worked with radium caused us to have blood tests made of all the workers in the roentgen-ray department of the Manchester Royal Infirmary, where at that time the conditions of work were far from ideal. We had numerous tests made from time to time, but none of them suggested that our staff was working under conditions of danger. Eventually, as the tests on all the workers gave negative results, they were abandoned. The two workers who were most exposed and whose radiation risks have been assessed (see p. 366) had, however, the advantage of fresh air, the operator always working beside an open window and the roentgenologist moving about constantly in an open car.*

In all the medium-voltage treatment that we have carried out in the last twenty years or more, we do not recollect a single case in which we noted the onset of anaemia or anything that indicated a blood count. Many of these

---

* The striking variations in the blood picture of normal persons shown by recent experiments (see p. 48) suggest that the blood-changes supposed in the past to be due to small intensities of radiations were probably within normal limits

patients were under treatment for very long periods and in the aggregate must have received an immense dose of primary and quite a substantial quantity of secondary radiations, since no precaution was taken at any time to cut these off.

If such large quantities of radiation can be tolerated without any clinical suggestion of blood change, it is hardly logical or just, unless other and more likely causes are eliminated, to attribute the indefinite changes that have been found from time to time in roentgen-ray workers to the effect of the very small quantities of rays they have received as compared with the enormous doses tolerated for years by patients undergoing treatment. We are, therefore, of the opinion that the very rare cases of blood changes in roentgen-ray workers are due to some other influence, most likely to effect of vitiated air, lack of fresh air and other conditions which inevitably accompany work in the obviously inadequate and ill-ventilated housing that has only too frequently been the lot of the roentgen-ray department in the past.

Our opinion is becoming stronger and stronger that there are not necessarily any risks attached to roentgen-ray work *provided* the roentgenologist is suitably equipped both with apparatus and with accommodation. In a modern department, with reasonable air space, etc., there is certainly nothing in the way of radiation risks, so far as we can measure, to suggest that ordinary operatives should be placed on a different footing from other hospital workers in hours of work or holidays. Some of the old departments were not fit for any person to live and work in; it is useless to legislate for such places.

There is, however, one worker whose claim to special treatment we would persistently urge. In spite of the best intentions, the dark room can never be healthy, and workers here should have special hours and holidays.

Measuring the safety limit in practice

The object of our research has been to find, if possible, a definite foundation, a tolerance dose, on which to base protective measures in the *diagnostic* roentgen-ray services only. We believe we have succeeded, and out of our observations, if they are corroborated from other sources, we think that it will now be possible to evolve an ionisation or photographic test* that will tell whether the average

* Fifteen members of a local society of roentgenographers have kindly submitted films that they have worn during an ordinary day of routine work. On development of the films we find that six are well within the safety limit; five are on the border line; four are far beyond what we should regard as the limit of safety. All those working within the safety limit and those on the border line were using modern apparatus. Of the bad results two were in workers whose conditions of work were bad and where there was no qualified roentgenologist in charge. The apparatus itself was reasonably good. One of the worst results was obtained from a worker in a modern and exceedingly well-equipped diagnostic department where, on the surface at any rate, the protective measures were carried almost to excess. Another was from a worker in a skin hospital. For more than twenty years it has been the habit of this worker, assisted by nurses, to hold restless ringworm patients during the whole of the exposure—the cubicles inside which he worked were perfectly protected! All these bad results were in the region of three times the safety limit.

position of the operator is or is not one of safety under normal working conditions. A test of this type, in addition to its simplicity, would at once reveal the presence of chinks in the protective armour, for it is the weak links in the chain that are the danger. Apart from the accidents due to the wanton exposure from ignorance in the early days, it is probable that the many tragedies that have occurred have been due to chance exposure to the primary beam through leaks and not to deficiency in the general strength of the armour. To be effective the protection need not be great, but it must be complete. Leaks and weak spots will be just as dangerous with massive as with light but effective protection. We very much doubt if anyone could be harmed in practice if so little as 0·5 mm. of lead was always interposed, as the following simple figures indicate:

Distance in.	Time for U.S.D. unfiltered, min.	Time for U.S.D. with 0·5 mm. lead interposed
9	8·0	13 hr. 40 min.
20	39·5	2 days 17 hr. 50 min.

Comparison

As far as we are aware, this is the first attempt to arrive at a tolerance dose from recorded observations on the human subject as a basis for protective measures. Mutscheller[4], however, has assumed that $\frac{1}{100}$ or 0·01 U.S.D. sustained in thirty days is harmless. Our estimate, stated in a similar way, shows that 0·008 U.S.D. in thirty days is harmless. Glocker and Kaupp[5] and Glocker[6] have based their investigations on the working hour, assuming that 1·0 U.S.D. in 1000 hours will be safe. We carried out our investigations in entire ignorance of their calculations, and it is a very striking fact that our deductions, arrived at by such different methods, should approximate so closely to those of these three workers.*

* In the following table we have attempted to compare results:

Mutscheller	Glocker	Our figures
$\frac{1}{100}$ U.S.D. in 30 days	1 U.S.D. in 1000 working hours	
0·00005 U.S.D. per working hour	0·0001 U.S.D. per working hour	0·00005 U.S.D. per working hour
0·00033 U.S.D. per day	0·0005 U.S.D. per day	0·00028 U.S.D. per day
A working month is roughly 200 hours	No estimate of the number of working hours per day is given. Our estimation of 5 hours is applied for the sake of comparison	A working day is roughly from 4 to 6 hours

The following table gives the protective figures arrived at:

			Roentgenography	Roentgenoscopy
Our figures	...	...	1·0 mm. lead	2·0 mm. lead
Mutscheller	...	...	1·2 ,,	1·8 ,,
Glocker	...	...	1·5–2·0 ,,	2·0 ,,

Conclusions

It will be seen that our conclusions do not differ very widely from the recommendations of the English Radium and X-ray Protection Committee as regards roentgen diagnostic work. They seem to indicate, however, several points in which it is likely that these go beyond what is necessary.

In framing protective measures we believe that our conclusions may, if corroborated, be used as a basis. No system of protection can, however, render roentgen-ray work fool-proof; any attempt to cater for folly must fail, yet it inevitably places a very serious handicap on the progress of roentgenology. We suggest that the first protective measure should be that no person be allowed to use a roentgen apparatus who is ignorant of electrical and radiation dangers and how to avoid them.

We wish to acknowledge our indebtedness to Prof. W. L. Bragg for suggestions and also for providing facilities for the preliminary calibration work, and to Dr G. W. C. Kaye of the National Physical Laboratory for pointing out fallacies and for granting the use of the lead absorption curve from which our figures are calculated.

References

1. MacKee, G. M. *X Rays and Radium in the Treatment of Diseases of the Skin.* Lea and Febiger, Philadelphia, 1927.
2. Barclay, A. E. "The dangerous art of palpation." *Brit. Jour. Radiol.* 1926, xxxi, 385.
3. Mottram, J. C. "Red cell blood content of those handling radium for therapeutic purposes." *Arch. Radiol. and Electroth.* 1920, xxv, 194.
4. Mutscheller, A. "Physical standards of protection against roentgen-ray dangers." *Amer. Jour. Roentgenol. and Rad. Therapy*, 1925, xiii, 65.
5. Glocker, R. and Kaupp, E. "Ueber den Strahlenschutz und die Toleranzdosis." *Strahlentherapie*, 1925, xx, 144.
6. Glocker, R. "Internationale Strahlenschutzbestimmungen." *Strahlentherapie*, 1926, xxii, 193.

APPENDIX III

NOTE ON SECONDARY RAYS

By G. STEAD, M.A.

*University Lecturer in Physics as Applied to Medical Radiology
in the University of Cambridge*

When X rays pass through matter, secondary rays of the following types may be produced:

1. *Scattered X rays of the same quality as the primary beam.* This process is analogous to the scattering in all directions of a beam of light from a motor head-lamp on a foggy night.

2. *Scattered X rays that are softer than the primary beam.* The process which gives rise to scattered rays of greater wave length than the primary beam is called the *Compton effect,* and there is no analogy to it in the optical region. The amount by which the wave length increases depends upon the direction of scattering, but for a given direction it is the same for all wave-lengths and for all scattering substances. The increase of wave length (in Ångstrom units) for different directions is indicated in Fig. 294, from which it will be seen that there is no change for rays scattered in the forward direction, and a maximum change of 0·048 Å. for rays scattered backwards in the direction of the source of the primary rays.

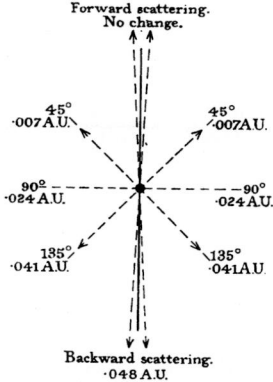

Fig. 294. Chart showing increase of wave length of
scattered rays according to direction.

Since the increase in wave length for a given direction of scattering is the same for all waves, it follows that the percentage change increases as the wave length diminishes. This is shown in the table on p. 380 for waves scattered backwards.

The numbers in the last column give the kilovoltage required to produce a primary beam in which the shortest wave length is equal to that of the scattered ray. Comparison of columns 1 and 5 gives some idea of the amount of softening.

K.V. on X-ray tube	Shortest wave length in primary beam (in Å.U.)	Wave length of corresponding scattered ray	Percentage change in wave length	Corresponding potential in K.V.
50	0·246	0·294	19·5	42
75	0·164	0·212	29·3	58
100	0·123	0·171	39·0	72
125	0·098	0·146	49·0	84
150	0·082	0·130	59·5	95

The relative importance of scattering without change of wave length and Compton scattering depends upon the atomic weight of the scattering material. For light elements such as carbon, nitrogen and oxygen Compton scattering predominates, whereas for heavy elements the reverse is the case. This is illustrated in Fig. 295,

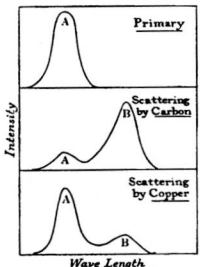

Fig. 295. Relative importance of scattering without change of wave length (A) and Compton scattering (B).

which, however, is not drawn to scale. The upper diagram is the spectrum of a nearly homogeneous primary beam; the lower diagrams show the spectrum of the rays scattered by carbon and copper. In each case peak A represents a scattered ray of the same wave length as the primary, and peak B the Compton scattering. It will be clear, therefore, that the rays scattered by soft tissues consist mainly of waves which are longer, and more easily absorbed, than the primary beam. Moreover, when a wide-angled primary beam is used to irradiate a large volume of tissue, the secondary scattered rays are themselves subject to scattering within the tissue, thus giving rise to still softer tertiary scattered rays, and so on.

3. *Secondary characteristic X rays.* These rays have definite wave lengths which are characteristic of the chemical elements that produce them and independent of the quality of the primary beam, provided that this is hard enough to excite the characteristic rays at all. The process resembles fluorescence in optics, and the rays are often called fluorescent X rays. Characteristic rays are always softer than the primary beam, but their hardness increases with the atomic weight. Thus, for copper the wave length is in the neighbourhood of 1·5 Å., and for tungsten about 0·2 Å.

4. *Secondary electrons.* These correspond to photo-electrons emitted by metals under the influence of light. They have high velocities but low penetrating power. Thus, the secondary electrons produced by X rays from a tube running at 100 K.V. are almost completely stopped by 0·1 mm. of aluminium, and at 200 K.V. by 0·2 mm. of aluminium. From the physical point of view it seems very probable that the biological effect of X rays is produced by secondary electrons liberated in the tissues.

APPENDIX IV

NOTE ON THE EFFECTS OF POSTURE ON THE BLOOD SUPPLY TO THE ABDOMEN

When an animal changes from the horizontal to the erect position or vice versa, the alteration in relation to gravity affects the distribution of blood throughout the body. When the trunk is horizontal, gravity plays no part, but when it is vertical, with the head up, gravity naturally tends to increase the blood pressure in the lower part of the trunk and to decrease it in the head. If no adjustment took place the blood supply to the abdomen would be increased and that to the head diminished, with the inevitable results: anaemia of the brain and loss of consciousness. It has long been known, however, that a compensating mechanism is provided by the vaso-motor system. The vaso-motor centre, situated in the medulla, is exquisitely sensitive to the amount of blood supplying it. When this is diminished the centre sends out vaso-motor impulses which constrict the arterioles—mainly in the splanchnic area—with the result that the blood supply in this region is diminished while that of the cerebral arteries is increased. The blood pressure in the carotid artery therefore suffers a momentary fall followed by recovery. This adjustment is less efficient in some individuals than in others; its poor development is probably the cause of the feeling of faintness which some people, especially sufferers from Glénard's disease, experience on suddenly standing upright after lying down. This, at any rate, is the generally-accepted view.

It occurred to Dr Ffrangcon Roberts, however, that too little attention had been paid to the venous side of the circulation. The veins differ from the arteries in that they readily undergo dilatation and considerable increase in their capacity with very little alteration in venous pressure. This is especially true of the veins of the abdominal cavity where the external support is poor and depends upon the variable state of distension of the viscera. It appeared to him that, if a subject with a lax abdominal wall changes from the horizontal to the upright position, blood will stagnate in the abdominal veins and the amount of blood returning to the heart will diminish. The heart, receiving less blood, has less to pump out; hence the fall in blood pressure.

In order to test this hypothesis Roberts carried out some experiments, the results of which he described at a meeting of the Physiological Society some years ago but did not publish. A cat was anaesthetised lightly with urethane and the blood pressure was recorded by tying a cannula into a carotid artery and taking a tracing on a smoked drum. When the cat was turned feet down there was a drop in the blood pressure followed by recovery which was only partial; the carotid pressure remained permanently lower in the upright than in the horizontal position. He then tied the armlet of an ordinary sphygmomanometer around the cat's trunk and distended this with air sufficiently to compress the abdomen with a pressure of the same order as the venous pressure—that is, 30–50 mm. of water. He found that, when the position of the cat was changed, the blood pressure remained almost unaltered, the reason being that dilatation of the abdominal veins was prevented by the external pressure.

He also tried the effect of internal pressure. He passed about 300 c.c. of water through a rubber oesophageal tube into the stomach (the cat having been starved before the experiment), and found again that the compensation against gravity was much improved, although it was not as good as when external pressure was applied.

He concluded therefore that alteration in the capacity of the abdominal veins played the major part in enabling an animal to maintain a steady central blood pressure in the face of alterations due to gravity.

APPENDIX V

INTERNATIONAL RECOMMENDATIONS FOR X-RAY AND RADIUM PROTECTION

(Promulgated at the Second International Congress of Radiology, Stockholm, July, 1928)

1. The dangers of over-exposure to X rays and radium can be avoided by the provision of adequate protection and suitable working conditions. It is the duty of those in charge of X-ray and radium departments to ensure such conditions for their personnel. The known effects to be guarded against are:

   (a) Injuries to the superficial tissues;
   (b) Derangements of internal organs and changes in the blood.

I. Working hours, etc.

2. The following working hours, etc., are recommended for whole-time X-ray and radium workers:

   (a) Not more than seven working hours a day.
   (b) Not more than five working days a week. The off-days to be spent as much as possible out of doors.
   (c) Not less than one month's holiday a year.
   (d) Whole-time workers in hospital X-ray and radium departments should not be called upon for other hospital service.

II. General X-ray recommendations

3. X-ray departments should not be situated below ground floor level.

4. All rooms, including dark rooms, should be provided with windows affording good natural lighting and ready facilities for admitting sunshine and fresh air whenever possible.

5. All rooms should be provided with adequate exhaust ventilation capable of renewing the air of the room not less than ten times an hour. Air inlets and outlets should be arranged to afford cross-wise ventilation of the room.

6. All rooms should preferably be decorated in light colours.

7. X-ray rooms should be large enough to permit a convenient lay-out of the equipment. A minimum floor area of 250 sq. ft. (25 sq. metres) is recommended for X-ray rooms and 100 sq. ft. (10 sq. metres) for dark rooms. Ceilings should be not less than 11 ft. (3·5 metres) high.

8. A working temperature of about 18° C. (65° F.) is desirable in X-ray rooms.

9. Wherever practicable, the X-ray generating apparatus should be placed in a separate room from the X-ray tube.

III. X-ray protective recommendations

10. An X-ray operator should on no account expose himself unnecessarily to a direct beam of X rays.

11. An operator should place himself as remote as practicable from the X-ray tube. It should not be possible for a well-rested eye of normal acuity to detect in the dark appreciable fluorescence of a screen placed in the permanent position of the operator.

12. The X-ray tube should be surrounded as completely as possible with protective material of adequate lead equivalent.

13. The following lead equivalents are recommended as adequate:

X rays generated by peak voltages	Minimum equivalent thickness of lead (mm.)
Not exceeding 75 K.V.	1·0
100	1·5
125	2·0
150	2·5
175	3·0
200	4·0
225	5·0

14. In the case of diagnostic work, the operator should be afforded protection from scattered rays by a screen of a minimum lead equivalent of 1 mm.

15. In the case of X-ray treatment the operator is best stationed completely outside the X-ray room behind a protective wall of a minimum lead equivalent of 2 mm. This figure should be correspondingly increased if the protective value of the X-ray tube enclosure falls short of the values given in paragraph 13. In such event the remaining walls, floor and ceiling may also be required to provide supplementary protection for adjacent occupants to an extent depending on the circumstances.

16. Screening examinations should be conducted as rapidly as possible with minimum intensities and apertures.

17. The lead glass of fluorescent screens should have the protective values recommended in paragraph 13.

18. In the case of screening stands the fluorescent screen should, if necessary, be provided with a protective "surround" so that adequate protection against direct radiation is afforded for all positions of the screen and diaphragm.

19. Screening stands and couches should provide adequate arrangements for protecting the operator against scattered radiation from the patient.

20. Inspection windows in screens and walls should have protective lead values equivalent to that of the surrounding screen or wall.

21. Efficient safeguards should be adopted to avoid the omission of a metal filter in X-ray treatment.

22. Protective gloves, which should be suitably lined with fabric or other material, should have a protective value not less than $\frac{1}{2}$ mm. lead throughout both back and front (including fingers and wrist). Protective aprons should have a minimum lead value of $\frac{1}{2}$ mm.

IV. ELECTRICAL PRECAUTIONS IN X-RAY ROOMS

23. The floor-covering of the X-ray room should be of insulating material such as wood, rubber or linoleum.

24. Overhead conductors should not be less than 9 ft. (3 metres) from the floor. They should consist of stout metal tubing or other corona-less type of conductor. The associated connecting leads should be of corona-less wire kept taut by suitable rheophores.

25. Wherever possible, earthed guards should be provided to shield the more adjacent parts of the high tension system. Unless there are reasons to the contrary, metal parts of the apparatus and room should be efficiently earthed.

26. The use of quick-acting double-pole circuit breakers is recommended. Over-powered fuses should not be used. If more than one apparatus is operated from a common generator, suitable overhead multi-way switches should be provided.

27. Some suitable form of kilo-voltmeter should be provided to afford a measure of the voltage operating the X-ray tube.

V. RADIUM PROTECTIVE RECOMMENDATIONS

(A) *Radium Salts*

28. Protection for radium workers is required from the effects of:
   (a) Beta rays upon the hands;
   (b) Gamma rays upon the internal organs, vascular and reproductive systems.

29. In order to protect the hands from beta rays, reliance should be placed, in the first place, on distance. The radium should be manipulated with long-handled forceps, preferably made of wood, and should be carried from place to place in long-handled boxes, lined on all sides with about 1 cm. of lead. All manipulations should be carried out as rapidly as possible.

30. Radium, when not in use, should be stored in a safe as distant as possible from the personnel. It is recommended that radium tubes or applicators be inserted into separate lead blocks in the safe, giving a thickness of protective wall amounting to 5 cm. of lead per 100 milligrammes of radium element.

31. A separate room should be provided for the "make-up" of screened tubes and applicators, and this room should only be occupied during such work.

32. In order to protect the body from the penetrating gamma rays during handling of the radium, a screen of not less than one inch thickness of lead should be used, and proximity to the radium should only occur during actual work and for as short a time as possible.

33. The measurement room should be a separate room and it should contain the radium only during its actual measurement.

34. Nurses and attendants should not remain in the same room as patients undergoing radium treatment.

35. All unskilled work, or work which can be learnt in a short period of time, should preferably be carried out by temporary workers, who should be engaged on such work for periods not exceeding six months. This applies especially to nurses and those engaged in "making-up" applicators.

36. Discretion should be exercised in transmitting radium salts by post. In the case of small quantities it is recommended that the container should be lined throughout with lead not less than 3 mm. thick. It is more satisfactory to transport large quantities by hand in a suitably designed carrying case.

(B) *Emanation*

37. In the manipulation of emanation, protection against the beta and gamma rays has likewise to be provided.

38. The handling of emanation should be carried out, as far as possible, during its relatively inactive state.

39. The escape of emanation should be very carefully guarded against, and the room in which it is prepared should be provided with an exhaust fan.

40. Where emanation is likely to come in direct contact with the fingers, thin rubber gloves should be worn to avoid contamination of the hands with active deposit. Otherwise, the protective measures recommended for radium salts should be carried out.

41. A separate pumping room should be provided with a connecting tube from the special room in which the radium is stored in solution. The radium in solution should be heavily screened to protect people working in adjacent rooms. This is preferably done by placing the radium in solution in a lead-lined box, the thickness of lead recommended being according to the following table:

Quantity of radium element	Thickness of lead
0·5 g.	6 in. (15 cm.)
1·0	6·6 (16·5 „)
1·5	6·8 (17 „)
2·0	7·2 (18 „)

N.B. Reference may also be made to the Recommendations of the British Protection Committee, copies of which may be obtained from the Director, The National Physical Laboratory, Teddington, Middlesex.

APPENDIX VI

THE LEGAL OWNERSHIP OF X-RAY FILMS*

By D. H. KITCHIN, of Gray's Inn, Barrister-at-Law

The question of who is the legal owner of an X-ray film does not seem ever to have been settled in an English court. It can therefore only be answered tentatively from a study of the principles of law which seem to be involved. The answer seems to depend on the nature of the contract which exists between the patient and the person or persons who make the film.

When a court of law has to interpret a doubtful contract, one of the most important problems before it is to discover what the parties meant their bargain to include when they made it. When a patient goes to a medical man for X-ray examination, the contract is not only unwritten but also largely unspoken. The general practitioner may have told the patient what the fee will be and arranged an hour for the examination; otherwise the conditions are all "implied", which means in this instance that no one has bothered much to consider what they are. If, therefore, a patient ever goes to an English court claiming possession of radiograms, or is sued for the radiologist's fee and says in defence that he has not received the films, the court will have to decide what contract the parties really intended to make. In making this decision it will first inquire into the usual custom in the profession, since if the parties have not expressed any particular intention and the transaction seems to be a usual one, they will generally be thought to have intended to follow the current custom in their dealings with one another. The court will therefore inquire: Is it the custom of the profession to hand over the X-ray films to the patient as part of the service for which he pays? If the court found that such a custom did not exist, it would be very slow to suppose that the parties intended, at the time they made their bargain, to do something unusual. It would only infer an unusual condition from evidence that the parties had expressly agreed to it—evidence either of an actual agreement in so many words, or of some behaviour by one or both parties which clearly showed that they had agreed to this condition. Moreover, if the patient declares that he and the radiologist agreed that he was to have the films, he must prove it; and if he declares that it is the custom for films to be handed to the patient, he must prove that before he can win his case. It is not for the radiologist to prove the contrary; though, of course, he would be well advised to bring evidence that it is customary for radiologists to retain films. As far as legal

* Abstracted from *Legal Problems in Medical Practice.* London, 1936, Edward Arnold.

ownership is concerned, the court would probably find that it remained with the radiologist or other medical man who took the films. As there seems to be no doubt that this is really the custom of the profession, it does not seem at all likely that any patient could succeed in establishing a claim to own films taken in the ordinary course of medical practice.

Notwithstanding this, the patient may conceivably have some say in the use to which films are put. If a patient breaks the head of a femur and is examined by a radiologist, and several years afterwards fractures the bone again, he certainly seems to have some right to benefit by the information which the earlier films contain. The original fee which he paid surely includes the future use of the films—irrespective of who owns them—at any time when they might be of use. Again, if a patient, after being examined by a radiologist, changes his surgical or medical adviser, he is surely justified in expecting the radiologist to give his new doctor full information about his case and to show him the films, if not without further fee, then at least for a minor one commensurate with the slight trouble of preparing and sending a duplicate report. This right may not be one which the patient could enforce in a court of law, but it would probably be granted to him by the radiologist as a matter of medical expediency and ordinary courtesy.

It has sometimes been suggested that the general practitioner owns the films, since they are part of the confidential report made to him by the radiologist. It seems fairly certain that the general practitioner cannot claim to be the owner of the films, for he is not one of the parties to the contract and has given no consideration for the film. It is just possible, however, that, if the radiologist sends the films attached to his report without reservation, the property contained in them passes to the general practitioner.

The British Medical Association has stated an opinion that films taken in hospital belong to the hospital and should be kept there and treated as confidential documents. This view is almost certainly sound in law. The patient who pays nothing to the hospital obviously has no claim to any film which may be taken in it. A patient who pays a weekly sum obviously pays for board, maintenance and service and perhaps pays for skilled treatment and nursing, but can no more claim to be paying for his radiograms than for his temperature charts. A patient in a nursing-home which possesses an X-ray installation may be in a slightly different position. Sometimes a diagnostic X-ray examination is a service for which he is charged specially. In this instance he pays a fee for the use of the apparatus and the help it gives in diagnosis. Although the films are part of the apparatus and do not become his property unless there is an express agreement that they shall, it seems probable that, having paid for the special service, he could claim the use of them if at a later date a medical adviser wished to see them. He is probably in the same position as if he had paid a radiologist's fee as a private patient.

To sum up, the question of who owns an X-ray film depends for its answer on the intentions of the parties to the contract. When the contract is between a patient and a medical practitioner, the parties will probably be taken, in the absence of an express agreement to the contrary, to have intended to follow the custom of the profession. It is almost certainly the custom that the films remain the property of the medical man who takes them, or under whose direction they are taken. Although many radiologists recognise an informal right in the patient to have the films lent to a practitioner who may at a future time have charge of the case for his guidance in its treatment, it is unlikely that the patient could enforce such a right at law.

APPENDIX VII

THE PHOTOGRAPHIC METHOD OF ESTIMATING EXPOSURE TO X-RAYS

While this book has been passing through the press, two papers dealing with the photographic method of X-ray measurement have been published by G. E. Bell,* who points out that in order to use the photographic action for measuring (in r units) quantities of radiation, we must know:

(1) How the blackening (or "photographic density")† of the film depends on the quantity of X rays falling on it.

(2) To what extent the blackening is influenced by the intensity of the radiation, as distinct from the quantity, which is, of course, the product of the intensity and time of irradiation.

(3) How the sensitivity of the film depends on the quality or hardness of the radiation.

The influence of these three factors was studied in some detail for most of the common makes of films (used, of course, without intensifying screens) and the more usual developers (Ilford, Kodak and Agfa formulae), and it was found that up to densities of unity the blackening is nearly proportional to the exposure, while for densities greater than 1·5 the blackening increases much less rapidly than the exposure. It was further found that at least over the range of intensities of 10,000 to 1, it is quite immaterial whether the exposure is made with an intense beam for a short time or with a weak beam for a correspondingly longer time.

The sensitivity of the film varies, of course, considerably with the quality of the radiation, and the paper includes curves showing the nature of this variation. In Fig. 296 the number of r units required to give a blackening of 0·5 is plotted against the half-value-layer in copper of the radiation. This curve indicates that the film shows a maximum sensitivity for a fairly soft radiation (H.V.L. 0·25 mm. Cu) and that for harder and softer radiations the sensitivity is lower. Thus to produce a given blackening requires three times as much radiation of H.V.L. 1·8 mm. Cu as of radiation having a H.V.L. of 0·25 mm. Cu.

In assessing the amount of radiation to which an X-ray worker has been subjected, the half-value-layer of the radiation is rarely known since there is a

* *British Journal of Radiology*, Vol. IX, No. 105, Sept. 1936, p. 578.

† The density of a film is determined by finding the fraction of incident light (I_0) transmitted by the film. If the transmitted intensity is I_1, the "density" (D) is given by

$$D = \log_{10} \frac{I_0}{I_1}.$$

mixture of very hard rays which have passed through the protective material and fairly soft rays which have been scattered by the patient and apparatus. In the range of X rays used for diagnostic purposes, Bell points out that the radiation is fairly soft and the blackenings produced on films worn by operators can

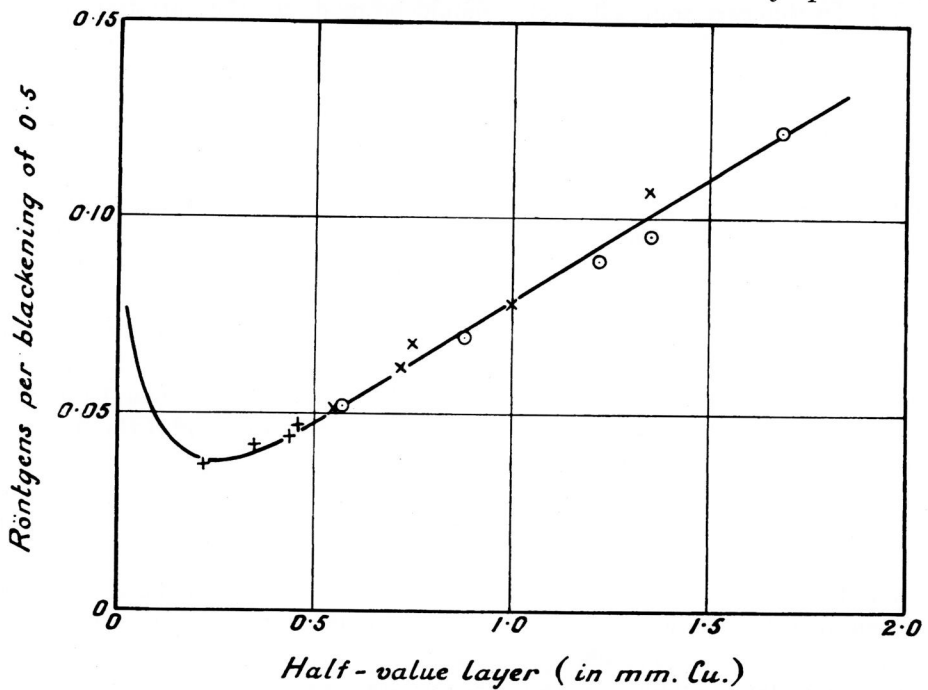

Fig. 296. Exposures (in r units) of various qualities of X rays necessary to produce a blackening of 0·5.

be compared with standard blackenings obtained by the method described on p. 35 of the paper. If such tests are carried out in a hospital not equipped with means of measuring the U.S.D. a less accurate but still serviceable estimate of the amount of radiation can be found by assuming that for ordinary films developed in standard developers under normal conditions, a blackening of unity* corresponds to about 0·1 rontgen (i.e. about 0·0002 U.S.D.). If the blackening of a film carried by an operator during a working day does not exceed unity, the exposure is safe, judged by any reasonable standard. If the blackening exceeds unity, or in extreme cases 1·5, it is not correct to assume that it is proportional to the

---

* There are several ways of measuring the density, but the simplest is to compare it with "standard tints" of known density. Such standard tints can be bought quite cheaply. Tints of densities 0·1, 0·2, 0·3, 0·5 and 1·0 serve to give densities up to 2·1 since they are additive, i.e. 0·7 may be obtained by adding 0·2 and 0·5.

exposure, and the film should be worn for half a day, or even a normal hour, and the daily exposure calculated by multiplying by the appropriate factor.

In therapy departments the stray radiation may be very hard, particularly if the operator works in a cubicle towards which the direct beam of X rays is pointed. In this case some allowance should be made for the variation in film sensitivity with the hardness of the radiation. To this end Bell suggests that two-thirds of the film should be covered by copper sheet about 1 mm. thick. After development, the portion of the film behind the copper is, of course, less dense. If this part is cut, and the two portions are superimposed, it can be seen at once whether the H.V.L. of the radiation is less than, equal to or greater than, 1 mm. Cu, since if the H.V.L. is *greater* than 1 mm. the two superimposed parts are together *denser* than the part of the film not shielded by the copper, while if the two superimposed parts are *lighter* than the unshielded portion, the H.V.L. is *less* than 1 mm. Cu.

By this means it is possible to estimate the exposure in rontgens since, if the H.V.L. is less than 1·0 mm., the amount of radiation may be found by direct comparison with the standard tint while for H.V.L.'s much greater than 1 mm. Cu the apparent dose should be increased by three or four times and if the H.V.L. is about 1 mm. Cu the apparent dose should be increased by 50%.

This method of correction is only a refinement, and a rough working rule for estimating the exposure in terms of the density of a film is "*A density of unity corresponds to an exposure of about* 0·1 *rontgen* (*or* 0·0002 U.S.D.)." If, however, the radiation is known to contain little scattered radiation, and the X-ray tube has been operated at high voltages, as in treatment, it is well to err on the side of safety and take the blackening of unity as corresponding to an exposure of about 0·3 r or 0·0006 U.S.D.

BIBLIOGRAPHY

AARON. *See* Levyn.

ABBE, R. *See* Wald (326).

(1) ABERLE, A. *Med.-chir. Zeitung*, Salzburg and Innsbruck, 1826, IV, 253.

ADAM. *See* Sauerbruch.

(2) ADAMS, J. E. *Brit. Med. Jour.* 1925, II, 1041.

(3) ADAMS, T. W., CLARKE, D. J., LEES, J. M., PEMBREY, M. S. and VINE, R. S. *Brit. Jour. Radiol.* 1932, V, 824, 869.

ADAMSON. *See* Knight.

ADIE. *See* Cabot.

(4) ÅKERLUND, A. Röntgenologische Studien über den Bulbus Duodeni. *Acta Radiol.* Suppl. I, Stockholm, 1921, I. Marcus.

(5) —— *Acta Radiol.* 1927, VIII, 538.

(6) —— *Amer. Jour. Surg.* 1931, XI, 233, 504.

(7) ALBRECHT, H. U. *Das Ulcusproblem im Lichte moderner Röntgenforschung.* Leipzig, 1930, Georg Thieme.

(8) —— *Forts. Geb. Rönt.* 1929, II, 374.

(9) ALLBUTT, T. CLIFFORD. *On Visceral Neuroses.* London, 1884, J. and A. Churchill.

ALLEN. *See* Smith.

(10) ALTSCHUL, W. *Brit. Jour. Radiol.* (B.I.R. Sect.), 1925, XXX, 465.

(11) ALVAREZ, W. C. *The Mechanics of the Digestive Tract.* 1928, 2nd ed. William Heinemann, Ltd.

(12) —— *Jour. Amer. Med. Assoc.* 1917, LXIX, 2018.

(13) —— *Amer. Jour. Roent.* 1921, VIII, 1.

(14) —— and FREEDLANDER, B. L. *Jour. Amer. Med. Assoc.* 1924, LXXXIII, 576.

(15) —— and GIANTURCO, C. *Proc. Staff Meet. Mayo Clinic,* 1932, VII, 669.

(16) —— and JUDD, E. S. *Proc. Staff Meet. Mayo Clinic,* 1934, IX, 433.

(17) —— —— WILBUR, D. L. and BAKER, C. P. *Proc. Staff Meet. Mayo Clinic,* 1934, IX, 433.

(18) —— and VANZANT, F. K. *Proc. Staff Meet. Mayo Clinic,* 1931, VI, 419.

(19) ANDERSON, A. G., LOCKHART, R. D. and SOUTER, W. C. *Brain,* 1931, LIV, 460.

(20) ANDERSON, C. C. *Brit. Jour. Radiol.* 1928, I, 428.

(21) ANDERSON, W. K. *Radiography and Clin. Phot.* 1934, IX, 15.

ANDREWS. *See* Miller, T. G.

(22) ANSELL, P. L. *Amer. Jour. Roent.* 1919, VI, 459.

(23) ARISZ, L. *Acta Radiol.* 1932, XIII, 41.

(24) ASCHNER, P. W. and GROSSMAN, S. *Surg. Gyn. and Obst.* 1933, LVII, 334.

(25) BAASTRUP, C. I. *Acta Radiol.* 1924, III, 180.

(26) BAILLIE, MATTHEW. *Lond. Med. Reposit.* 1825, XXIV, 515.

BAKER. *See* Alvarez.

(27) BALFOUR, D. C. *Proc. Staff Meet. Mayo Clinic,* 1931, VI, 55.

(28) BARCLAY, A. E. *Proc. Roy. Soc. Med.* 1909, II (Sect. Electrotherapy), 53.

(29) —— *Brit. Med. Jour.* 1910, II, 540.

(30) —— *Arch. Roent. Ray,* 1912, XVI, 422.

(31) —— *Med. Chron.* 1913, CLXXXVII, 249.

(32) —— (and RAMSBOTTOM). *Arch. Roent. Ray,* 1913, XVIII, 167.

(33) —— *Proc. Roy. Soc. Med.* 1913, VI (Sect. Electrotherapy), 138.

(34) —— *Proc. Roy. Soc. Med.* 1914, VII (Sect. Electrotherapy), 15.

BIBLIOGRAPHY

(35) BARCLAY, A. E. *Arch. Roent. Ray*, 1914, XIX, 172.

(36) —— *Proc. Roy. Soc. Med.* 1915, VIII (Sect. Electrotherapy), 96.

(37) —— *Jour. Anat.* 1920, LIV, 260.

(38) —— *Amer. Jour. Roent.* 1922, IX, 792.

(39) —— *Acta Radiol.* 1926, IV, 135; *Brit. Jour. Radiol.* 1926, XXXI, 385.

(40) —— *Quart. Jour. Med.* 1932, XXV, 257.

(41) —— *Brit. Jour. Radiol.* 1927, XXXII, 446.

(42) —— *Brit. Jour. Radiol.* 1930, III, 534; *Proc. Staff Meet. Mayo Clinic*, 1930, V, 251.

(43) —— *Brit. Jour. Radiol.* 1930, III, 295.

(44) —— *The Alimentary Tract: A Radiographic Study.* Manchester, 1915, Sherratt and Hughes.

(45) —— The Rockefeller Foundation, *Methods and Problems of Medical Education*, 12th Series, 1929.

(46) —— *The Lancet*, 1922, II, 261.

(47) —— *Arch. Roent. Ray*, 1910, XV, 167.

(48) —— *Brit. Jour. Surg.* 1915, II, 638.

(49) —— *Brit. Med. Jour.* 1928, II, 671.

(50) —— *Brit. Med. Jour.* 1928, II, 1026.

(51) —— *The Lancet*, 1934, II, 1258.

(52) —— *Brit. Jour. Radiol.* 1935, VIII, 652.

(53) —— *Brit. Jour. Radiol.* 1935, VIII, 373.

(54) —— and Cox, S. F. *Amer. Jour. Roent.* 1928, XIX, 551.

BARGEN. *See* Wesson.

BARRET. *See* Leven.

(54a) BÁRSONY, A. *Forts. Geb. Rönt.* 1928, XXXVIII, 629.

BARTLE. *See* Lyon.

BECK. *See* Levyn.

(55) BÉCLÈRE, H. and MERIEL, E. *Ann. internat. de chir. gastro-intest.* 1912, VI, 132, 190.

(56) BEDINGFIELD, H. *Quart. Jour. Med.* 1928–9, XXII, 611; and 1929–30, XXIII, 1.

(57) BELL, J. R. and MacADAM, W. *Quart. Jour. Med.* 1923–4, XVII, 215.

(58) BERG, H. H. *Roentgenuntersuchungen am Innenrelief des Verdauungskanals.* Leipzig, 1930, Georg Thieme.

(59) —— *Über das klinische und röntgendiagnostische Bild der Hiatusbrüche und der Divertikel des Magendarmkanals.* Proc. 10th Conference, 1930, Gesellschaft für Verdauungs- und Stoffwechselkrankheiten. Leipzig, 1931, Georg Thieme, p. 68.

(60) —— *Brit. Jour. Radiol.* (B.I.R. Sect.), 1925, XXX, 372.

(61) BERGLUND, NILS. *Acta Paed.* 1928–9, VIII, 323.

(62) BERGMANN, G. VON. In *Spez. Path. u. Therap. innerer Krankh.* 1921, Kraus und Brugsch, V, 367.

(63) BIGELOW, W. A. *Canad. Med. Assoc. Jour.* 1930, XXIII, 22.

(64) BLAND-SUTTON, J. *The Lancet*, 1914, II, 931.

(65) BOLDIREFF, W. Quoted by A. J. Carlson, *The Control of Hunger in Health and Disease.* Chicago, 1916, p. 75.

BOLLMAN. *See* Caylor.

(66) BOLTON, C. and SALMOND, R. W. A. *The Lancet*, 1927, I, 1230.

(67) BRAILSFORD, J. F. *Proc. Roy. Soc. Med.* 1932, XXV, 1249.

(68) BRAITHWAITE, L. R. *Brit. Jour. Surg.* 1923, XI, 7.

BROWN. *See* Goldthwait.

(69) BUCKSTEIN, J. *Amer. Jour. Roent.* 1932, XXVII, 59.

(70) —— *Peptic Ulcer, Annals of Roentgenology.* New York, 1933.

(70a) —— *Amer. Jour. Roent.* 1934, XXXII, 171.

(71) BURCH, H. A. *Proc. Staff Meet. Mayo Clinic*, 1935, X, 471.

(71a) BURKITT, F. T. *The Lancet*, 1933, II, 728.

(72) BUZZARD, T. *Trans. Path. Soc. Lond.* 1889, XL, 347.

(73) CABOT, H. and ADIE, G. C. *Ann. Surg.* 1925, LXXXII, 86.

(74) CAMPBELL, J. M. H. and CONYBEARE, J. J. *Guy's Hosp. Rep.* 1924, LXXIV, 354.

(75) CANDY, T. I. *The Lancet*, 1926, I, 15.

(76) CANNON, W. B. *Amer. Jour. Physiol.* 1898, I, 359.

(77) CANTANI. *Virchows Jahresbericht*, 1879, II, 180.

(78) CANTIERI, C. *Arch. Sci. Med., Turin*, 1910, XXXIV, 439.

(79) CARLSON, A. J. *The Control of Hunger in Health and Disease.* Chicago, 1916, p. 75.

(80) CARMAN, R. D. and MILLER, A. *The Roentgen Diagnosis of Diseases of the Alimentary Canal.* Philadelphia, 1917, W. B. Saunders Co.

(81) —— *Acta Radiol.* 1926, VI, 224.

(82) —— and FINEMAN, S. *Radiology*, 1924, III, 26.

(83) CARSLAW, R. B. *The Lancet*, 1927, I, 287; and *Brit. Jour. Surg.* 1927-8, XV, 545.

(84) CARSON, H. W. *Post-Grad. Med. Jour.* 1926, II, 33.

(85) CARTER, L. J. *Canad. Med. Assoc. Jour.* 1921, XI, 256; 1924, XIV, 212.

(86) CASE, J. T. *Amer. Jour. Roent.* 1929, XXI, 217.

(87) —— *Amer. Jour. Roent.* 1915, II, 654.

(88) —— *Amer. Jour. Roent.* 1916, III, 314.

(89) —— *Proc. 17th Internat. Congress of Medicine*, London, 1913 (Sect. Radiol.), "X-ray Observations on Colonic Peristalsis, etc."

(90) —— *Arch. Roent. Ray*, 1915, XIX, 375.

(91) —— *Acta Radiol.* 1926, VI, 230.

(92) —— *Jour. Amer. Med. Assoc.* 1920, LXXV, 1463.

(93) CAYLOR, H. D. and BOLLMAN, J. L. *Arch. Path. and Lab. Med.* 1927, III, 993.

(94) CERNÉ, A. and DELAFORGE. *La radioscopie clinique de l'estomac.* Paris, 1908, J.-B. Baillière et fils.

CHAMBERLAIN. *See* Moody.

(95) CHAOUL, H. *In* Stierlin: *Klinische Röntgendiagnostik des Verdauungskanals.* Berlin, 1928, J. Springer.

CHAOUL, H. *See* Sauerbruch.

(96) CHURCH, G. T. and WALTERS, W. *Proc. Staff Meet. Mayo Clinic*, 1933, VIII, 733.

(97) CILLY, E. I. L., LEDDY, E. T. and KIRKLIN, B. R. *Amer. Jour. Roent.* 1934, XXXII, 360, 805; 1935, XXXIII, 88.

CLARKE. *See* Adams.

(98) CLAESSEN, G. *The Roentgen Diagnosis of Echinococcus Tumours.* Acta Radiol. Supp. VI, 1928.

(99) CLAYTON-GREEN, W. H. and HARRIS, W. *Proc. Roy. Soc. Med.* 1911-12, V (Clin. Sect.), 153.

(100) COFFEY, R. C. *Gastroenteroptosis.* D. Appleton and Co. 1923.

(101) COLE, L. G. *Arch. Roent. Ray*, 1911-12, XVI, 242, 425; XVII, 172.

(102) —— *The Lancet*, 1914, I, 1239.

COLE, W. H. *See* Graham.

(102a) COLE COLLABORATORS. *The Radiological Exploration of the Mucosa of the Gastrointestinal Tract*, 1934. Bruce Pub. Co.

(103) —— —— *Radiology*, 1932, XVIII, 221, 471.

(104) CONRAN, P. C. *Quart. Jour. Med.* 1921-2, XV, 144.

CONYBEARE. *See* Campbell.

COPHER. *See* Graham.

COX. *See* Barclay.

(105) CRANE, A. W. *Amer. Jour. Roent.* 1927, XVII, 416.

(106) CRUVEILHIER, J. *Traité d'anatomie pathologique générale.* Paris, 1849, Baillière et fils.

CRYMBLE. *See* Smith.

(107) DALTON, N. and REID, A. D. *Trans. Clin. Soc. Lond.* 1905, XXXVIII, 122.

(108) DAVIS, K. S. and PARKER, C. *Radiol. Rev.* 1930, LII, 317.

DELAFORGE. *See* Cerné.

(109) DIETRICH, H. A. *Münch. med. Woch.* 1912, LIX, 638.

(110) DUNHILL, T. *Brit. Jour. Surg.* 1935, XXII, 475.

(111) DURET, H. *Rev. de chir.* Paris, 1896, XVI, 421.

(112) EINHORN, M. *N.Y. Med. Rec.* 1888, XXXIV, 751.

(113) —— *Arch. Roent. Ray*, 1907, XI, 265.

(114) ELLIOT SMITH, G. Cunningham's *Anatomy*, 1922, 5th ed. p. 594.

ELLISON. *See* Lyon.

(115) EWING, J. *Ann. Surg.* 1918, LXVII, 715.

(116) FABER, K. *Arch. de mal. de l'app. digestif*, 1926, XVI, 969.

FELDMAN. *See* Friedenwald.

FINEMAN. *See* Carman.

(117) FINZI, N. S. *Proc. Roy. Soc. Med.* 1916, X (Sect. Electrotherapy), 63.

(118) FLINT, E. R. *Brit. Med. Jour.* 1921, II, 257.

(119) —— *The Lancet*, 1921, I, 903.

(120) FORSSELL, G. *Archiv und Atlas der normalen und pathologischen Anatomie in typischen Röntgenbildern.* Hamburg, 1913, Gräfe und Sillem.

(121) —— Normale und pathologische Reliefbilder der Schleimhaut. *Proc. 7th Conference, Gesellschaft für Verdauungs- und Stoffwechselkrankheiten*, 1927, p. 199. Leipzig, 1928, Georg Thieme.

(122) —— *Forts. Geb. Rönt.* 1928, XXXVII, 393.

(123) —— *Amer. Jour. Roent.* 1923, X, 87.

FREEDLANDER. *See* Alvarez.

(124) FRIEDENWALD, J. and FELDMAN, M. *Radiology*, 1933, XXI, 162.

(125) GAGE, H. C. *Brit. Jour. Radiol.* 1932, V. 282.

(126) —— and HUNT, T. C. *Brit. Jour. Radiol.* 1932, V, 718.

GAGE. *See* Miller.

(127) GEHUCHTEN, VAN and MOLHANT. *Le Névraxe*, 1912, XIII, 55.

(128) GEORGE, A. W. and LEONARD, R. D. *The Roentgen Diagnosis of Surgical Lesions of the Gastro-Intestinal Tract.* Boston, 1915.

(129) —— —— *The Pathological Gall-Bladder*, vol. II. *Annals of Roentgenology.*

(130) —— and GERBER, I. *Amer. Jour. Roent.* 1914, I, 287.

GERBER. *See* George.

GERSHON-COHEN. *See* Shay.

(131) GIANTURCO, C. *Proc. Staff Meet. Mayo Clinic*, 1933, VIII, 737.

(132) —— *Proc. Staff Meet. Mayo Clinic*, 1933, VIII, 784.

GIANTURCO. *See* Alvarez.

(133) GIBBON, W. H. *Radiology*, 1933, XXI, 491.

(134) GLÉNARD, F. *Sem. méd.* Paris, 1886, VI, 211. *Les ptoses viscérales.* Paris, 1899.

(135) GOLDTHWAIT, J. E. and BROWN, L. T. *Surg., Gyn. and Obst.* 1913, XVI, 587.

(136) GOLOB, M. *Radiology*, 1933, XXI, 277.

(137) GOODALL, A. *Edin. Med. Jour.* 1932, XXXIX, 85.

(138) GRÅBERGER, G. *Acta Radiol.* 1931, XII, 164.

(139) GRAHAM, E. A., COLE, W. H. and COPHER, G. H. *Jour. Amer. Med. Assoc.* 1925, LXXXIV, 14.

(140) GRAY, E. D. *Brit. Jour. Radiol.* 1932, V, 640.

(141) GRIER, G. W. *Radiology*, 1924, II, 265.

(142) GROEDEL, F. M. *Berl. klin. Woch.* 1908, XLV, 742.

(143) —— *Deuts. med. Woch.* 1910, XXXVI, 701.

(144) GROEDEL, F. M. "Die Magenbewegungen" in *Archiv und Atlas der normalen und pathologischen Anatomie in typischen Röntgenbildern*. Leipzig, 1912, Georg Thieme; *Forts. Geb. Rönt.* Suppl. 27.

GROSSMAN. *See* Aschner.

(145) HACKWOOD, J. F. *Brit. Med. Jour.* 1934, I, 1030.

(146) HAËN, ANTONIUS DE. *Ratio medendi in nosocomio practico.* Vienna, 1747, X, 372.

HARRIS. *See* Clayton-Green.

(147) HASSELWANDER. *Sitzungsberichten der Phys.-med. Soz. zu Erlangen*, 1934, LXV, 35.

HASTINGS. *See* James.

(148) HAUDEK, M. *Arch. Roent. Ray*, 1911, XVI, 6.

(149) —— *Wien. med. Woch.* 1913, LXIII, 1251.

(150) HAUSMANN, T. *Berl. klin. Woch.* 1904, XLI, 1153.

(151) HEALY, T. R. *Amer. Jour. Roent.* 1925, XIII, 266.

HECK. *See* Priestley.

(152) HENNING, N. *Die Entzündung des Magens.* Leipzig, 1934, J. A. Barth.

(153) HERRNHEISER, G. *Forts. Geb. Rönt.* 1924, XXXI, 702.

HIGGINS. *See* Mann.

(154) HIRSCH, I. SETH. *Med. Jour. Rec.* 1924, CXIX, 541.

(155) HJELM, R. *Acta Radiol.* 1931, XII, 146.

HODGSON, GRAHAM. *See* Lockhart-Mummery.

(156) HOLLAND, C. THURSTAN. *Clin. Jour.* 1914, XLIII, 199.

(157) —— *Arch. Roent. Ray*, 1913, XVIII, 46

(158) —— *Arch. Roent. Ray*, 1914, XVIII, 373.

(159) HOLMES, G. W. and SCHATZKI, R. *Amer. Jour. Roent.* 1935, XXXIV, 145.

(160) HOLZKNECHT, G. *Mitteil. aus dem Lab. für radiol. Diag. und Ther.* Wien, 1906, I, 72.

(161) —— *Münch. med. Woch.* 1909, LVI, 2401. Translated in *Arch. Roent. Ray*, 1910, XIV, 273.

(162) HORTON, B. T. *Amer. Jour. Anat.* 1928, XLI, 197.

(163) —— and MUELLER, S. C. *Proc. Staff Meet. Mayo Clinic*, 1932, VII, 185.

HUNT. *See* Gage.

(164) HUNTER, RICHARD H. *Jour. Anat.* 1934, LXVIII, 264.

(165) —— *Ulster Med. Jour.* 1933, II, 104.

(166) —— *Jour. Anat.* 1928, LXII, 297.

(167) HURST, A. F. *The Sensibility of the Alimentary Canal.* London, 1911, Oxf. Med. Pub. p. 47.

(168) —— *Constipation and Allied Intestinal Disorders.* London, 1909, Oxf. Med. Pub.

(169) —— *Guy's Hosp. Rep.* 1927, LXXVII, 22.

(170) —— *Brit. Med. Jour.* 1913, II, 918.

(171) —— *Proc. Roy. Soc. Med.* 1914, VII (Sect. Electrotherapy), 10.

(172) —— *Proc. Roy. Soc. Med.* 1909, II (Sect. Electrotherapy), 73.

(173) —— *Arch. Radiol. and Electrol.* 1915, XX, 143.

(174) —— *Medical Essays and Addresses.* London, 1924, W. Heinemann. (Medical Books.)

(175) —— *Brit. Med. Jour.* 1933, II, 89.

(176) —— *Guy's Hosp. Rep.* 1934, LXXXIV, 43.

(177) —— *Brit. Med. Jour.* 1935, I, 1002.

(178) —— *Price's Text-book of Medicine*, 1933.

(179) —— and NEWTON, A. *Jour. Phys.* 1913–14, XLVII, 57.

(180) —— and RAKE, G. *Quart. Jour. Med.* 1929–30, XXIII, 491.

(181) —— and STEWART, M. J. *Gastric and Duodenal Ulcer.* London, 1929, Oxf. Med. Pub.

(182) JACKSON, CHEVALIER. *Jour. Amer. Med. Assoc.* 1929, XCII, 369.

(183) JAMES, W. W. and HASTINGS, S. *Proc. Roy. Soc. Med.* 1932, XXV, 1343 (Sect. Odont.), 39.

(183a) JANKER, R. *Forts. Geb. Rönt.* 1931, XLIV, 658
(184) JARRE, H. A. *The Science of Radiology*, 1933, p. 198
(185) JEFFERSON, G. *Arch. Roent. Ray*, 1915, XIX, 414.
(186) —— *Brit. Jour. Surg.* 1916–17, IV, 209.
(187) JORDAN, A. C. *Arch. Roent. Ray*, 1911, XVI, 26.
(188) —— *Arch. Roent. Ray*, 1914, XVIII, 328.
JUDD. *See* Alvarez.
(189) KAESTLE, K. *Lehrbuch der Roentgenkunde*, 1913, I, 504, 516, 531.
(190) —— RIEDER, H. and ROSENTHAL, J. *Arch. Roent. Ray*, 1910, XV, 3.
(191) KAHN, H. *Strahlentherapie*, 1930, XXXVII, 751.
(192) KANTOR, J. L. *Amer. Jour. Roent.* 1927, XVII, 405.
(193) KEITH, A. *The Lancet*, 1903, I, 631, 709.
(194) —— *Brit. Med. Jour.* 1923, I, 451, 499.
(195) KELLOGG, J. H. *Surg., Gyn. and Obst.* 1913, XVII, 563.
(196) KERLEY, P. *Recent Advances in Radiology.* London, 1931, J. and A. Churchill.
(197) KIENBÖCK, R. *Forts. Geb. Rönt.* 1913, XX, 231.
(198) KILLIAN, G. *Ann. de mal. de l'oreille,* 1908, XXXIV (2), 1.
(199) KIRKLIN, B. R. *Amer. Jour. Roent.* 1931, XXV, 46.
(200) —— *Proc. Staff Meet. Mayo Clinic*, 1933, VIII, 629.
(201) —— *Brit. Jour. Radiol.* 1935, VIII, 170.
(202) —— *Proc. Staff Meet. Mayo Clinic*, 1932, VII, 728.
(203) —— *Proc. Staff Meet. Mayo Clinic*, 1935, X, 309.
(204) —— *Amer. Jour. Roent.* 1933, XXIX, 437.
KIRKLIN. *See* Cilly.
(205) KITCHIN, D. H. *Brit. Med. Jour.* 1934, I, 80, and *Legal Problems in Medical Practice*, p. 127. London, 1936, Ed. Arnold.
(206) KLASON, T. *Acta Radiol.* 1930, XI, 444.
(207) KNIGHT, G. C. and ADAMSON, W. A. D. *Proc. Roy. Soc. Med.* 1935, XXVIII, 891.
(208) KNOEPP, L. F. *Proc. Staff Meet. Mayo Clinic*, 1933, VIII, 765.
(209) KNUTSSON, F. *Acta Radiol.* 1931, XII, 157.
(210) KONJETZNY, G. E. *Die entzündliche Grundlage der typischen Geschwürsbildungen im Magen und Duodenum.* Berlin, 1930, J. Springer.
(211) KRETSCHMER, E. *Physique and Character.* London, 1925, H. K. Lewis.
(212) KRONECKER, H. and MELTZER, S. *Arch. Physiol.* 1880, CCXCIX, 446; 1883, Suppl. p. 328.
(213) KUENZEL, WILHELMINE and TODD, T. W. *Jour. Lab. and Clin. Med.* 1930, XVI, 141.
KUENZEL. *See* Sommerfield.
(214) LANGMEAD, F. S. *Brit. Jour. Child. Dis.* 1929, XXVI, 1.
(215) LAURELL, H. *Acta Radiol.* 1931, XII, 455.
LEDDY. *See* Cilly.
LEES. *See* Adams.
LEONARD. *See* George.
(216) LEVEN, G. *L'aérophagie: syndromes gastriques, intestinaux, circulatoires et respiratoires.* Paris, 1926, Gaston Down. 2nd ed.
(217) —— and BARRET, G. *C.R. Soc. de biol.* 1903, LV, 1218; *Presse méd.* 1906, XIV, 503.
(218) LEVYN, L., BECK, E. C. and AARON, A. H. *Amer. Jour. Roent.* 1933, XXX, 774.
LE WALD. *See* Wald.
(219) LEXER, E. *Münch. med. Woch.* 1911, LVIII, 1548.
LOCKHART. *See* Anderson.
(220) LOCKHART-MUMMERY, J. P. and HODGSON, H. G. *Brit. Med. Jour.* 1931, I, 525.
(221) LÖNNERBLAD, L. *Acta Radiol.* 1932, XIII, 551.
(222) LUFF, A. P. *Brit. Med. Jour.* 1929, II, 1125.

(223) LYON, B. B. V., BARTLE, H. J. and ELLISON, R. T. *Med. Jour. New York*, 1921, CXIV, 272.

MACADAM. *See* Bell.

MACCARTY. *See* Wilson.

M'CORMICK. *See* Stuart.

(224) M'CREA, E. D'A. *Brit. Jour. Surg.* 1926, XIII, 621.

(225) —— McSWINEY, B. A. and STOPFORD, J. S. B. *Quart. Jour. Exp. Physiol.* 1925, XV, 201.

(226) McGIBBON, J. E. G. and MATHER, J. H. *Brit. Med. Jour.* 1933, II, 1013.

(227) McINTYRE, J. *Arch. Skiag.* 1897, I, 37.

(228) MacKEE, G. M. *Amer. Jour. Roent.* 1916, III, 293.

(229) MACKEITH, N. W., SPURRELL, W. R., WARNER, E. C. and WESTLAKE, H. J. *Guy's Hosp. Rep.* 1922, LXXII, 479.

MACMILLAN. *See* Mosher.

McNEE. *See* Rolleston.

(230) McROBERTS, J. W. *Proc. Staff Meet. Mayo Clinic*, 1933, VIII, 685.

M'SWINEY. *See* M'Crea.

(231) MAGEE, H. E. *Brit. Jour. Exp. Biol.* 1932, IX, 409.

(232) MANN, F. C. and HIGGINS, G. M. *Proc. Soc. Exp. Biol. and Med.* 1927, XXIV, 930.

MARXER. *See* Spriggs.

MATHER. *See* McGibbon.

(233) MAYER, E. *Med. Rec. N.Y.* 1910, LXXVIII, 10.

(234) MECKEL, J. F. *Handbuch der pathol. Anatomie.* Leipzig, 1816–18.

MELTZER. *See* Kronecker.

MENGIS. *See* Rosselet.

MERIEL. *See* Béclère.

(235) MEULENGRACHT, E. *Proc. Roy. Soc. Med.* 1935, XXVIII, 841.

(236) MILLER, R. and GAGE, H. C. *Arch. Dis. Child.* 1930, V, 83; 1932, VII, 65.

(237) MILLER, T. G., PENDERGRASS, E. P. and ANDREWS, K. S. *Amer. Jour. Med. Sci.* 1929, CLXXVII, 15.

MILLER. *See* Carman.

(238) MILLS, R. W. *Amer. Jour. Roent.* 1917, IV, 155.

(239) —— *Amer. Jour. Roent.* 1922, IX, 199.

(240) —— *Amer. Jour. Roent.* 1922, IX, 731.

(241) MIXTER, S. J. *Jour. Amer. Med. Assoc.* 1915, LXV, 1607.

MOLHANT. *See* Gehuchten.

(242) MOODY, R. O. *Jour. Anat.* 1927, LXI, 223.

(243) —— CHAMBERLAIN, W. E. and VAN NUYS, R. G. *Jour. Amer. Med. Assoc.* 1923, LXXXI, 1924.

(244) —— —— —— —— *Amer. Jour. Anat.* 1926, XXXVII, 273.

(245) —— and VAN NUYS, R. G. *Amer. Jour. Roent.* 1928, XX, 348.

(246) MOORHEAD, T. G. *Medical Diseases of the War.*

(247) MORGAGNI, J. B. *The Seats and Causes of Disease investigated by Anatomy* (in five books). Translated from the Latin *De Sedibus* (1761) by Benjamin Alexander. London, 1769, II.

(248) MORISON, J. M. WOODBURN. *Arch. Radiol. and Electrol.* 1922, XXVII, 353; 1923, XXVIII, 72, 111, and *Proc. Roy. Soc. Med.* 1930, XXIII (Sect. Electrotherapy), 23.

(249) —— *Brit. Jour. Radiol.* 1927, XXXII, 388.

(250) MORLEY, JOHN. *Brit. Med. Jour.* 1920, II, 542.

(251) —— *Abdominal Pain.* Edinburgh, 1931.

(252) —— *Brit. Med. Jour.* 1928, I, 887 and 1085.

(253) MORLEY, JOHN and TWINING, E. W. *Brit. Jour. Surg.* 1931, XVIII, 397.

(254) MOSHER, H. P. and MACMILLAN, A. S. *Laryngoscope*, 1927, XXXVII, 235.

(255) MOTTRAM, J. C. *Brit. Jour. Radiol.* 1932, V, 156.

(256) MOYNIHAN, BERKELEY. *Two Lectures on Gastric and Duodenal Ulcer.* Bristol, 1923, J. Wright.

MUELLER. *See* Horton.

(257) MUIR, J. *Brit. Jour. Radiol.* 1930, III, 391.

(258) NEWCOMB, W. D. *Brit. Jour. Surg.* 1932, XX, 279.

NEWTON. *See* Hurst.

(259) O'BRIEN, F. W. *Radiology*, 1928, X, 226.

(260) OGLE, J. W. *Trans. Path. Soc. Lond.* 1865–6, XVII, 141.

(261) OKA, MITSUTOMO. *Forts. Geb. Rönt.* 1930, XLI, 892.

OLSON. *See* Walters.

(262) ORR, J. BOYD. *Brit. Med. Jour.* 1927, II, 788.

(263) PALUGYAY, J. *Forts. Geb. Rönt.* 1922–3, XXX, Kongressheft I, 35; and *Röntgenuntersuchung und Strahlenbehandlung der Speiseröhre.* Vienna, 1931, Julius Springer.

(264) PANCOAST, H. K. *Amer. Jour. Cancer*, 1933, XVII, 373.

PARKER. *See* Davis.

(265) PAYNE, W. W. and POULTON, E. P. *Quart. Jour. Med.* 1923–24, XVII, 53.

(266) —— —— *Jour. Physiol.* 1927, LXIII, 217; 1928, LXV, 157.

(267) PEDEMONTIUM, FRANCISCUS DE. In Mesue, *Opera de Medicamentorum purgantium delectu, castigatione, et usu.* Venice, 1589.

PEMBREY. *See* Adams.

PENDERGRASS. *See* Miller, T. G.

(268) PERRY, E. C. and SHAW, L. E. *Guy's Hosp. Rep.* 1893, L, 171.

(269) PIRIE, A. HOWARD. *Amer. Jour. Roent.* 1921, VIII, 75.

(270) PIRIE, G. A. *Arch. Roent. Ray*, 1908, XIII, 41.

(271) PITRES, A. and TESTUT, L. *Les nerfs en schémas, anatomie et physiopathologie.* Paris, 1925, p. 219.

(272) PLUMMER, H. S. *Jour. Amer. Med. Assoc.* 1908, LI, 549.

(273) POTTER, R. P. *Radiology*, 1930, XV, 685.

(274) POULTON, E. P. *The Lancet*, 1928, II, 1223 and 1277.

POULTON. *See* Payne.

(275) PRIESTLEY, J. T. and HECK, F. J. *Proc. Staff Meet. Mayo Clinic*, 1933, VIII, 315.

(276) PURTON, T. *Lond. Med. and Phys. Jour.* 1821, XLVI, 540.

(277) RADT, P. *Med. Klin.* 1930, XXVI, 1888.

RAKE. *See* Hurst.

RAMSBOTTOM. *See* Barclay.

(278) RATKÓCZI, N. *Amer. Jour. Roent.* 1924, XII, 246 and *Brit. Jour. Radiol.* 1926, XXXI, 253.

(279) RAVEN, R. W. *Brit. Jour. Surg.* 1933, XXI, 235.

(280) REDDING, J. MAGNUS. *X-ray Diagnosis.* London, 1926, Cassell and Co.

REID. *See* Dalton.

(280a) REYNOLDS, RUSSELL J. *Brit. Jour. Radiol.* 1934, VII, 415; 1935, VIII, 135.

(281) RIEDER, H. *Münch. med. Woch.* 1904, LI, 1548.

RIEDER. *See* Kaestle.

(282) ROLLESTON, H. D. *Trans. Path. Soc. Lond.* 1896, XLVII, 37.

(283) —— *Trans. Path. Soc. Lond.* 1899, L, 69.

(284) —— *The Lancet*, 1901, I, 1121.

(285) —— and MCNEE, J. W. *Diseases of the Liver, Gall-bladder and Bile-ducts.* London, 1929, Macmillan and Co.

ROSENTHAL. *See* Kaestle.

(286) Rosselet, A. and Mengis, O. *Acta Radiol.* 1934, xv, 438.
(287) Rovsing, T. *Ann. Surg.* 1913, lvii, 1.
Salmond. *See* Bolton.
(288) Sampson, H. H. *Brit. Jour. Surg.* 1933, xx, 447.
(289) Saralegui, J. A. *Amer. Jour. Roent.* 1934, xxxii, 167.
(289a) Sauerbruch, F., Chaoul, H. and Adam, A. *Deuts. Med. Woch.* 1932, lviii, 1391.
(290) Schatzki, R. *Acta Radiol.* Supp. 1933, No. xviii.
(291) Schlesinger, E. *Berl. klin. Woch.* 1910, xlvii, 1977.
(292) —— *Deuts. Arch. klin. Med.* 1912, cvii, 552.
(293) Schreiber, J. *Arch. exp. Path.* 1912, lxvii, 72.
(294) Schwarz, G. *Klinische Roentgendiagnostik des Dickdarms und ihre physiologische Grundlagen.* Berlin, 1914, p. 61.
(295) Scott, S. Gilbert. *The Lancet,* 1926, ii, 222.
(295a) Sear, H. R. *Med. Jour. Austral.* Supp. 1927, ii, 225.
(296) Sebening, Walter. *Proc. Staff Meet. Mayo Clinic,* 1932, vii, 139.
(297) Shanks, S. C. *Brit. Med. Jour.* 1934, ii, 1032.
(298) Shay, H. and Gershon-Cohen, J. *Surg., Gyn. and Obst.* 1934, lviii, 935.
Shaw. *See* Perry.
(299) Sherrington, C. S. *Brain,* 1915, xxxviii, 191.
(300) Smith, M. Brice, Crymble, P. T. and Allen, F. M. *Brit. Med. Jour.* 1934, i, 1074.
(301) Sommerfield, W. A., Kuenzel, W. M. and Todd, T. W. *Jour. Lab. and Clin. Med.* 1931, xvii, 151.
Souter. *See* Anderson.
(302) Spriggs, E. *The Lancet,* 1931, ii, 31.
(303) —— and Marxer, O. A. *Quart. Jour. Med.* 1925–6, xix, 1.
Spurrell. *See* Mackeith.
Stewart. *See* Hurst.
(304) Stierlin, E. *Zeits. klin. Med.* 1912, lxxv, 486.
Stopford. *See* M'Crea.
(305) Ström, S. *Acta Radiol.* 1923, ii, 468.
(306) Stuart, T. P. Anderson and M'Cormick, A. *Jour. Anat. and Physiol.* 1891–2, xxvi, 231.
(306a) Stumpf, P. *Forts. Geb. Rönt.* 1936, liii, 356.
(307) Sutherland, C. G. *Radiology,* 1927, viii, 111.
(308) Taylor, A. E. *Digestion and Metabolism.* London, 1912, p. 152.
(309) Telford, E. D. *See Amer. Jour. Roent.* 1922, ix, 792.
(310) Telling, W. H. M. *The Lancet,* 1908, i, 843, 929.
(311) —— *Brit. Med. Jour.* 1908, ii, 1346.
Testut. *See* Pitres.
(312) Todd, T. Wingate. *Behaviour Patterns of the Alimentary Tract.* Baltimore, 1930, The Williams and Wilkins Co.
(313) —— *The Clinical Anatomy of the Gastro-Intestinal Tract.* Manchester, 1915.
(314) —— *Inter-State Post-grad. Assembly N. Amer.* 1931, p. 549.
Todd. *See* Kuenzel and Sommerfield.
(315) Treves, F. *Brit. Med. Jour.* 1885, i, 415.
(316) Twining, E. W. *Brit. Jour. Radiol.* 1933, vi, 644.
Twining. *See* Morley.
(317) Uspensky, A. E. and Wichert, M. O. *Brit. Jour. Radiol.* 1928, i, 197.
(317a) Van de Maele. *Jour. Belge de Rad.* 1935, xxiv, 265.
Van Nuys. *See* Moody.
Vanzant. *See* Alvarez.
(318) Vietor, Agnes C. *Boston Med. Surg. Jour.* 1906, clv, 139, 168.

VINE. *See* Adams.

(319) VINSON, P. P. *Proc. Staff Meet. Mayo Clinic*, 1933, VIII, 370.

(320) VIRCHOW, R. *Arch. path. Anat.* 1853, V, 348.

(321) WALD, L. T. LE. *Amer. Jour. Roent.* 1928, XX, 423.

(322) —— *Arch. Surg.* 1927, XIV, 332.

(323) —— *Radiology*, 1926, VI, 138.

(324) —— *Radiology*, 1924, III, 91.

(325) —— *Amer. Jour. Roent.* 1917, IV, 76.

(326) —— *Med. Rec.* 1914, LXXXVI, 190. (In paper by Robert Abbe.)

(327) WALTERS, WALTMAN. *Proc. Staff Meet. Mayo Clinic*, 1932, VII, 143.

(328) —— and OLSON, P. F. *Proc. Staff Meet. Mayo Clinic*, 1935, X, 287.

WALTERS. *See* Church.

(329) WALTON, HENRY. *Amer. Jour. Roent.* 1924, XI, 420.

(330) WALTON, A. J. *The Lancet*, 1931, I, 1071.

WARNER. *See* Mackeith.

(330a) WATSON, J. R. *Proc. Staff Meet. Mayo Clinic*, 1933, VIII, 735.

(331) WAUGH, G. E. *Brit. Jour. Surg.* 1919–20, VII, 343.

(332) —— *Brit. Jour. Surg.* 1928, XV, 438.

(333) WEBER, F. PARKES. *Brain*, 1904, XXVII, 170.

(334) WESSON, H. R. and BARGEN, J. A. *Proc. Staff Meet. Mayo Clinic*, 1934, IX, 789.

WESTLAKE. *See* Mackeith.

(335) WESTPHAL, K. *Zentralbl. für Chir.* 1934, LXI (1), 370.

(336) WETTERSTRAND, G. A. *Acta Radiol.* 1926, V, 105.

WICHERT. *See* Uspensky.

(337) WILBUR, D. L. *Proc. Staff Meet. Mayo Clinic*, 1933, VIII, 609.

WILBUR. *See* Alvarez.

(338) WILLIAMS, F. H. *Trans. Assoc. Amer. Phys.* 1899, XIV, 168.

(339) WILLIAMSON, BRUCE. *Vital Cardiology.* Edinburgh, 1934, p. 3.

(340) WILSON, L. B. and MacCARTY, W. C. *Amer. Jour. Med. Sci.* 1909, CXXXVIII, 846.

(341) WOLF, G. *Forts. Geb. Rönt.* 1928, XXXVII, 890.

(342) WOODS, R. R. *The Lancet*, 1931, I, 1137.

(342a) WRIGHT, A. D. *Trans. Med. Soc. Lond.* 1935, LVIII, 94.

(343) ZENKER, F. A. *Berl. klin. Woch.* 1882, XIX, 657; *Handbuch der speziellen Pathologie und Therapie*, 1874–7, VII, 1.

(344) ZUPPINGER. *In* Schinz, Baensch and Friedl: *Lehrbuch der Röntgendiagnostik.* Vol. I, p. 26, tables 5–7.

(345) EDITORIALS. *Brit. Jour. Radiol.* 1932, V, 486, 742.

(346) —— *The Lancet*, 1932, I, 781.

(347) —— (British Empire Cancer Campaign), *The Lancet*, 1933, II, 138.

(348) ABSTRACT. *Brit. Jour. Radiol.* 1932, V, 789.

(349) EDITORIAL. *The Lancet*, 1933, II, 728.

"I also will here make an end of my book, and if I have written well and to the point in my story, this is what I myself desired; but if meanly and indifferently, that is all I could attain unto."

Apocrypha, II Maccabees, xv, 37, 38, R.V.

AUTHORS' INDEX

GENERAL INDEX

Printed in the United States
By Bookmasters